Understanding Diseases in Skin of Color

Inyang Ukot

Understanding Diseases in Skin of Color

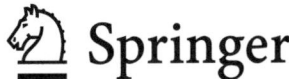 Springer

Inyang Ukot
Impact Clinics Ltd.
Uyo, Nigeria

ISBN 978-3-031-97502-8   ISBN 978-3-031-97503-5   (eBook)
https://doi.org/10.1007/978-3-031-97503-5

This Springer imprint is published by the registered company Springer Nature Switzerland AG
The registered company address is: Gewerbestrasse 11, 6330 Cham, Switzerland

If disposing of this product, please recycle the paper.

This book is dedicated to my family (Mrs. Sarah Ukot and daughters Mrs. Grace Inyang Alegeh, Elor Ukot, Sarah Ukot, Jr., and Joy Ukot). This dedication is for the great contributions they have made over the years that this project spanned despite none of them being a physician. Not only regarding the making of this book did they provide immense support to go on but also joined in prayers and gave sundry input to maintain and enhance my not-so-wonderful health to arrive at this desirable point.

The book is also dedicated to Emmanuel Edem Ukot, my young nephew. Right from his teenage years, Emmanuel showed an intense interest in medicine and went further to promise to specialize in dermatology. Although he changed his mind along the way, this book is dedicated to him for his unusual interest in dermatology at such a young age. I believe that this book will achieve at least what he would have accomplished in the lives of patients with dermatological conditions.

Foreword

Dr. Inyang Ukot, a 1981 graduate of College of Medicine of the University of Lagos, Nigeria, is a Fellow in Family Medicine of the National Postgraduate Medical College of Nigeria (1991) and the West African College of Physicians (1995). He also obtained the Postgraduate Diploma in Occupational Medicine from the Royal College of Physicians of London in 2005.

In the wide range of medical facilities where Dr. Ukot has worked over the years pre- and post-fellowship, he has garnered extensive experience which includes dermatology in primary, secondary, and tertiary healthcare medical facilities located in rural areas, semi-urban areas, and cities in Nigeria. Inyang is therefore the non-dermatologist who is qualified to author *Understanding Diseases in Skin of Color*.

This dermatology book contains more than 250 figures in natural color in 10 of its chapters. The book commences with an Introduction that contains 60 highly illustrated figures that take the reader to gross human anatomy and its relationship with dermatology; this chapter is a sine qua non for the reader's understanding of the rest of the book as it not only takes the busy non-dermatologist and the clinical years medical student back to the basics but also provides a solid basis on how to approach any dermatological condition with confidence. The remaining chapter titles cover dermatological conditions as follows: bacterial infections, fungal infections, viral infections, parasitic infestations of the skin, common disorders of skin appendages—hair, sebaceous gland, and nail disorders, inflammatory disorders, papulosquamous disorders, cutaneous neoplasms—benign and malignant, and cutaneous manifestations of systemic diseases. Each of these chapters has five multiple-choice questions (MCQs) of the single best answer (SBA) format with each MCQ having four answer options, the best of which is the answer. Two peculiar chapters end the book; they are: "Medications in Dermatology" and "Answers and Notes for MCQs." Every chapter of the book has appropriate references. A robust index provides a veritable and a quick reference guide for the reader.

Apart from the contents described in the previous paragraph, the book's reach is for a global audience, and the style is unique as it takes the approach of a case study/report followed by MCQs that form a self-assessment tool. The book is written in a simple, easy-to-read, and easy-to-understand way. Its usefulness for the medical community and general healthcare community is indubitable.

This is a must-read book that I recommend to medical students, residents in family medicine, and general medical practitioners who need to confidently navigate skin conditions in patients with skin of color. I have known Inyang since September 1976 when we were roommates in the first year in College of Medicine of the University of Nigeria in Lagos, Nigeria.

Associate Clinical Professor   Ikechukwu Uzoaru
Department of Pathology
University of Illinois
Chicago, IL, USA

Preface

Why another book on dermatology, you may ask? *Understanding Diseases in Skin of Color* is a needed addition to medical literature. This book is a good resource for clinicians and their patients; it is a product of unwarranted superficiality regarding the way some physicians approach dermatology, just because they are not dermatologists. The book is good for patients because the author has observed that when doctors provide their patients with accurate information in a way that their level of education is immaterial for absorbing the information, they become partners with their doctors in the business of solving or minimizing such health challenges. This book is an attempt to give these two partners information from the same source. This is therefore a book that a patient who listens carefully to the clinician who has read and thoroughly internalized the contents will satisfactorily explain any dermatological condition to the patient or the patient's parents (and, sometimes, accompanying relatives or caregivers of elderly patients). It sometimes happens that doctors have no clear idea how patients think and feel until they are in the same shoes as patients by becoming patients—with dermatological conditions or a myriad other conditions in medicine. There are not enough textbooks that have enough (or have created enough) space to attend to the multitude of needs of the clinician and the patient satisfactorily.

As you are reading this book, people are battling with recent skin conditions. There are more people who should prevent preventable skin conditions, and there are yet people whose skin conditions should not be allowed to get worse or develop offshoots that doctors call complications. In his practice, this author prefers to use "offshoots" and similar words when discussing clinical conditions because such words tend to make the buck stop at the patient—at least at the time of presentation for the first consultation. In his area of practice, "complications" tend to make the patient look for a scapegoat that may be the clinical condition that they brought to meet the doctor, another person (like parents, colleagues, and work environment). When a patient relieves themselves of carelessness, inappropriate care for their skin, going to the wrong sources for treatment, postponing a visit to the hospital with a skin condition to consult a doctor, or engaging in self-treatment using medications readily procured over the counter, and the like, the word "complication" is self-absolving. When a doctor makes the patient take responsibility for the decisions and actions they have taken (having now experienced the results), they are very likely to want to stem further "offshoots." These may not only be "deeper more serious" forms of the original (or initial) disease entity, but also additional conditions. Melanoma is a good example, for it does not only get wider and more inconveniencing but may also become metastatic and involve other parts of the body.

As indicated in the first paragraph, "Why another book on the skin?" might be your question. It is also because the skin is the largest organ in the human body; being the gatekeeper of the body, its integrity and good health frequently reflect what happens to the hidden, unseen, internal organs and, furthermore, what happens to the intangible part of our bodies—our minds. Many skin conditions impact our minds, and our minds direct a lot of what we accept, understand, and do—or refuse to do.

This book is divided into 11 main chapters. The 12th chapter consists of all the answers and notes for the MCQs that appear at the end of each of Chaps. 1, 2, 3, 4, 5, 6, 7, 8, 9, 10, and 11.

- Chapters 2, 3, 4, 5, 6, 7, 8, 9, and 10 are treated using a case studies format. The order for every topic in Chaps. 2, 3, 4, 5, 6, 7, 8, 9, and 10 is: First Figure > Symptoms > Signs > Diagnosis > Treatment > Etiology > Prognosis > Follow-up care > Discussion. Differential diagnoses are generally not included unless the author considers that there is a good reason to do so in a few cases—in dermatology, the differential diagnoses could be up to ten or more—this is because there are plenty of conditions that look alike. The reader is encouraged to read on some of these conditions in standard dermatology textbooks for their differential diagnoses and other details.
- The only place that the reader will find the topics in each chapter is conspicuously listed.
- Unlike other textbooks on dermatology, the approach of this book is to keep the reader in suspense. This simulates the general medical practitioner's daily experience in the general outpatient clinic. Therefore, the topic is nameless (without a title at the top). The reader is welcomed by a figure followed by the symptoms and signs. It is after the signs that a provisional diagnosis is provided—this is what we do daily; you listen to the patient, ask them questions because you are thinking of the likely diagnoses, then you examine the patient for signs before making a diagnosis. Thereafter, you start an empirical treatment at the same time that you think of what could have caused this (etiology) and request for investigations to help you narrow down the possibilities (the look-alike conditions) when you obtain and study the investigation results (or reports). You engage your patient by providing information on the condition when you are certain of the results, including the prognosis. Thereafter, you discuss the appointment for follow-up care; sometimes you negotiate and arrive at a common ground of an acceptable day and time for the first follow-up care and subsequent one at every such review consultation until you get to the point of giving the patient "an all clear." The patient now determines when to return to the

hospital or when to return to the hospital with another illness or health challenge.

- Each chapter also has ten relevant references. The references are neither unwieldy nor distractive but just adequate to draw the reader's attention to their propriety. The contents of this book have the clinician in focus. The references appear at the end of each chapter.
- The first 11 chapters contain multiple-choice questions (MCQs). The MCQs are limited to the conditions in the respective chapter. The MCQs are of the single best answer (SBA) format, and they are particularly of the best-of-four options. Currently, this is the most preferred type of MCQs for medical schools, and during the residency program, the clinician will definitely benefit from the content.
- Chapter 11 summarizes medications in groups. The contents are designed in a way that enables the physician to know from which category of drugs they should choose the most appropriate drugs to obtain the best efficacy for their patients.
- Answers and Notes for MCQs are provided in the back matter after Chap. 11 but just before the index. The answers are backed with robust notes that indicate why one option is the answer—and, sometimes, why the other three are not.
- The book has an elaborate Index. The index is a useful tool for the reader to quickly identify and refer to any index listing in the book.

In summary, this book uses its Chap. 1 to introduce the reader to the contents of the book and concomitantly transport them back to the basics that we all studied in medical school. The selection of topics is highly illustrated to flow with what the reader will read in the rest of the book. The remainder of the book simply empowers you to handle the consultation with your patient with dermatology conditions in the same professional way you give them good service without knowing beforehand what conditions brought them to the clinic, emergency room, or the ward. Finally, this author is a proponent for making the reader grasp the basics of any area in medicine and "run with it." Your patient should have good memories of consulting with you, many months (nay, many years) after the encounter—this book will contribute to your attaining this laudable goal.

Uyo, Nigeria   Inyang Ukot
February 13, 2025

Acknowledgments

The author's acknowledgments go to Dr. Charles Nga, MBBS, FWACP. This senior lecturer at the University of Uyo, Nigeria, and Honorary Senior Consultant Dermatologist in its University of Uyo Teaching Hospital, Uyo, Nigeria, is the colleague who caught the project idea of this author and provided the author with a selection of the dermatological images he obtained from his primary patients. The images are as follows: Chapter 3: Figures 3.3, 3.4, 3.5, 3.6, 3.7, 3.11, 3.12, 3.13, 3.14, 3.15, and 3.16. Chapter 4: Figures 4.4, 4.5, 4.6, 4.7, 4.8, 4.9, 4.10, and 4.11. Chapter 6: Figures 6.1 and 6.2. Chapter 7: Figures 7.10, 7.11, 7.17, 7.18, 7.22, 7.27, 7.28, 7.29, 7.34, 7.35, 7.36, 7.37, 7.38, 7.39, 7.40, 7.41, and 7.42. Chapter 8: Figures 8.1, 8.2, 8.3, 8.4, 8.5, 8.6, 8.7, 8.8, 8.9, 8.10, 8.11, 8.12, 8.13, 8.14, 8.15, and 8.16. Chapter 9: Figures 9.7, 9.8, 9.15, 9.16, 9.17, 9.18, 9.20, 9.21, 9.22, and 9.23. Chapter 10: Figures 10.2, 10.3, 10.4, 10.5, 10.6, 10.7, 10.8, 10.9, 10.10, 10.11, and 10.12.

The author's appreciation also goes to Dr. Adamu Onu, MBBS, FWACP, MS, PhD, a consultant in family medicine and the Medical Director of Garki Hospital, Abuja, Nigeria. He understood the potential of the then-proposed project's contribution to knowledge in this invaluable specialty (dermatology) and approved the author's application containing the request to obtain anonymized images from patients who gave their consent in writing.

The next colleague is Dr. Izuchukwu Benerdin Achusi, MBBS, FMCPath, Consultant Histopathologist at the Federal Medical Center, Abuja. Dr. Achusi, despite his busy schedule, provided the author with suitable selections of photomicrographs on the skin. These images, available in Chap. 1, are as follows: Figures 1.48, 1.49, 1.50, 1.51, 1.52, 1.53, 1.54, 1.55, 1.56, 1.57, 1.58, 1.59, and 1.60.

Contents

About the Author

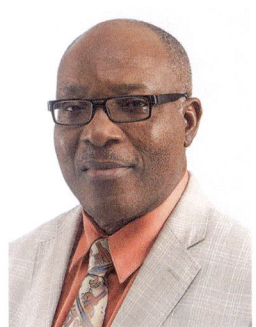

Inyang Ukot graduated from College of Medicine of the University of Lagos, Nigeria, with Bachelor of Medicine and Bachelor of Surgery (M.B. and B.S.) in 1981. He completed a residency in Family Medicine and is a Fellow in Family Medicine of the National Postgraduate Medical College of Nigeria (1991) and the West African College of Physicians (1995). He obtained the postgraduate Diploma in Occupational Medicine from the Royal College of Physicians of London in 2005. He was the coordinator of training in Family Medicine in the National Postgraduate Medical College of Nigeria between 1995 and 1999.

Dr. Inyang Ukot has extensive experience as a family medicine specialist and first contact specialist in the healthcare system, a career spanning over 40 years in Nigeria. This extensive experience and exposure cover healthcare facilities in North, South, East, and West of Nigeria, a highly populated country in Sub-Saharan Africa. In the first year of his career, Inyang worked in Eku Baptist Hospital located in a rural area in the South-South part of Nigeria. During his year of compulsory service (NYSC) to Nigeria, he worked in a State government-owned secondary care medical facility in Birnin-Gwari in the North-Central part of Nigeria. During his residency in Family Medicine, he spent some time in a Presbyterian Church hospital in the South-South part of Nigeria, NKST Hospital, and two Catholic Church hospitals in Benue State (North-Central Nigeria). Dr. Inyang Ukot was the first family physician to head the General Outpatients' Department of the University of Port Harcourt Teaching Hospital in the capital city of the oil-producing Rivers State in the early 1990s. Later, he worked alongside a surgeon colleague to run a smooth staff medical services for one of the largest commercial banks in Nigeria—United Bank for Africa (UBA). He also worked in two private hospitals in Ikeja, Lagos State, between 1992 and 1996. Thereafter, he also served in the petroleum industry as a staff physician for ExxonMobil in Nigeria between 1998 and 2006. He spent 5 years as the most senior family physician in the University of Uyo Teaching Hospital, Uyo, Nigeria. Only recently he has worked on contract with the foremost Nigerian national oil corporation in its medical services arm.

In the wide range of medical facilities depicted in the previous paragraph, Inyang Ukot's extensive experience has included dermatology in the said primary, secondary, and tertiary healthcare medical facilities in hospitals located in rural areas, semi-urban areas, and cities in Nigeria. He has shown consistent interest in dermatology without specializing in the specialty the way I did. His first book in medicine is dated 1996, and the last book known to me is on Amazon.com with ISBN-13: 978-1961507739 and a publishing date of November 2023. Inyang is therefore the nondermatologist who is qualified to author *Understanding Diseases in Skin of Color*, a must-read book that is recommended to medical students, residents in family medicine, and general medical practitioners who need to confidently navigate skin conditions in patients with skin of color.

Introduction

Dermatological conditions affect people of all ages, sparing neither the neonate nor the older person. A medical student or doctor should, therefore, be armed with adequate information and ready with various levels of training and expertise to attend to skin diseases—at least the common ones. The others should be referred promptly to dermatologists. Skin lesions may appear on one side of the body or both sides. When they appear only, or principally, on one side, it could be significant and assist in making the diagnosis, e.g., herpes zoster; at other times, one-sided presentation could just be due to an early stage of the disease process. The number may not be significant unless it is related to the patient's habits, e.g., picking the lesions on one side of the face (rather, or more, than the other.) Skin rashes may also appear on certain parts of the body and not the others, e.g., scabies and tinea corporis; in other instances, rashes may start from one part of the body but eventually affect others, e.g., chicken pox and measles. These, and other, features may help in arriving at a diagnosis or making differential diagnoses.

During history, taking the medical student or the doctor is also interested in knowing the following:

- The onset of the rashes (whether sudden or insidious).
- The duration (whether hours, days, weeks, months, or longer).
- The first episode or a recurrent episode (and if recurrent, the actual or approximate number of times as it indicates the order [first, third, fifth, etc.] of the index episode).
- A description of features of the lesion, for example:
  - Whether painless or painful (in which case the intensity of pain. The pain score that the patient assigns should be documented although it is a subjective assessment by the patient and the doctor may not agree with the score).
  - Non-pruritic or pruritic (if the latter case the degree of pruritus and time-relatedness).
  - Associated symptoms, e.g., fever (and if fever, if it preceded the onset of lesions and by how long, or no fever).
  - Other constitutional symptoms that may point to the onset of a systemic disease or indicate a concomitant systemic disease, or indicate that the skin condition is a manifestation of a systemic disease. In such cases, the consultation tends to be longer, involve more investigations, and may require a referral by even a dermatologist to other specialists—occasionally for co-management. An example is late consultation with melanoma (a common situation)

Supplementary Information The online version contains supplementary material available at https://doi.org/10.1007/978-3-031-97503-5_1.

in which a dermatologist, surgeon, and oncologist may co-manage the patient.

- The patient's feelings or reaction towards the rashes, e.g., unconcerned, embarrassed, bitter, and hopeless.
- What idea does the patient or patient's parents have about the condition, e.g., its etiology, progress, prognosis, etc.?
- Does the lesion affect the functioning of the patient, e.g., attendance at school, work in the office, taking care of home duties, or enjoyment of a vacation?

The answers to these and other questions, e.g., the expectations that the patient and their family members have from medical and other hospital personnel, may determine/explain the reason and the timing of the patient's visit to the clinic for consultation. Answers that the doctor obtains during a detailed and focused history taking usually help in making a diagnosis when matched with clinical findings; the answers may also enable the physician to understand the patient, their family background, financial background, experiences in the index or other hospitals, and more.

The author ends this part by mentioning what may be safely excluded during a typical consultation in some parts of the world. The topic is spirituality. In Africa (and specifically in the most populous African country which is where this author currently practices and has been practicing), the patient's spirituality may take the center stage. This is usually not initiated by the doctor but by the patient or patient's relative(s). The initial reaction in the usually busy clinics is to dismiss such "unnecessary" and unrequested information or opinion to attend to other patients waiting to be attended to. In this short paragraph, the doctor who "successfully dismisses" the patient and their beliefs/concerns may not see the patient again as the patient may conclude that the physician is uncaring. The patient may even go to another hospital, unless there is no other in the community. Spirituality in clinical conditions is another topic but it is broached here to draw the physician's attention to the fact that with some patients, the doctor may go the extra mile. How

do you go the extra mile when you have no idea of the patient's spirituality slant, you do not agree with the patient's perspective, or you are certain that there is no connection whatsoever between lichen simplex chronicus at the neck, melanoma on the sole of the foot, or fixed drug eruption on the anterior chest wall close to the breast or on the upper thigh and the spiritual causation, progress, or approach to treatment that the patient suggests?

Examination findings of skin rashes must include a description of their appearance on inspection and palpation. Rashes could be macules, papules, nodules, pustules, vesicles, plaques, etc.

- Macules are flat and at the same level with surrounding skin, cannot be palpated, and are individually not more than 10 mm (1 cm) in diameter; they can coalesce and form larger lesions of various sizes and shapes.
- Papules are small elevations that are usually less than 10 mm but could be up to 10 mm in diameter; they are palpable.
- Pustules are like papules in size, but they contain pus.
- Vesicles are like papules in terms of size, but they are filled with fluid that is usually clear.
- Nodules are larger than 10 mm, may be up to 20 mm, and are elevated above the skin; they could be depressed below the skin surface because they also have a base within the skin/beneath the skin surface.
- Plaques are lesions that are raised above the skin; they are usually similar in size with nodules but could be wider than nodules. Plaques are well circumscribed and are generally plateau-like (i.e., have a flat surface/top) [1, 2].

The skin rashes just mentioned above could become secondary lesions over time, e.g., ulcers, scars, etc. Ulcers are the result of a break in the continuity of skin and may take different sizes, shapes, bases, and borders. Scars are the result of healing of certain rashes—just like they can be caused by other disease processes, e.g., from trauma. This introductory description is on dermatological diseases generally.

This book cannot address all dermatological conditions or even all the common ones. What the book does is attend to a selection of dermatological conditions. It was difficult to determine which condition to include in a book that has only a limited number of pages especially when it necessarily contains many images for illustration and clarification. The author also ensured that some conditions have two to five photographs to satisfactorily "paint the picture" regarding them—good examples are toxic epidermal necrolysis and lichen planus in Chap. 7.

Depending on which part of the globe the reader is, some of the conditions in this book are so common that a medical student in the clinical years is unlikely to fail to encounter them before graduation from the medical school. With respect to medical practitioners, virtually every experienced practicing doctor would have encountered patients who have such conditions. Other conditions that are in this book may prove difficult to diagnose when a doctor comes across them in a patient the first time. With others, if a diagnosis is attempted it would only be a provisional (tentative, unconfirmed) diagnosis and the definitive diagnosis of such conditions is best left for dermatologists—to whom such cases should be referred for further investigations, evaluation, and management.

If the medical practice is in a low- or middle-income country (LMIC), the patient may additionally live in one of the remote or poor communities with limited utilities and facilities. There may be insufficiency or absence of potable water, unstable electricity or electricity of poor voltage, poor road networks, poor and expensive means of transportation, insecurity, and others—in addition to paucity of medical personnel. Even such disadvantaged patients may need to return to the referring doctor for continuing or follow-up care, and this may be a nightmare—not because they do not want to cooperate with their doctor for their desired well-being. This does not happen in the developed parts of the world where patients are given reminders to visit the hospital

or clinic to keep follow-up appointments. In either case, it is important for the doctor who referred such patients to the specialist to request a feedback from the specialist. The referring doctor and their colleagues and the returning patients benefit from back-referral by the dermatologist as they all get equipped with information to guide in adequate care of patients with skin and skin-related conditions.

The chapter contains the following subtopics:

- Skin Structure and Function—this topic consumes at least 80% of the chapter
- Immune System of the Skin (Stratum Corneum/Cellular/Molecular)
- Skin Protection
- Skin of Color/Indigenous

Skin Structure and Function

Most of the chapter is devoted to this subtopic, with emphasis on skin structure. The author presents skin structure with multiple images, starting with gross anatomy and inserting histological and histopathological features in appropriate photomicrographs.

All the images in this book are images pertaining to Black skin in health and disease. They all are original images obtained from primary sources of whom the author is among. The images that have further illustration are the additional work done by the author.

This illustration shows a non-glabrous skin (hair-bearing skin). There are parts of the body that are glabrous skin (hair does not grow on them; good examples are the palms and the soles).

Going clockwise from the top right:

White line arrow = Pore on the surface of the skin

Blue line arrow = The epidermis with the following layers from the surface down:

- Stratum corneum—This is the cornified layer of the epidermis. The stratum corneum has

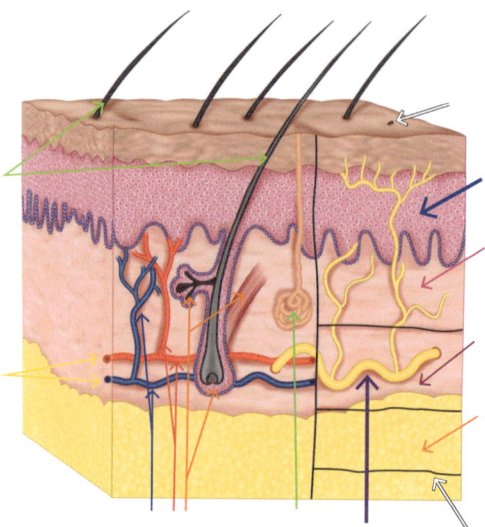

Fig. 1.1 Diagrammatic representation of cross-section of the skin (skin layers)

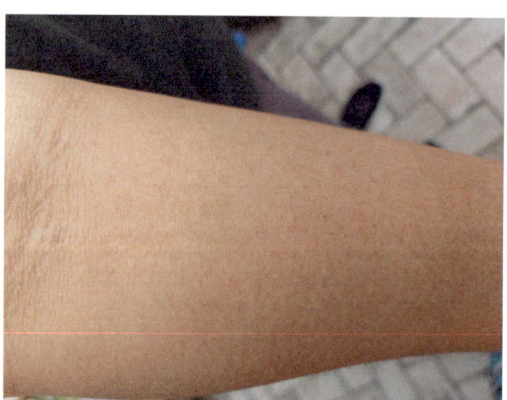

Fig. 1.2 Skin tones (light tone in Black skin)

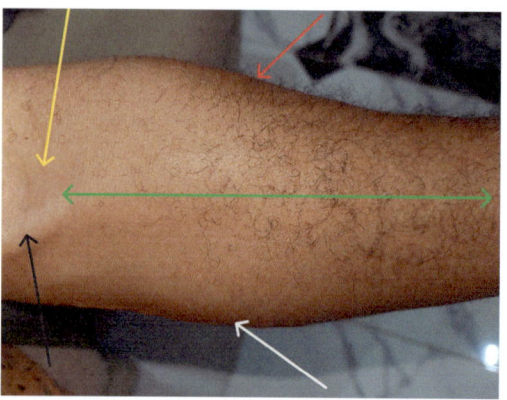

Fig. 1.3 Skin tones (moderate tone in Black skin)

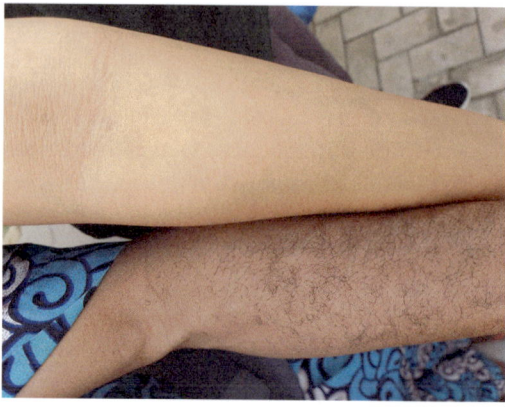

Fig. 1.4 Skin tones (light and moderate tone in Black skin side-by-side, for comparison)

Fig. 1.5 Skin tones (deep tone in Black skin)

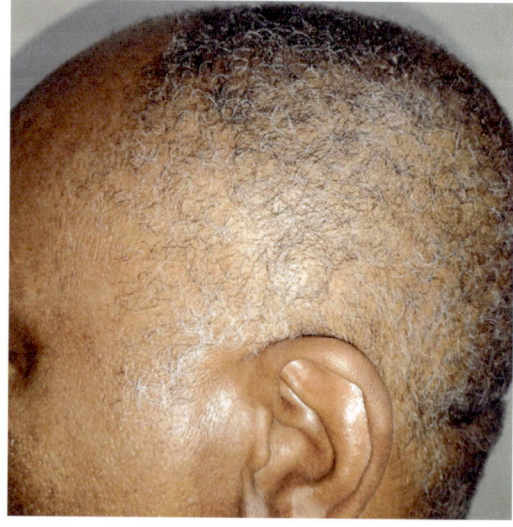

Fig. 1.6 Features of facial image may guide in assessing a person's age

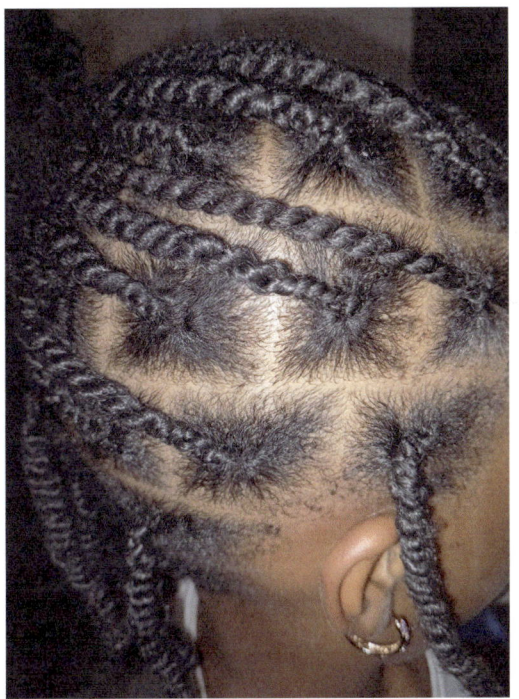

Fig. 1.7 Scalp skin and hair of a 6-year-old girl

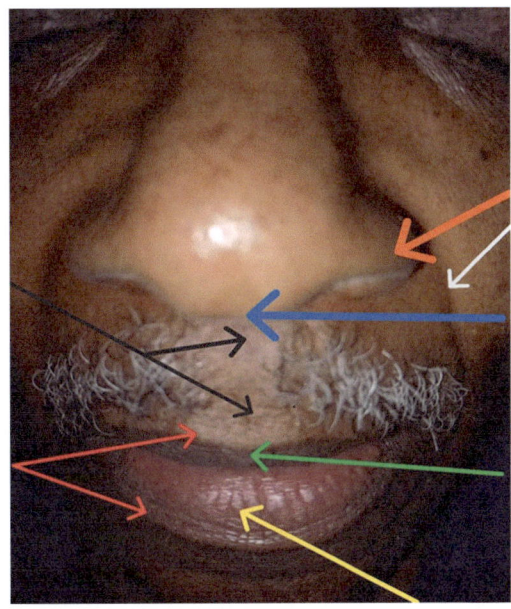

Fig. 1.9 Frontal view of the face

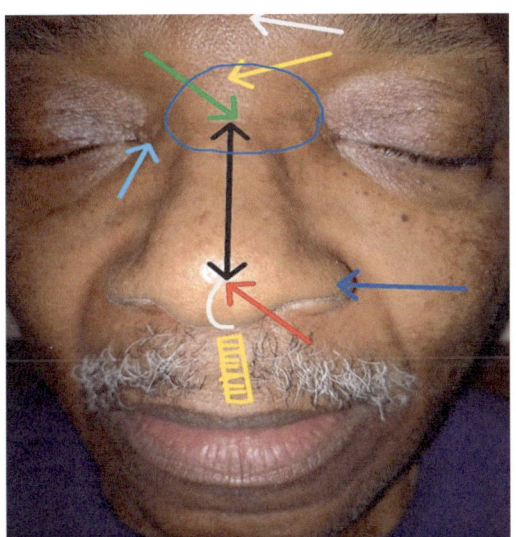

Fig. 1.8 Frontal view of the face

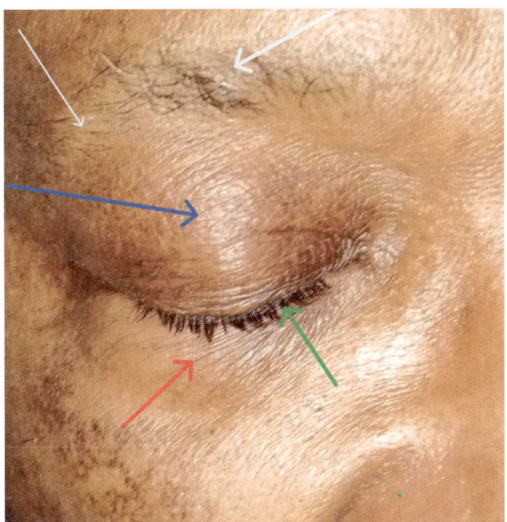

Fig. 1.10 Right eye basics

layers of nonviable epithelial cells corneocytes. Corneocytes are rich in keratin which keratinocytes form. Keratinocytes are present in the stratum basale of the epidermis. Corneocytes have lost the potential to differentiate and proliferate, unlike the keratinocytes that are their precursors. Having been programmed to do so, corneocytes are regularly shed when they get to the outermost part of the skin [3]. The stratum corneum has thickness that differs from one location of the body to another—using a selection of parts of the body to illustrate, the stratum corneum is

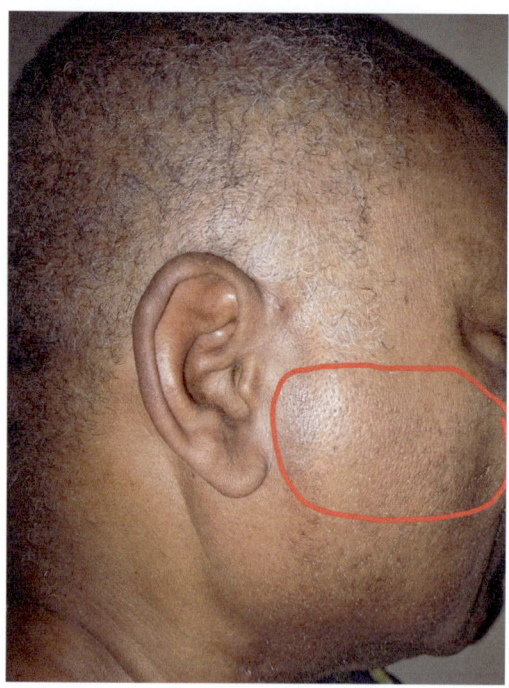

Fig. 1.11 Malar area of the face

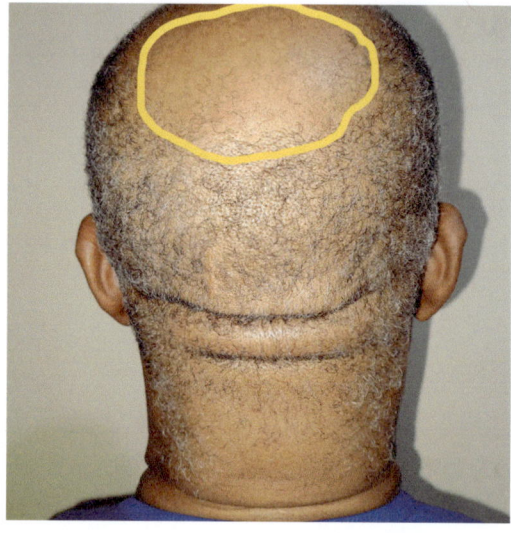

Fig. 1.13 A general description of this patient would include baldness

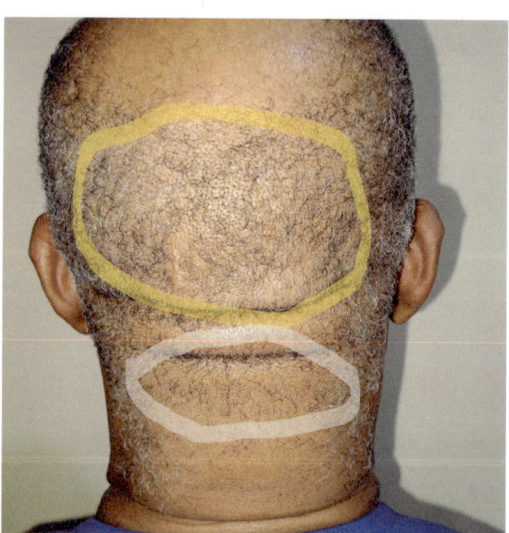

Fig. 1.14 Posterior surface of the head and neck

thin at the upper eyelid compared to the anterior abdominal wall which is also thinner than the back of the torso and which itself is thinner than the inferior surface of the foot at the heel.

- Stratum granulosum.
- Stratum spinosum.
- Stratum basale,

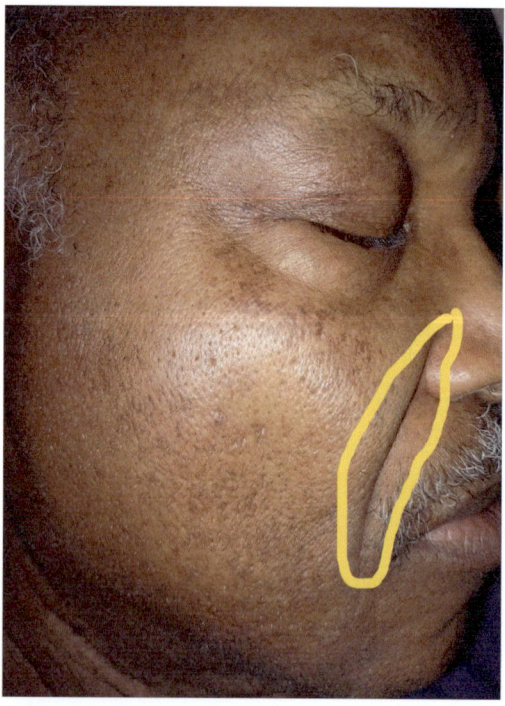

Fig. 1.12 Right side of the face

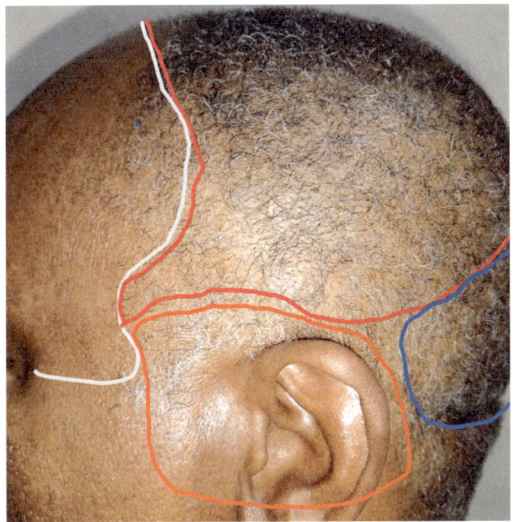

Fig. 1.15 Left side of the scalp

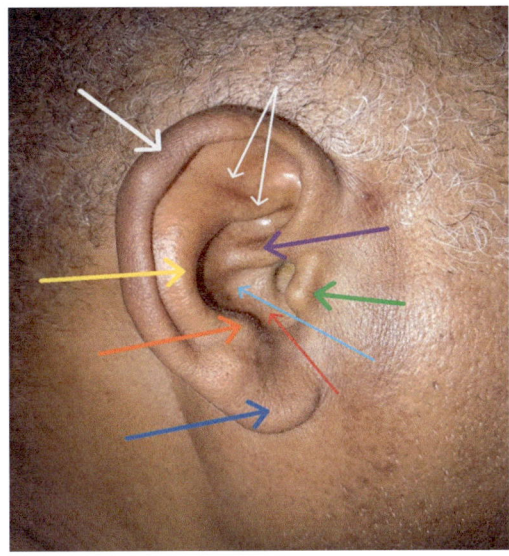

Fig. 1.17 The right outer ear (also called auricle or pinna)

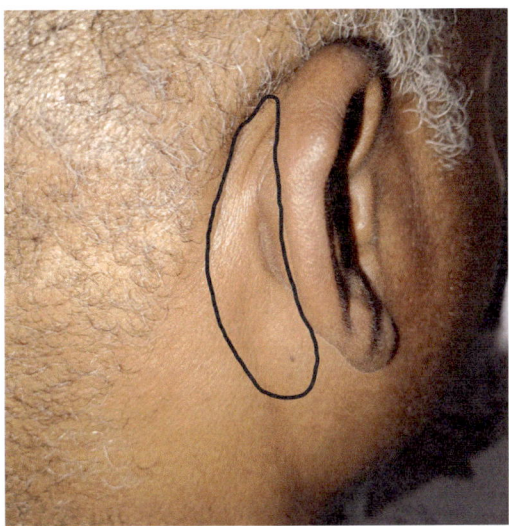

Fig. 1.16 Right side of the face

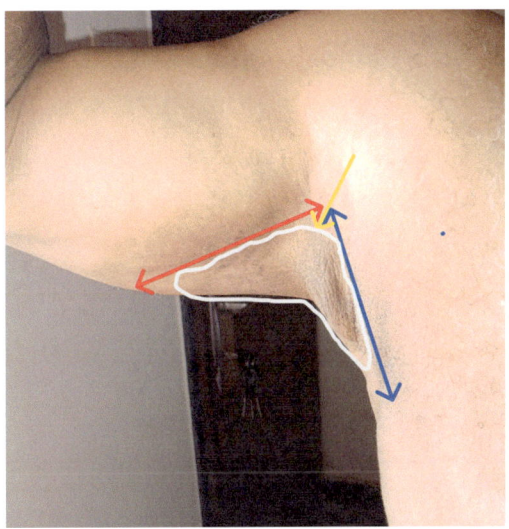

Fig. 1.18 The right axilla

The function of the stratum corneum is to assist in the hydration of the skin by encouraging water retention—the layer achieves this by preventing water loss, which would otherwise result in skin cracking.

Magenta line arrow = The dermis showing a rich network of structures shown mainly in the left part of the illustration

Dark red line arrow = The hypodermis (subcutaneous layer, adipose tissue layer) showing a rich network of structures shown mainly in the left part of the illustration

Orange red line arrow = Muscle layer. This is strictly not a part of the skin, but it is shown to demonstrate the relationship between it and the skin covering superficial muscles.

Grey (Gray) line arrow = Bone. Bone is not a part of the layers of the skin, but it is included in the figure to demonstrate the relationship between it and the skin overlying superficial bones and muscles.

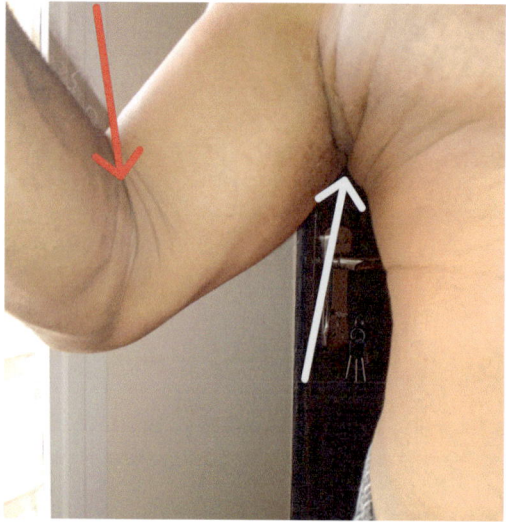

Fig. 1.19 Image showing two skin flexures

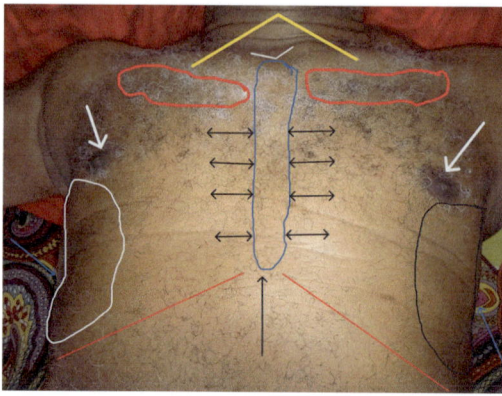

Fig. 1.21 The anterior chest wall

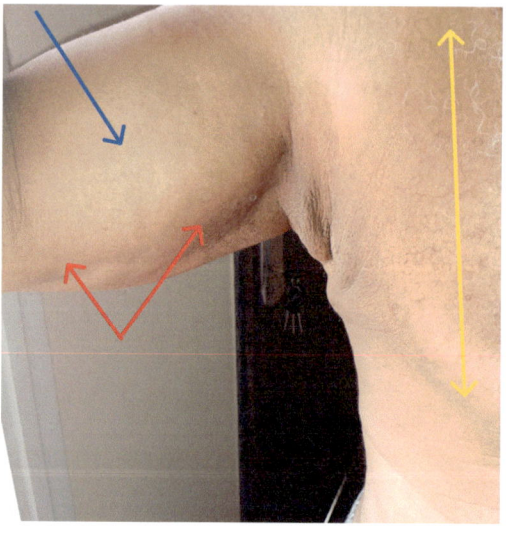

Fig. 1.20 Right arm and right lateral chest wall

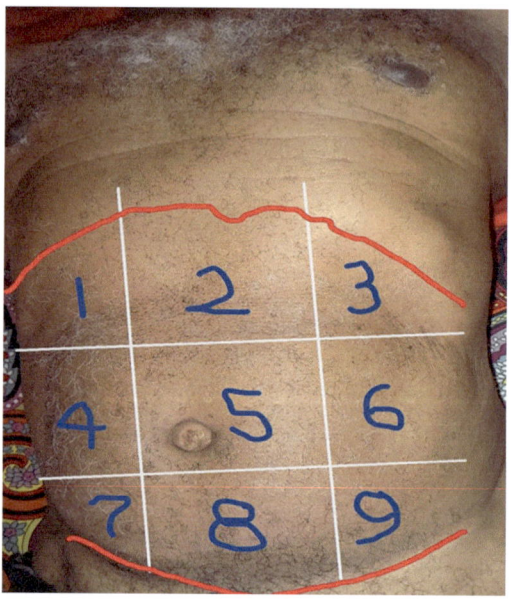

Fig. 1.22 The anterior abdominal wall showing nine regions

Purple line arrow = An illustration of the network of nerve supply to the skin. They terminate as tiny free nerve endings that are sensitive to pain and temperature but also have the following nervous receptors:

- Meissner's corpuscle (subserves light [or sensitive] touch)
- Pacinian corpuscle (subserve pressure and vibration sensations)
- Ruffini's corpuscle (subserve stretch, pressure sensation, and touch)

- Krause's corpuscle (subserves cold sensation)
- Merkel's disk (subserves touch)

Intraepidermal free nerve endings are the endings of the following sensory nerve fibers:

- Aδ-fiber
- Peptidergic C-fiber
- Non-peptidergic C-fiber

Dark green line arrow = Eccrine sweat gland with an opening on the surface of the skin

Fig. 1.23 The posterior trunk

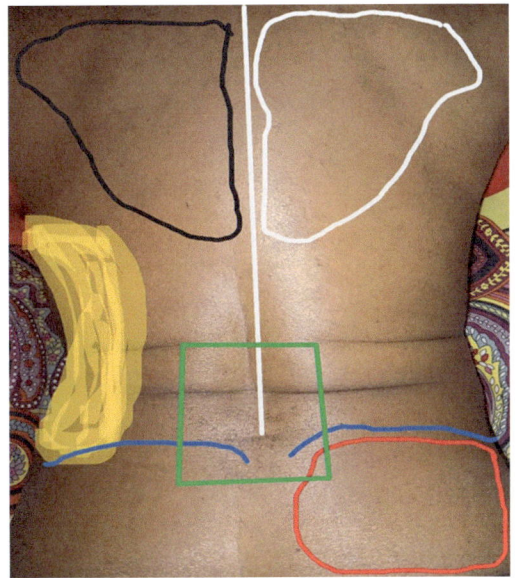

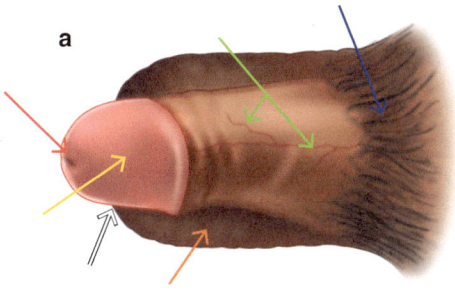

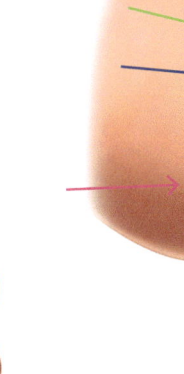

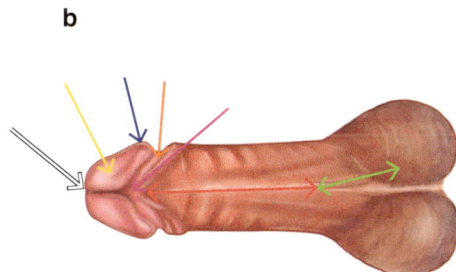

Fig. 1.24 The male perineum

Orange line arrow = The three arrows point at, first, a hair follicle; second, arrector muscle fibers; and, third, sebaceous gland.

Red line arrows = An artery and some of its branches

Blue line arrows = A vein and some of its tributaries

Yellow line arrows = The pores of a vein and an artery

Green line arrows = A hair filament growing form the hair follicle towards the skin surface and another hair above the skin surface

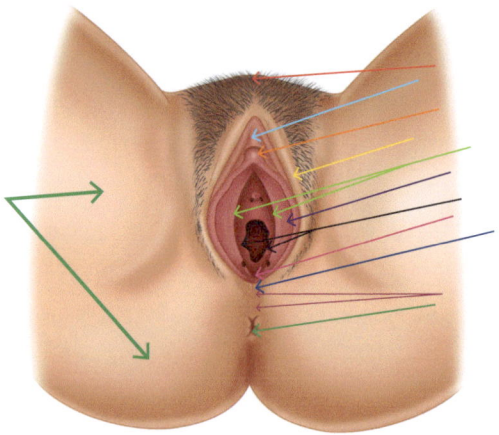

Fig. 1.25 The female perineum and external genitalia (vulva, pudendum)

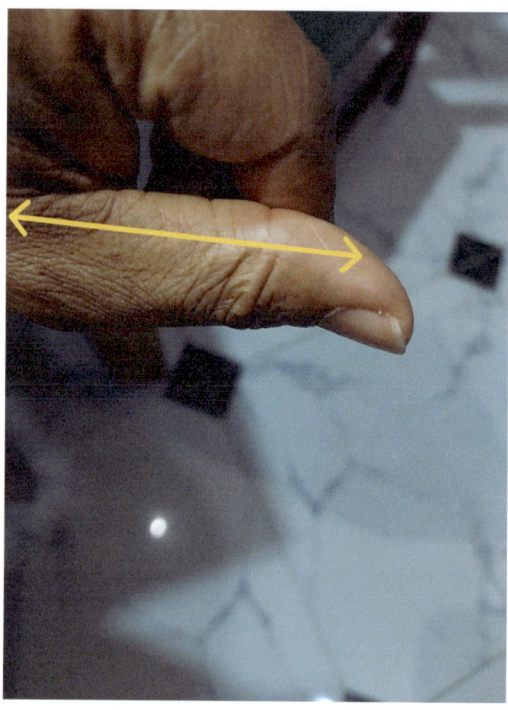

Fig. 1.28 The left thumb

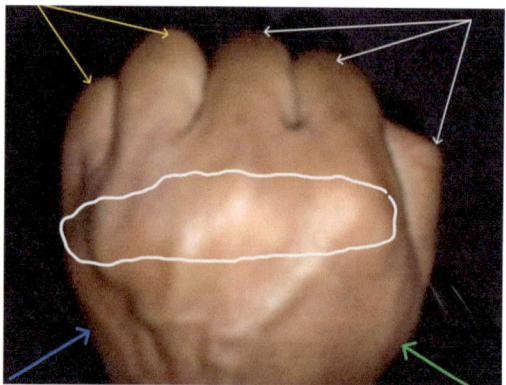

Fig. 1.26 Dorsal surface of the left hand (clenched)

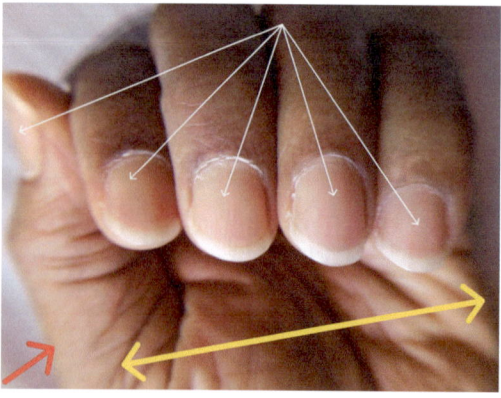

Fig. 1.27 The cupped left hand

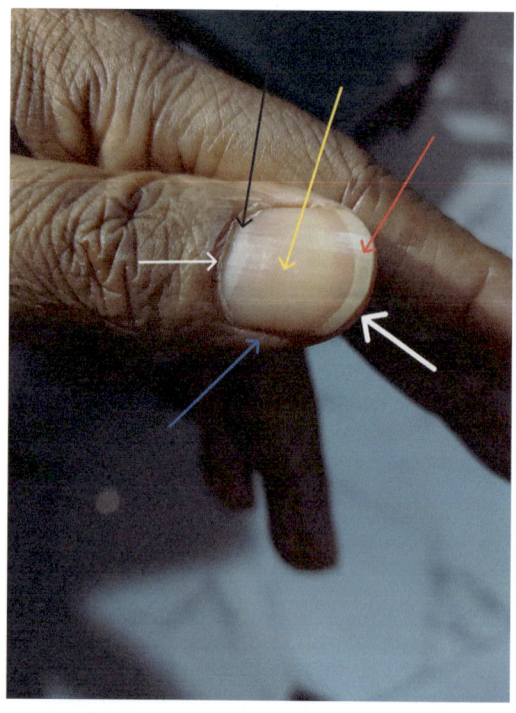

Fig. 1.29 The left thumb

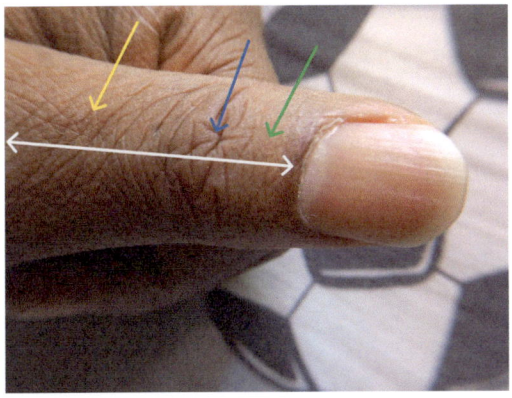

Fig. 1.30 The left thumb

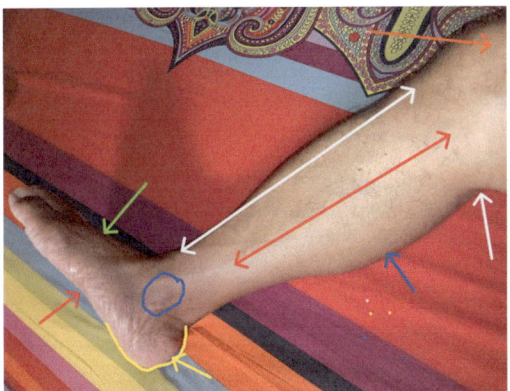

Fig. 1.31 The anterior and medial surfaces of the right leg and foot

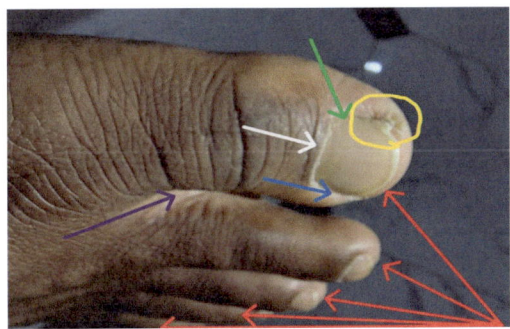

Fig. 1.32 The dorsal surface of the right foot

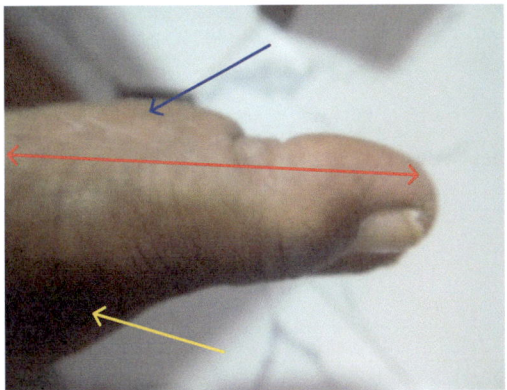

Fig. 1.33 The right foot

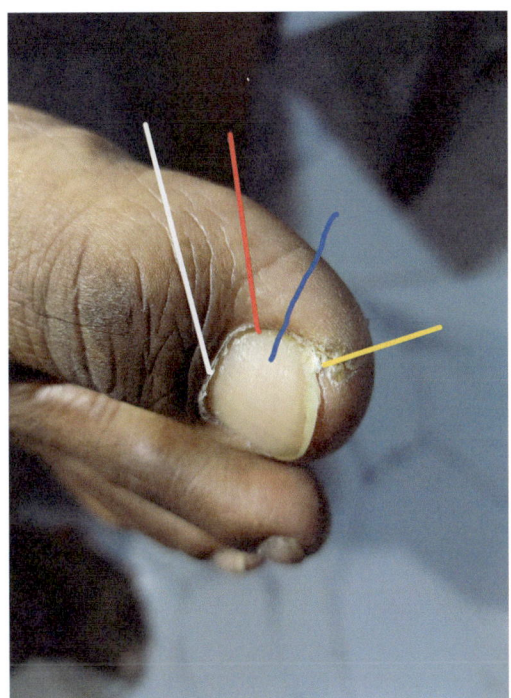

Fig. 1.34 The right foot

In the dermis, the skin also contains lymphatic vessels which are not indicated in this illustration.

Yellow line arrow = Skin over the antecubital fossa.

Red arrow = Lateral border of the left forearm.

Green double line arrow = The anterior surface of the left forearm.

White line arrow = Medial border of the right forearm.

Black line arrow = Median cubital vein. This vein is one of the three major veins in the antecubital fossa—the others are the cephalic vein (laterally) and the basilic vein (medially).

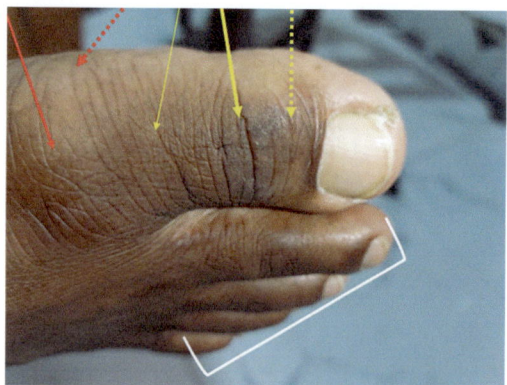

Fig. 1.35 The right foot

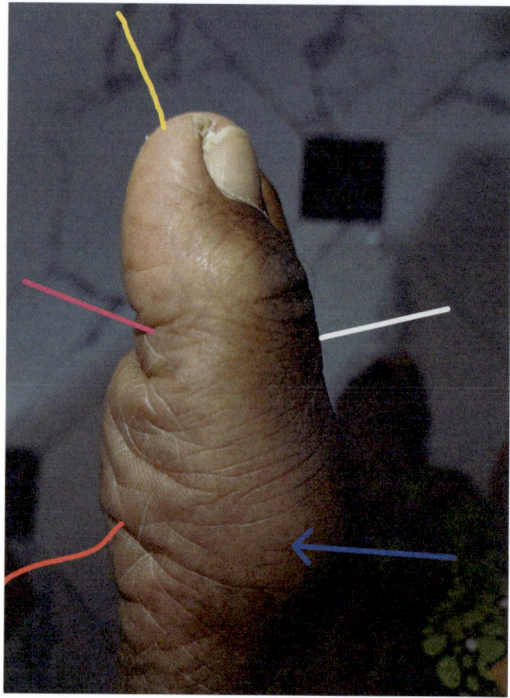

Fig. 1.37 The right foot

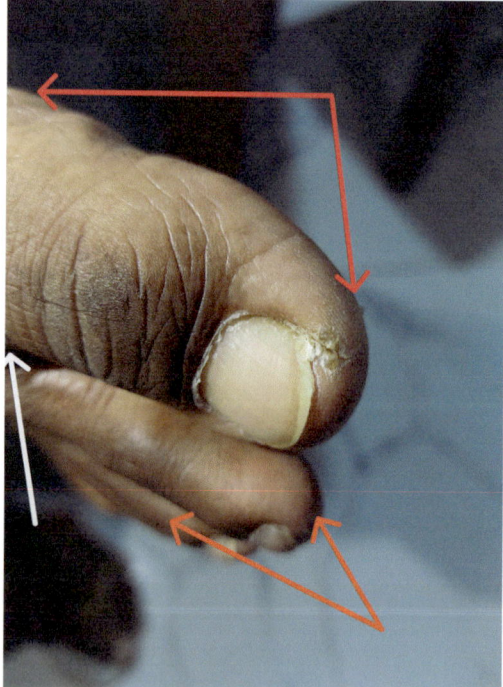

Fig. 1.36 The right foot

The features of a patient's face have the potential of unravelling various types of information to an observant physician. Usually, there is what this author calls a "clinical distance" during an outpatient consultation (and in-patient care). This safe and utilitarian distance is just close enough to enable a doctor with good natural or aided vision to be able to pick up information that can aid in making a "spot diagnosis," comparing with what the patient says during history taking, assessing

the patient's condition generally and level of care for their bodies (at least the skin), or having bases for asking certain questions to confirm suspicions or refute doubts in the clinician's mind.

A doctor may, for example, be able to place the patient's age within an age range/bracket. This is one of the skills that every physician who works in an environment where some employees use "official age" to enable them to remain in a "secure employment" beyond their actual retirement date. This documented "declaration of age" makes them "younger" by taking off some years; it enables them to work for more years. With practice, the doctor can determine that the patient is older than the age from the stated date of birth. For some female patients, they want to be "forever young," and stating 40 as their age when they are 53 (or the like) is not strange. In such cases, the doctor is wise enough to use clinical assessment of age for solving a clinical problem rather than engaging in an argument with the patient. The skill is also useful when some comatose patients are brought to the hospital for emergency care—the entry for age is better than nothing.

In this normal scalp in a child, note the smoothness and uniformity of the exposed scalp surface. There are no rashes, desquamation, crusting, or scaling of the scalp skin. There is a smooth transition between the scalp skin and facial/neck skin. The is no difference between the degree of pigmentation of the scalp skin and facial or neck skin. In older people who do not want "their age to show" and, therefore, use black dye to maintain the expected color of Black scalp hair, the scalp may become hyperpigmented after frequent hair dyeing.

White line arrow = Glabella

Yellow line arrow = Nasion

Green line arrow = Nasal root

Black double line arrow = Nasal ridge

Red line arrow = Tip of the nose

Black line arrow = Left ala of the nose

Area encircled in blue = Nasal bridge

Light blue line arrow = Inner canthus (right)

White curved line = Skin over columella

Orange design below the base of the nose = Philtrum

Orange line arrow = Left ala (wing) of the nose

White line arrow = Left nasolabial fold

Blue line arrow = Tip of the nose

Black double line arrows = Philtrum

Green line arrow = Tubercle of the superior lip

Yellow line arrow = Lower lip

Red double red arrows = Vermillion borders of upper and lower lips

White bold line arrow = Normal density of eyebrows medially

White line arrow = Sparse eyebrows laterally

Blue line arrow = Upper eyelid

Green line arrow = Upper eyelashes

Red line arrow = Infraorbital margin

Area encircled in red = Malar area of the right side of the face; the left side of the face has a mirror image.

Area encircled in yellow = The right nasolabial fold

Area encircled in yellow highlight = Occipital scalp skin

Area encircled in white highlight = Nape

Area delineated with white = Frontal scalp

Area outlined with red = Parietal scalp

Area demarcated with blue = Occipital scalp

Area encircled in orange = Temporal scalp

When describing a rash, e.g., of tinea capitis, or a carbuncle, or an enlarged lymph node due to an infective process, it is important to indicate precisely where it is—not just "macule on scalp."

Area encircled in black = Right posterior auricular area

Blue line arrow = Lobule of the right auricle

Orange line arrow = Antitragus

Yellow line arrow = Antihelix

White line arrow = Helix

Double white arrows = Crura of the antihelix (superior and inferior [or posterior and anterior])

Purple line arrow = Crus of helix

Green line arrow = Tragus

Light blue line arrow = Cavum of concha of the right auricle

Red line arrow = Intertragic notch (incisura)

Red double line arrows = The lateral border of the right axilla

Blue double line arrows = The medial border of the right axilla

Yellow line arrow = The apex of the right axilla

Area encircled in white = Skin of the right axilla

Red line arrow = Skin flexure over the right elbow

White line arrow = Skin flexure at the right axilla

Blue line arrow = Anterior surface of the right arm

Red double line arrows = Medial surface of the right arm

Yellow double arrows = Lateral aspect of the right chest wall

Blue line arrows = Lateral aspect of the chest wall

Area encircled in white = Right anterolateral chest wall (roughly)

Area encircled in black = Left anterolateral chest wall (roughly)

White line arrows = Right and left breasts

Areas encircled in red = Infraclavicular areas (Right and left)

V-shaped area = Jugular (suprasternal) notch

Two yellow line arrows = Clavicles (Right and left)

Area encircled in blue = Skin over the sternum

Black double arrows = Skin over anterior abdominal wall lateral to the right and left sternal borders

Two red lines = Inferior margins of the chest wall

Black line arrow = Skin over the position of the xiphisternum

1 = Right hypochondriac

2 = Epigastric

3 = Left hypochondriac

4 = Right lumbar

5 = Umbilical

6 = Left lumbar

7 = Right iliac

8 = Hypogastric

9 = Left iliac

Area encircled in black = Skin over the left scapula

Area encircled in white = Skin over the right scapula

Area depicted in yellow highlight = Skin over the left flank

White straight line = Skin over the midline depression formed by the spine

Area enclosed by green quadrangle = The lower back (From L1 to L5)

Blue curved lines = Skin approximately over the iliac crests (L4/L5 intervertebral disk space)

Area enclosed in red = Skin over the right buttock (gluteal area). This is not a part of the back but a part of the posterior trunk.

(A)

Red line arrow = External urethral orifice

Green double line arrows = Superficial dorsal veins of the penis

Blue line arrows = Pubic hairs. Some patients who do close skin shaving. Scrotal skin is thin and relatively loose of pubic hair may develop furuncles. Pediculosis pubis (or pthiriasis pubis), the parasitic infestation Pthirus pubis causes, preferentially affects the hairs at this site. Much less commonly, the crab lice may infest hair on the mustache, axilla, eyebrows, anterior chest wall, or beards. The causative organism is called crab louse because when viewed under the microscope it is reminiscent of the shape of a crab. This parasitic infestation is frequently transmitted by sexual contact or direct bodily contact. The infection may be transmitted by fomites like clothing, towels, and bedding used by an infested individual.

Red line arrow = Scrotal skin. Scrotal skin in thin and relatively loose compared with the skin in most parts of the body.

White line arrow = Prepuce. The prepuce is a continuation of the penile shaft skin; it covers glans penis and the external urethral meatus [4]. Individuals who have not been circumcised still have the prepuce (foreskin). The prepuce is retractable but it is not so at birth; retractability of the prepuce occurs as a boy grows, and when there are no problems, it is complete by about age 18 years [5]. There is an association between the penile cancer and the human papillomavirus (HPV) [6]. While there is no clear-cut link between the role of circumcision and the development of penile cancer, a male who did not undergo circumcision in childhood is at a greater risk of developing an invasive form of the cancer [6]. The study by Cooblal et al. showed that ignorance and misunderstanding are rife among parents regarding the role of the prepuce in boys; this is irrespective of the fact preputial pathology is common in the pediatric population in the practice setting of the study [7].

Yellow line arrow = Glans penis

(B)

White line arrow = External urethral orifice

Yellow line arrow = Glans penis

Blue line arrow = Corona of glans penis

Orange line arrow = Neck of glans penis

Magenta line arrow = Frenulum (This part that is present only on the ventral surface of the penis)

Red double line arrows = Shaft of the penis: This illustration demonstrates the ventral surface of the penis although the shaft circumference is covered by penile skin. A description of a rash on the penile shaft should be specific and indicate if it is at the distal end of the dorsal surface, right or left lateral surface, or ventral surface; the same should apply to the mid-shaft, or the proximal end which abuts with or in close proximity to the root of the penis.

Green double line arrows = Root of the penis

(C)

Dark purple line arrow = Scrotum

Red line arrow = Pubic symphysis

Yellow line arrow = Urogenital triangle

Orange line arrow = Anal triangle

Green line arrow = Anus

White line arrow = Tip of the coccyx

Magenta line arrow = Right buttock

Blue line arrow = Ischial tuberosity

Green line arrow = Ischiopubic ramus

Light purple line arrow = Right upper thigh

Commencing at the top of the image and going clockwise the parts illustrated are:

Red line arrow = Mons pubis

Light blue line arrow = Prepuce of clitoris

Orange line arrow = Glans of clitoris

Yellow line arrow = Left labium majus

Light green double line arrows = Vestibule of vagina. This is the space that the labia minora surround. This triangular space is the equivalent of the dorsal wall of the cavernosa urethra in males and where the paraurethral gland (Skene) ducts open bilaterally in addition to the external urethral orifice [8]. During female orgasm, Skene glands expel their secretion (which contains prostatic specific antigen) into the vestibule [8].

Purple line arrow = Left labium minus

Black double line arrows = Vaginal orifice and hymenal caruncle

Magenta line arrow = Vestibular fossa

Dark blue line arrow = Frenulum of the labia minora

Red double arrows = Posterior commissure of the labia minora and perineal raphe (skin covering the perineal body)

Green line arrow = Anus

Green double line arrows = Medial surface of the proximal part of the thigh and the right buttock.

Blue line arrow = Medial surface of the left hand

Area encircled in white = Knuckles (Skin over the metacarpophalangeal joints)

Two yellow line arrows = Knuckles (Skin over the proximal interphalangeal joints of the fourth (ring) and fifth (little) fingers

Three white line arrows = Knuckles of the third (middle) and second (index) and first finger

(thumb). Note that since the thumb has only two phalanges, its knuckle is formed by the interphalangeal joint—unlike the other four phalanges that each have three phalanges and consequently have proximal and distal interphalangeal joints.

Examination of the dorsum of the hand also yields useful information. On healthy, well-protected hands, the skin of the dorsi has little or no scars, is smooth, and has a uniform pigmentation. Some patients who have used creams, lotions, and soaps that contain bleaching agents (usually called skin lightening or skin toning agents) do not maintain the expected or usual uniformity of pigmentation and texture of the dorsi of the hands at the knuckles; what they have is hyperpigmentation (from bleaching) of the skin over the knuckles.

Red line arrow = Lateral border (side) of the left hand

Yellow double line arrows = Slightly oblique extent of the palmar (anterior) surface of the hand

Five white line arrows = The fingernails of the left hand

The fingernails have proved to be reliable indicators of health and disease. It is important for every medical student and general medical practitioner to pay close attention to the features of a patient's fingers even when the patient's complaints are not primarily dermatological. When the complaints are dermatological and particularly about the hands and fingers, the examination must be thorough and the description of the features and findings in the affected nail(s) should be detailed and precise. If the fingernail features cannot be appreciated by direct observation with the eyes, some magnification will serve the examiner a good purpose, and the simplest and most readily available tool is a magnifying glass. The doctor should look out for changes in shape or color (or both) when examining nails. The specific shape abnormalities are koilonychia, onycholysis, clubbing, Beau's lines, Mees' lines, longitudinal striations, and pitting. Color abnormalities include yellow nails, splinter hemorrhage, telangiectasia, dark longitudinal streaks, Terry's white nails, and half-and-half nails—half-and-half nails are pathognomonic for renal failure and present as a white nail plate proximally while the distal half has a different color like brown or red with a sharp demarcation between them [9].

Yellow double line arrows = The medial surface of the left thumb

Blue line arrow = Lateral skin fold of the left thumb

White line arrow = Eponychium (proximal skin fold of the thumb)

Black line arrow = Lunule. This whitish crescentic (half-moon shaped) proximal part of the nail plate is also called lunula with lunulae the name for the plural. Structurally, the lunule determines the shape of the free end of the nail plate. The lunule is the most distal part of the nail matrix which is further proximal and covered by the eponychium. Growth of the nail plate is from the matrix. There may be morphological changes or abnormalities of the lunule (lunula) in the form of absence (anolunula), too big (macrolunula), too small (microlunula), or abnormality in shape with loss of convexity of the distal end which is normally of a convex edge. The abnormality may also be in the form of color when there is a color other than white. A disruption of normal nail plate growth shows as a loss of the lunule and eventual disconnection of the nail plate from the nail bed; there is a proximal dislodgement of the affected nails as they are "lifted" from the bed from the proximal part of the nail towards the tip (distal end) of the nails. An example is discussed in Chap. 8.

Yellow line arrow = Nail plate

Red line arrow = Free distal end of the nail plate

Bold white line arrow = The convex edge of the free distal end of the nail plate

White double line arrows = Skin of the dorsum (dorsal surface) of the left thumb starting from the first metacarpophalangeal joint (not clearly shown) to the eponychium.

Yellow line arrow = Skin over the proximal phalanx of the first finger (thumb)

Blue line arrow = Skin over the interphalangeal joint of the thumb

Green line arrow = Skin over the distal phalanx of the thumb

Orange line arrow = Skin over the anterior surface of the knee (patella)

Double white line arrows = Skin over the "shin bone." The shin bone is the tibia which is covered by a layer of skin, the thickness of which does not protect the bone from significant trauma. Moreover, the vascularization of the skin over the shin is poor compared to that of the back of the leg. Injuries on this anterior part of the leg frequently leads to scars right from childhood. Many people feel dissatisfied with the appearance of multiple scarred feet and seek a solution from dermatologists and plastic surgeons.

White line arrow = Posterior surface of the knee. Skin over the popliteal fossa is one of the sites of flexural eczema in young teenagers and adults and atopic dermatitis (atopic eczema) in infants, toddlers, and older children.

Blue line arrow = Posterior surface of the leg. Note bulky tissue beneath the skin unlike the rigid structure beneath the skin over the anterior surface.

Area encircled in blue = Skin over the medial malleolus. Patients with sickle cell anemia tend to develop superficial ulcers at the malleoli. Injuries at the anterior and posterior malleoli require great care to ensure adequate healing.

Yellow line arrow and C-shaped illustrations = The heel of the right foot. The major weight-bearing bone that the thick skin of the foot covers at the heel is the calcaneus. Hyperkeratosis of the heel has a predilection for the heels although other parts of the plantar surface of the foot are affected.

Five red line arrows = The distal ends of first, second, and third digits and the dorsal surfaces of the fourth and fifth toes of the right foot

Purple line arrow = The web (interdigital space) between the right big toe and the right second toe. Note the description: It is wrong to write "the second right toe" as the meaning is totally different. All the toes (and fingers) are named by number and not by the side (right or left). It is the side that identifies which second toe. Therefore, in this figure, the foot and all its toes are right. The correct description is the second toe that is on the right side of the body—"the right second toe." On the other hand, "the second right toe" means that there is a right toe that has more than one of its type, i.e., that toe has a first, second, and even third or more. This apparently otiose detail is important because a dermatologist and every other specialist create a mental picture of what you tell them on phone or what they read on paper or laptop screen. Referral letters or notes (and descriptions on the phone) must be precise so that the mental image that the person you communicate with is on the same page with you.

Blue line arrow = Lateral skin fold of the right big toe

White line arrow = Proximal skin fold of the right big toe

Green line arrow = Medial skin fold of the right big toe

Area encircled in yellow = A healed area of ingrowing right big toe nail medially

Yellow line arrow = The dorsal surface (dorsum) of the right foot

Red double line arrow = The medial surface of the right foot

Blue line arrow = The plantar surface (sole) of the right foot

White line = The proximal nail fold

Red line = Medial nail fold

Blue line = Nail plate of the right thumb

Yellow line = Medial end of the right big toenail showing roughness and the skin demonstrating thickening (lichenification)

Red line arrow = Skin over the metatarsophalangeal joint of the right big toe

Red broken line arrow = Medial surface of the right big toe

Thin yellow line arrow = Skin over the dorsum of the metatarsophalangeal joint of the right big toe

Yellow broken line arrow = Skin over the dorsum of the distal phalanx of the right big toe

White bracket = The second, third, fourth, and fifth (little) toes of the right foot

White line arrow = Interdigital space between the big toe and the second toe (the first interdigital space of the right foot)

Double red line arrows = The medial surface (border) of the right big toe

Double orange line arrows = Distal end (tip) of the right second toe and the dorsum of the right third toe

Red curved line = Plantar surface of the distal half of the right foot

Magenta line = Plantar skin over the interphalangeal joint of the right big toe

Yellow line = The distal end (tip) of the right big toe

White line = Dorsum of the right big toe

Blue line arrow = Top of the medial surface of the right big toe over the metatarsophalangeal joint (formed by the base of the proximal phalanx and the head of the metatarsus) of the first (big) toe.

Ichthyosis Vulgaris

Symptoms

The patient, a young man of about 25 years of age, came to the hospital to consult the doctor with complaints of dry skin and multiple scaly rashes of many years; he could not specify his precise age at onset but indicated that he was a child. His parents also did not take the rashes as serious and could not pinpoint the onset but simply stated that they were from his early childhood, between ages 3 and 5. Attempts at obtaining a solution right from when his parents started feeling worried about the condition had proved abortive as the doctors in each hospital in his community (and nearby communities) almost consistently advised use of petroleum jelly and "to manage" with the condition. The young man was now feeling not only concern but embarrassment because of the poor aesthetics of his body and he had plans to marry in the near future but did not know who fair it would be to get married without finding and implementing a solution to this health challenge. He strongly hoped that the teaching hospital doctors would proffer a solution to the skin condition.

Signs

Figures 1.38, 1.39, and 1.40 are photographs of a young man in the mid-20s age group. Examination of the affected parts of the body showed that he

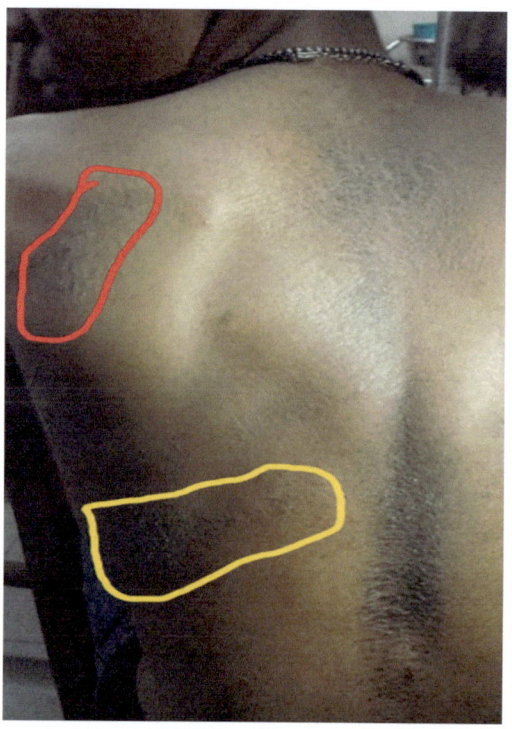

Fig. 1.38 Hyperpigmented scaly lesions on the midline of upper and mid-back

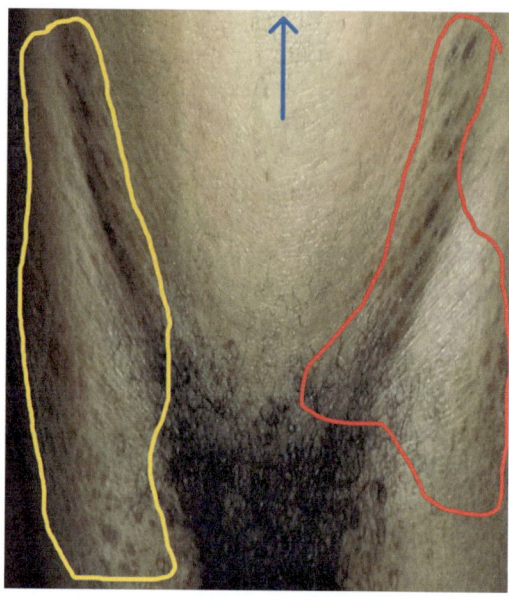

Fig. 1.40 Lesions on the abdomen and anterior thighs in the same patient in the two earlier figures

The above photograph, Fig. 1.38, shows the back. The extent was from the midline of the upper back, extending laterally on both sides, although falling short of the medial border of the scapula bilaterally. The lesions on the mid and lower back appeared to be more prominent, more hyperpigmented, more scaly, and more dense than the ones on the upper part of the back. These rashes were almost limited to the midline, barely encroaching on the skin over the erector spinae muscles.

There were similar, though less pronounced, rashes on the skin over the superolateral part of the left scapula (circled red) and a lateral strip inferior to the inferior angle of the left scapula (circled yellow).

The lesions on the neck and anterior upper chest were concentrated on the skin over the suprasternal notch and the supraclavicular fossae. Being larger hyperpigmented rashes, their separation by normal skin shows that many of them are discrete and are polygonal in shape. For the discrete lesions, there is a clear demarcation between them and the contiguous (separating) skin which is less hyperpigmented than the lesions but not of the normal pigmentation of unaffected skin just over and inferior to the left clavicle.

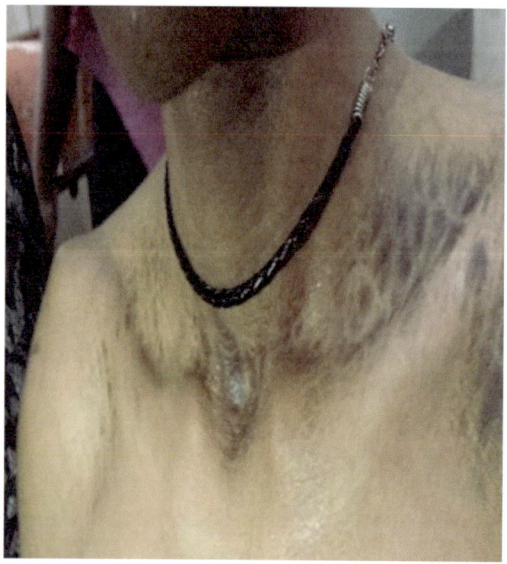

Fig. 1.39 Lesions on the neck and anterior upper chest

had had dry scaly skin. The lesions were thick and hyperpigmented, with polygonal scales separated by fissures.

Although this patient's anterior chest wall lesion on the lateral aspect of the left upper chest is not fully represented by Fig. 1.39, it extended to the lateral end of the upper chest wall at the anterior margin of the medial wall of the left axilla.

Examination findings were similarly multiple, rough, scaly rashes circled yellow and red. However, they were less hyperpigmented than the lesions on the back and neck shown in the two earlier figures. The up-pointing blue line arrow indicates the location of the umbilicus as higher and outside the upper limit of this photograph.

Diagnosis

On clinical grounds, this presumptive diagnosis of this patient was ichthyosis vulgaris.

This patient was referred to consult the dermatologist who took over the care of the patient.

Follow-Up Care

Follow-up care was provided by the dermatologist.

Discussion

Ichthyosis vulgaris may be inherited or acquired. The pediatric disease is transmitted by autosomal dominant inheritance and usually manifests first during infancy. The acquired form is the usual form in adult-onset disease. Acquired ichthyosis vulgaris usually has underlying diseases, e.g., diabetes mellitus, atopy, systemic lupus erythematosus, lymphoma, renal failure, thyroid disease, etc.; it could be consequent upon exposure to certain drugs, e.g., clofazimine used in treatment of leprosy; lipid-lowering drugs like statins (atorvastatin, simvastatin, and rosuvastatin) and fibrates (fenofibrate); and butyrophenone. History taking should attempt to identify the likely underlying condition.

Ichthyosis vulgaris is the commonest and mildest of ichthyosis which presents a picture reminiscent of fish scales. Skin cells are produced normally, but due to increased accumulation with minimal shedding of skin epithelium (stratum corneum), there is thickening, dryness, and scaling of the skin.

Pathophysiology The pathophysiology of ichthyosis vulgaris is mutation of the protein molecule filaggrin; it is responsible for the development of ichthyosis vulgaris. The correct level of hydration of the skin is regulated by the protein filaggrin. A defect in filaggrin allows excessive loss of water from the superficial layer of the skin, and this is responsible for the dryness.

Presentation Regarding severity, it varies from patient to patient—thus while it may be mild in one patient, another patient could present with severe symptoms and signs. Symptoms are various degrees of pruritus and skin dryness. Signs are obvious dryness, lichenification, and scaling. The scales are usually large. Large portions of the body may be affected. Moist, flexural parts of the skin tend to be spared, e.g., axillae, inframammary area, groin, etc. Literature indicates that lower limbs are most frequently affected with other parts being the abdomen and gluteal region while the face tends to be spared. Extensor surface of the skin at joints, e.g., knees and hip, tend to be affected more severely. The scaling produces tiny, whitish scales. In the patient whose photographs are shown, the thickening and scaling are concentrated on the following parts: central part of the back longitudinally (Fig. 1.38); the upper part of the chest especially the suprasternal notch, suprascapular fossa bilaterally, and the left infrascapular area (Fig. 1.39); and the inguinal area and anterior upper thighs bilaterally (Fig. 1.40). The areas of concentration described above have various degrees of hyperpigmentation. Warmth and moisture tend to ameliorate symptoms.

Investigations Investigations carried out on patients with ichthyosis vulgaris after history taking and physical examination which may provide a lead to the underlying cause may cover any of the following: Prenatally, ultrasonography may demonstrate polyhydramnios and excessive intraamniotic debris as a pointer to the inherited disease; full blood count with differential count and bone marrow aspirate analysis may be useful in cases of leukemia and myelodysplastic syndromes; skin biopsy—involved skin in ichthyosis vulgaris—demonstrates mild hyperkeratosis and a reduction in the granular layer of the epidermis, but there is no abnormality in the dermis; serum glucose shows characteristic elevation in diabetes mellitus; chest X-ray may prove useful in tuberculosis, HIV, lymphoma, and sarcoidosis. Other tests include HIV testing, serum cholesterol sulfate, CT scan, genetic testing, lipoprotein electrophoresis, etc.

Treatment Treatment should target moisturizing the skin with emollients; for this purpose, 10% of urea, glycerin, or lactic acid in the moisturizers is useful for most patients, or alphahydroxy acids. For patients with atopy who are allergic to alpha-hydroxy acids, another moisturizer that does not include these acids should be chosen. Oral retinoids are useful by virtue of their anti-keratinizing action; they produce results that mitigate depression, cosmetic disfigurement, and social isolation that patients also suffer from in very severe cases. In summary, medical, surgical, or other treatment recommended depends on the extent of disease and associated conditions.

Heel Hyperkeratosis (Cracked Heels)

Yellow line arrow = Dorsum of the foot (the skin over this surface is thinner than covering the rest of the foot

Green line arrow = Skin over the anterior surface of the ankle joint. Dorsiflexion reduces the angle at this joint while plantarflexion increases it to achieve an obtuse angle. Rashes on this flexural surface include neurodermatitis (lichen simplex chronicus).

Red double line arrows = Parts of the talus; the talus is located superior to the calcaneus.

Blue line arrow = The calcaneus. The calcaneus is the largest bone on the foot and is a principal bearer of the weight of the body at the foot.

Posteriorly and inferiorly, it is covered by skin that has thick cornified epithelium. The stratum corneum at the heel and the rest of the plantar surface of the foot is thickest in the body.

Three red line arrows = Depict the sole of the foot which is thick. This part of the skin is frequently involved in hyperkeratosis of the heel with consequent cracking or fissuring. Patients frequently visit the outpatient clinics with this condition during winter and harmattan.

Four yellow line arrows = Fissures on the sole of the heel of the right foot. The one on the central part of the heel is transversely disposed while the most medial is irregular although curved.

Symptoms

This patient is an elderly man over 65 years old. He is hypertensive but not diabetic. His blood pressure is well controlled. He is prediabetic with HbA1c of 6.1%; his last random blood glucose value in the previous 3 days was 7.7 mmol/L.

He complained of a recurrent, seasonal, cracking of the soles of his feet for "as many years as he could remember." There would always be cracking of his feet during the harmattan season which is usually between November and January in Nigeria. He said that at the beginning of the season, he would not bother about the beginning of the cracks, but within 2 weeks (like in this current episode), he would develop pain and examine the affected foot only to find that the "wound" on the foot was deeper just within 2 weeks. His observa-

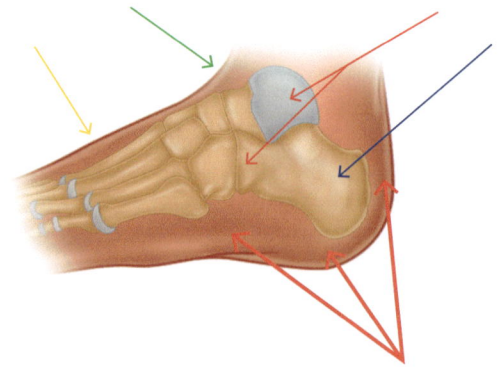

Fig. 1.41 Diagrammatic illustration of the foot

tion was that although the 2 feet were involved, only the right foot caused him greater concern for the cracks on that foot were not only more in number but also more painful, deeper, and occasionally caused bleeding. Bleeding usually occurred when he wore covered footwear to go to work or sneakers for his exercise walks. In this season, he experienced everything other than bleeding. The pain he experienced was not sufficient to prevent him from doing his normal work or carrying out any duties or functions outside his home as it used to happen when he was not retired; now he could control both his time and activities. Only rarely would he take a dose or two of paracetamol (Tylenol) for pain occasioned by this condition.

Relieving factors consisted of using a piece of stone to scrub the feet, particularly the affected parts, applying cream at the sides of the feet, and keeping his feet clean and uncovered. At bedtime, he usually applied any available "heel balm" to the soles of the feet, particularly the affected part and wore a pair of socks immediately thereafter, before lying down to sleep. For many years, he always ensured that he kept "heel balm" handy in anticipation of this recurrent problem during harmattan.

The patient had never experienced fever, malaise, or symptoms of systemic illness associated with the condition. He could not say that there was a family history but one of his siblings and one of their adult daughters experienced a milder form of the condition.

Two red lines arrows = Two longitudinal fissures on the lateral half of the plantar surface of the proximal part of the right foot

Black line arrow = Lateral surface of the right foot

Signs

On examination, the patient was an articulate, well-nourished elderly man who was well groomed and well dressed. He wore simple footwear (flip flops) and did not appear in any form of discomfort or pain while walking into the consulting room, unassisted.

Figure 1.42 is a photograph of the plantar surface of a clean right foot showing fissures on the sole of the heel of the right foot. The most lateral was superficial, longitudinal, and not tender. The fissure next to it was longer, the surfaces were not completely apposed, and the fissure appeared deeper, non-tender, and longitudinal like the first one. The one on the central part of the heel was transversely disposed and had surfaces that were satisfactorily apposed, and the fissure had the semblance of just a depression caused by a recently healed scar; like the other two, there was no tenderness. The fourth fissure is the most medial of the four; its shape was irregular although curved and somewhat oblique.

Figure 1.43 is an enlargement of the two lateral cracks on the patient's foot. The lateral crack still shows its longitudinal disposition. The second one shows a lateral extension (short) branching off from the middle of the length of the fissure; on the medial side, there is more of a thickening than a medial extension. Sensation of pain was intact on this patient's foot as there was neither tenderness, paresthesia, nor dysesthesia.

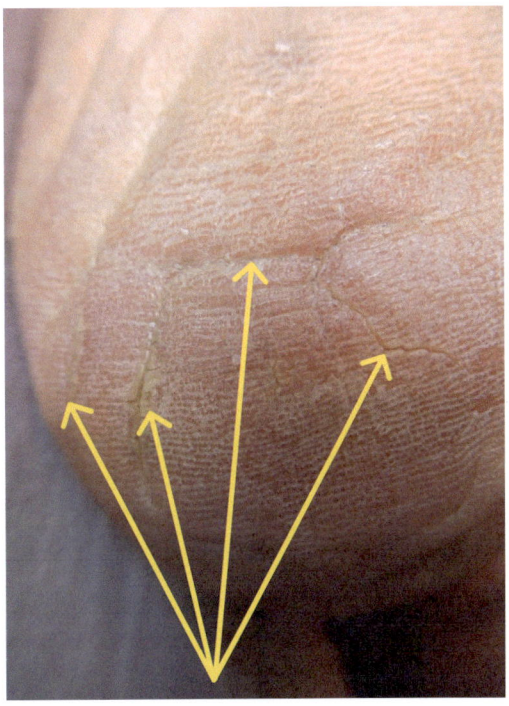

Fig. 1.42 Sole of the right foot

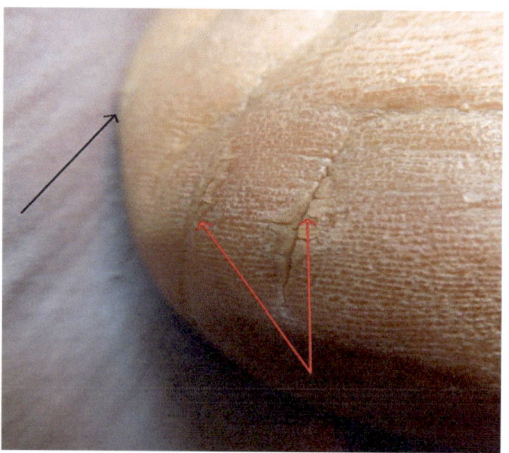

Fig. 1.43 Proximal part of the sole of the right foot; same patient as in Fig. 1.42

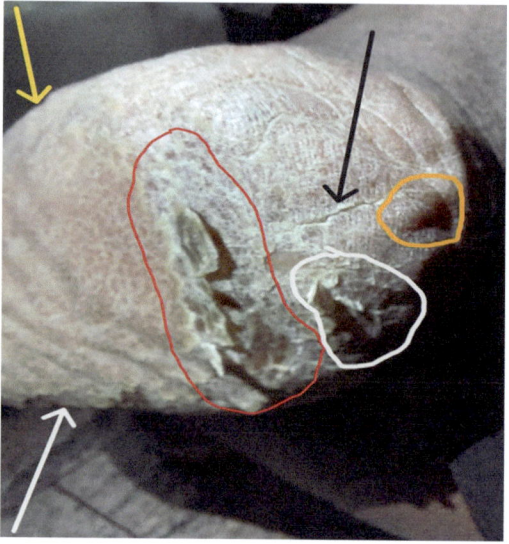

Fig. 1.44 The proximal part of the left heel of a 64-year-old patient

Yellow line arrow = The lateral surface of the left foot

White line arrow = The medial surface of the affected foot

Black line arrow = A longitudinal superficial fissure almost commencing from the proximal part of the heel

Area encircled in orange = An ovoid elevated part of the heel just abutting the beginning of the longitudinal crack

Area encircled in white = Scaly, superficial ulcerated medial aspect of the left heel

Area encircled in red = A deep and wide transverse disruption of the entire medial half of the plantar surface of the distal part of the heel. The affected part consisted of thick flaps of the stratum corneum of the epithelium.

Symptoms

The second patient, although having a diagnosis of obesity, did not have hypertension or diabetes mellitus. The symptoms of this elderly female patient were similar to those of the male patient described above. For this patient, the involvement was also on both feet, but the symptoms were more severe and more inconveniencing.

Signs

The signs are shown in Fig. 1.44. The photograph is of the left foot. The skin flaps (the part lifted off from the sole of the foot) were not tender, except at the points where they were still attached to the ulcerated, non-bleeding, portion of the heel. Figure 1.45 shows skin that is rough, dusky, and with multiple exaggerated creases some of which have formed superficial fissures.

Figures 1.44, 1.45, and 1.46 show that there was no debris and there was no bleeding in other parts of the heel.

The entire foot was thickened but the entire affected part was dry, scaly, and thick, but was clean.

The sole of the left foot was also thickened but the heel had less alarming lesions.

Diagnosis

Heel hyperkeratosis (cracked heels)

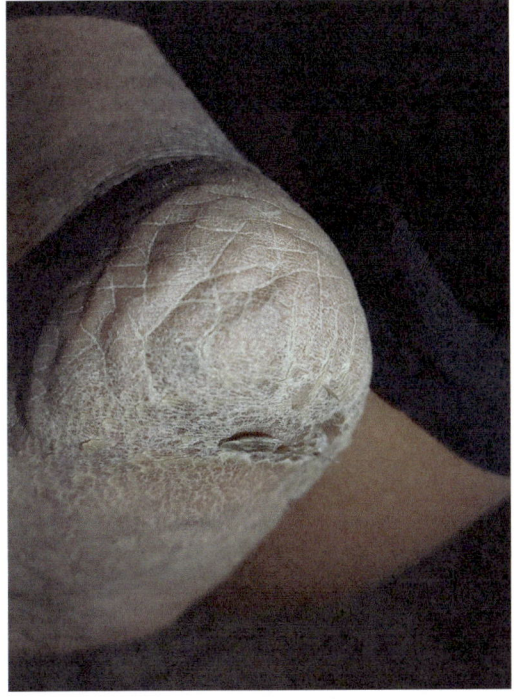

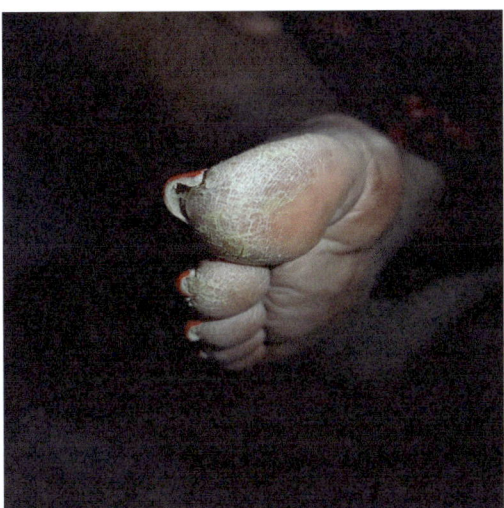

Fig. 1.47 In this severe case, the toes were also involved; the big toe was mostly affected

lesions cleared within 10 days of applying the prescribed heel balm.

Fig. 1.45 This image focuses on the posterior surface of the heel

Prognosis

The prognosis of heel hyperkeratosis (Cracked heels) is good although it is a predictable weather-based condition of the foot. A patient who cares for their feet is not expected to have complications of cracked feet like cellulitis, bleeding, and pain especially when walking.

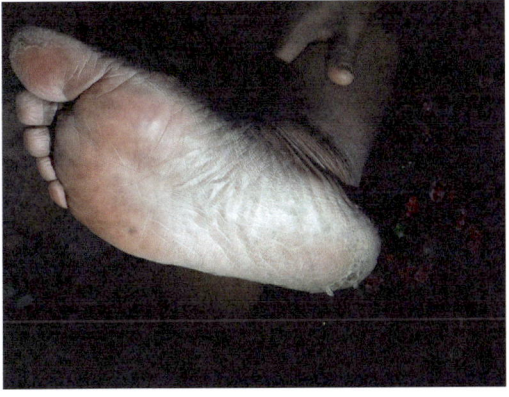

Follow-Up Care

For the first patient, there was no need for follow-up care.

Fig. 1.46 In this severe case of hyperkeratosis, the entire foot is affected

However, follow-up care for the second patient consisted of good foot care to carefully scrape off excess surface skin without injuring her feet and establishment of smooth plantar surfaces, all sides of the feet especially the posterior borders of the feet. The next steps were cultivating and maintaining a consistent lifestyle consisting of regular exercise, weight loss, dietary control to postpone or prevent the onset of diabetes, foot inspection to detect cracks early during the har-mattan, application of emollients, and mechani-

Treatment

The treatment for these two patients was a heel balm containing the active ingredient urea 25% concentration. For the second patient, the flaps were recommended for clipping off to maintain a reasonable semblance of smoothness for the heel balm to act as expected. Her extensive foot

cal and chemical removal of excess keratin in the stratum corneum of the soles of the feet.

In patients with diabetes mellitus or obesity, it may be necessary to provide them with follow-up care—to give them encouragement and objectively assess improvement or otherwise.

Discussion

In many patients, cracked heels is a condition that they experienced during harsh weather like harmattan and winter. In such patients who are old enough to have experienced it previously, there is a tendency to anticipate this condition and take measures to mitigate its effects if an episode cannot be avoided. Eating good food, covering the feet with socks all day (ensuring frequent change of socks for washed, dried, and ironed ones), and avoiding additional trauma to the feet, particularly the heels, is good practice. Ensuring good nutrition and carrying out mild to moderate exercises to maintain mobility appears to be good practice. It is important to keep a supply of any genuine heel balm that contains 25% urea.

Photomicrographs and Notes

This photomicrograph of atopic dermatitis (chronic eczema) shows mild epidermal acanthosis, mild dermal fibrosis, and hyperkeratosis.

A photomicrograph featuring superficial lymphocytic perivascular cellular infiltrate and dermal melanosis.

Eccrine poroma—Photomicrograph shows anastomosing bands of monomorphic, small, cuboidal cells replacing and extending into the dermis.

Eccrine poroma—Photomicrograph shows anastomosing bands of monomorphic, small, cuboidal cells replacing and extending into the dermis.

Melanoma—Photomicrograph of skin tissue shows sheets of polygonal cells that contain atyp-

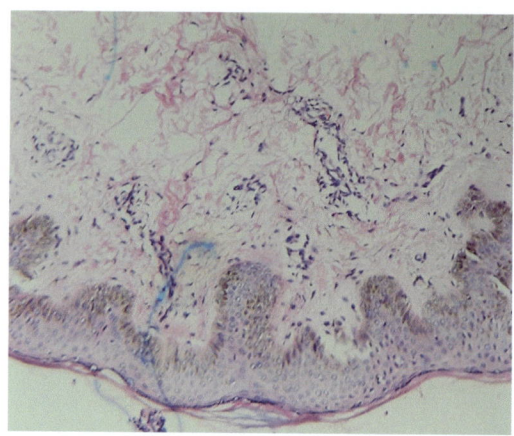

Fig. 1.48 Atopic dermatitis

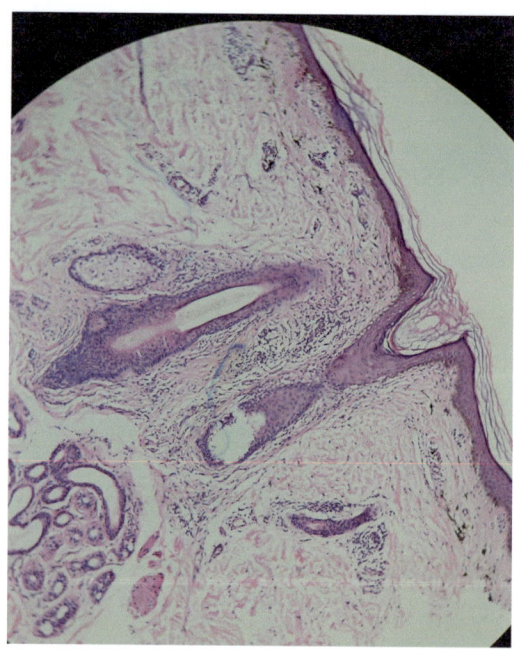

Fig. 1.49 Post inflammatory hyperpigmentation

ical nuclei, prominent nucleoli, and cytoplasm that contain pigments, ×40 magnification.

Melanoma—Photomicrograph of skin tissue shows sheets of polygonal cells that contain atypical nuclei, prominent nucleoli, and cytoplasm that contain pigments, ×40 magnification.

Lichen planus—Skin photomicrograph shows thickening of the epidermis, dense keratin surface, saw-tooth appearance of the rete pegs, and

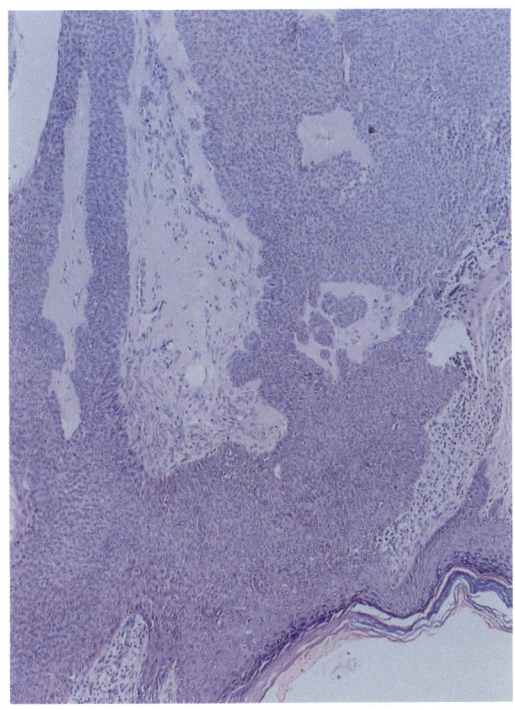

Fig. 1.50 Eccrine poroma

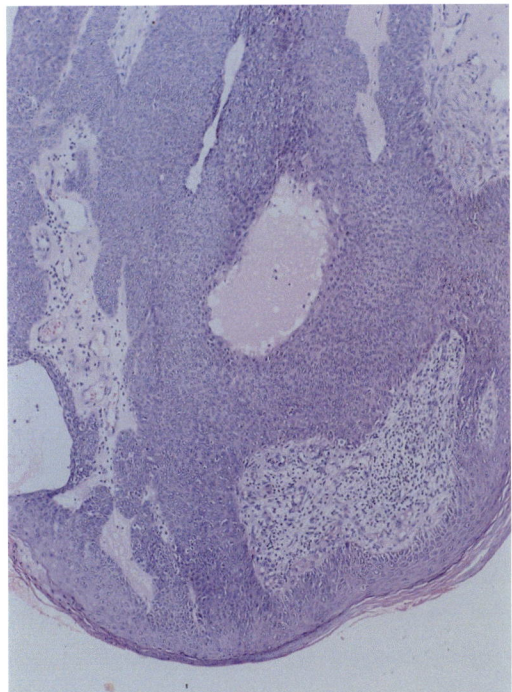

Fig. 1.51 Eccrine poroma

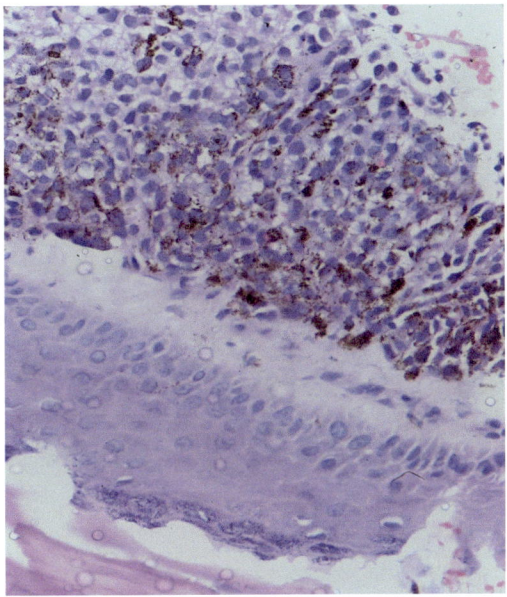

Fig. 1.52 Melanoma

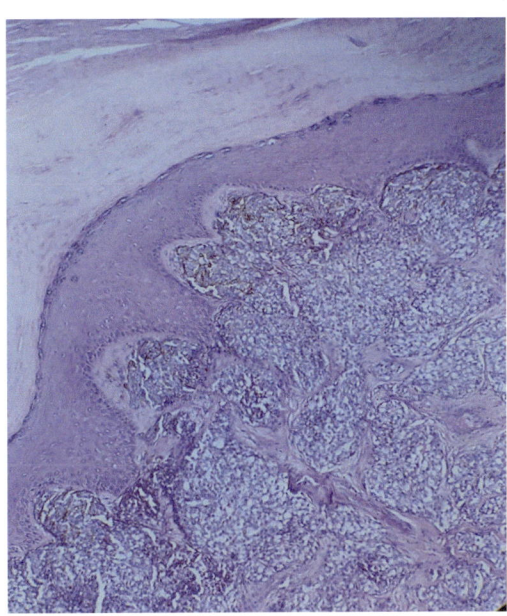

Fig. 1.53 Melanoma

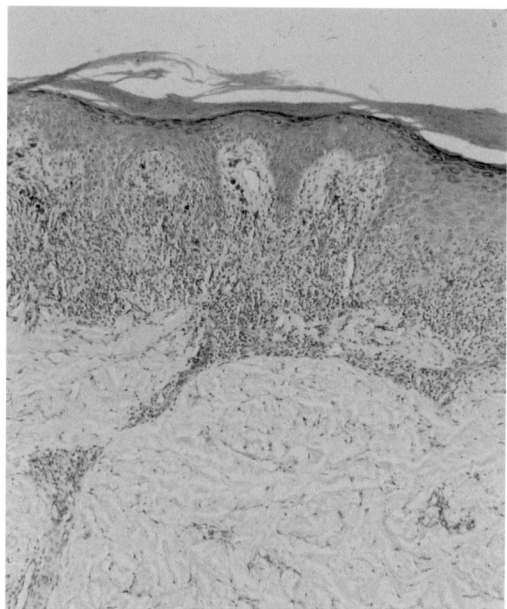

Fig. 1.54 Lichen planus

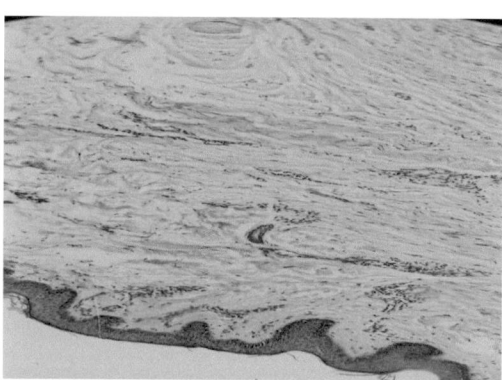

Fig. 1.55 Normal skin

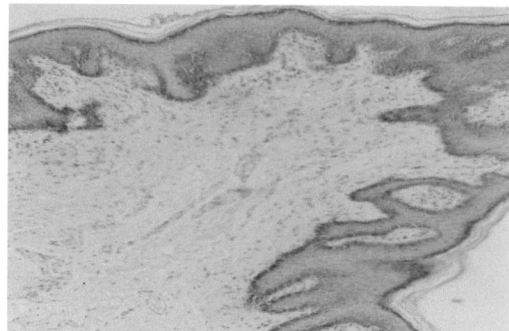

Fig. 1.56 Normal skin

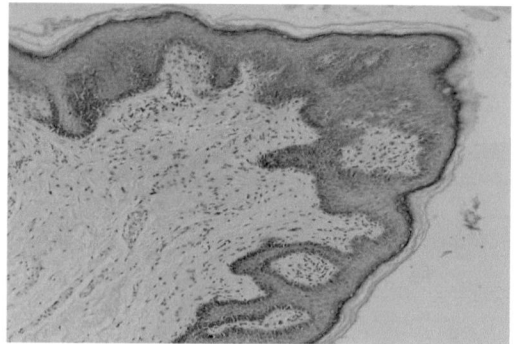

Fig. 1.57 Normal skin

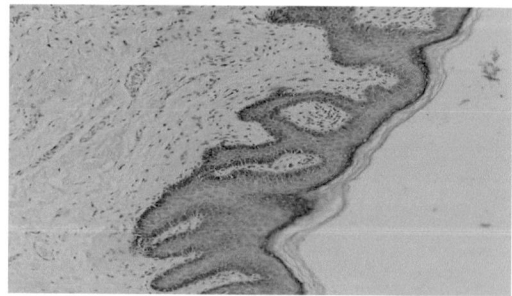

Fig. 1.58 Normal skin

band-like lymphocytic cellular infiltrate at the dermo-epidermal junction ×40 magnification.

The next six photomicrographs, Figs. 1.55, 1.56, 1.57, 1.58, 1.59, and 1.60, show normal skin, with skin tissue showing normal appearing epidermis, sweat glands a hair follicle ×10 magnification.

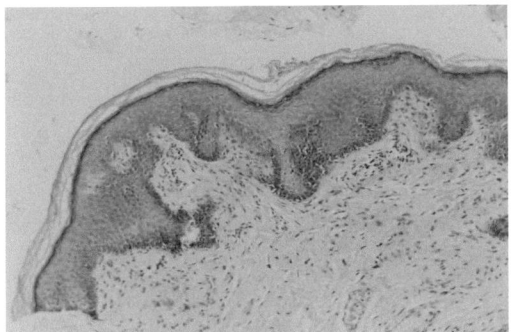

Fig. 1.59 Normal skin

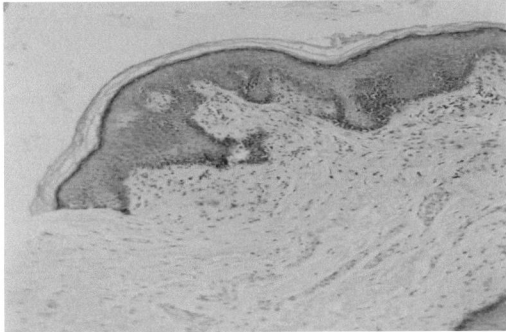

Fig. 1.60 Normal skin

Mechanical Protection by the Skin

The skin, and particularly the stratum corneum, is the first line of protection for the body from the external environment. The stratum corneum consists of corneocytes which are keratinocytes that have lost the capacity of differentiation; they are dead cells as they have lost their nuclei and organelles becoming filled with keratin. Corneocytes are the same cells that make up the nail plate. The stratum corneum forms a protective layer the thickness of which depends on the part of the body. These cells are vertically oriented and are held together by a matrix that is rich in lipids. The stratum corneum is semi-impenetrable. The stratum corneum in the eyelid and the sole of the foot are different in thickness. While the eyelids protect the eyes from injury, the sole of the foot protects the body not only from pressure injury but also from external noxious agents and infective agents. Cracked feet is evidence of the breach of the thick protective layer of the feet; in severe cases, the patient may develop bacterial infection, including cellulitis.

Skin Immune System and Immunological Protection by the Skin

The skin is rich in cells whose function is primarily or secondarily immunological. The cells protect the human body from external injury from microorganisms (bacteria, viruses, fungi, parasites) just as they protect from infestation by organisms that are visible to the eye like arthropods which are vectors to microorganisms; although the microorganisms that these vectors transport to the human skin occasionally cause damage or superficial and deep infections, it would have been worse if this natural barrier were absent or totally incompetent. The cells within the epidermis and the dermis of the human skin naturally recognize self but sometimes they do not; in such cases, rather than using their immunological capabilities to protect the body, they unleash an immunological offensive efforts against the body with the result of autoimmune disorders/diseases and hypersensitivity reactions, among others. Cells that are present in the skin and have immunological functions include stromal cells and bone marrow-derived cells. Stromal cells are keratinocytes, adipocytes, endothelial cells, and fibroblasts. Cells that are derived from bone marrow include mast cells, dendritic cells, T cells, natural killer cells, and macrophages. The populations of immunological cells that are derived from bone marrow are either innate or adaptive. The innate ones usually respond rapidly to immunological threats. The adaptive immune cell populations are slower, but they respond to specific threats using the antigen-antibody response.

Skin of Color/Indigenous

Skin of color refers to the skin of people whose skin pigmentation is darker than what applies to Caucasians [10]. It is, therefore, somewhat amorphous as a wide variety of skin colors is subsumed into this classification and it incorporates Africans, Asians, Native Americans, and those from the Pacific Islands.

This book describes diseases specifically to one of these groups, viz.: the Black skin. The black skin is the predominant skin color among people who reside in sub-Saharan Africa. This book's patients are all from this part of the world.

However, what is described in this book may apply to people in the parts of the world mentioned in the first paragraph whose dark skin is akin to the light tone, moderate tone, or deep tone of Black skin.

Multiple-Choice Questions

1. Of the functions of the skin, which of the following is *not* one?
   A. Prevention of loss of tissue fluids.
   B. Regulation of body temperature.
   C. Gluconeogenesis.
   D. Production of cholecalciferol.
2. Albinism is *not* characterized by which of the following?
   A. Absence of pigment from the iris.
   B. Absence of melanocytes.
   C. Deficiency of tyrosinase.
   D. Proneness to developing squamous cell carcinoma.
3. Which of the following relationships concerning vitiligo is correct?
   A. Clinical presentation—Hypopigmentation
   B. Association—Immunosuppression
   C. Late feature—Perioral distribution of lesions
   D. Histological feature—Total loss of epidermal pigmentation
4. An 18-year-old female presents in your clinic following the observation by her younger sister that she has "a couple of whitish rashes" on her back. You consider pityriasis versicolor as the tentative diagnosis. Which of the following associations is correct?
   A. Etiology—Gram-positive bacterium
   B. Site of pathology—Stratum corneum
   C. Presentation—Multiple, achromic macules
   D. Treatment—Third-generation cephalosporins
5. A 15-year-old secondary school (high school) student who, 8 weeks earlier, moved into the school residential facility for students recently observed sleeplessness from pubic hair itching and itching of axillary hair. The itching is worse at night but during classes the urge to scratch is also distracting and embarrassing. What is the likely diagnosis?
   A. Pthiriasis pubis
   B. Tinea pubis
   C. Pityriasis rosea
   D. Folliculitis

References

1. Linton CP. Essential morphologic terms and definitions. J Dermatol Nurses Assoc. 2011;3(2):102–3. https://doi.org/10.1097/JDN.0b013e318211c6f0. Available from: https://journals.lww.com/jdnaonline/fulltext/2011/03000/essential_morphologic_terms_and_definitions.10.aspx.
2. Benedett J. Description of skin lesions. In: MSD manual. Professional version; 2024. Available from: https://www.msdmanuals.com/professional/dermatologic-disorders/approach-to-the-dermatologic-patient/description-of-skin-lesions.
3. Murphrey MB, Miao JH, Zito PM. Histology, stratum corneum. In: StatPearls [Internet]; 2022. Available from: https://www.ncbi.nlm.nih.gov/books/NBK513299/#:~:text=.
4. World Health Organization and Joint United Nations Programme on HIV/AIDS (UNAIDS). Male circumcision: global trends and determinants of prevalence, safety and acceptability. Geneva: World Health Organization; 2007. [Google Scholar][Ref list].
5. Esposito C, Centonze A, Alicchio F, Savanelli A, Settimi A. Topical steroid application versus circumcision in pediatric patients with phimosis: a prospective randomized placebo controlled clinical trial. World J Urol. 2008;26:187–90. https://doi.org/10.1007/s00345-007-0231-2. [DOI] [PubMed] [Google Scholar][Ref list].
6. Daling JR, Madeleine MM, Johnson LG, Schwartz SH, Shera KA, Wurscher MA, et al. Penile cancer: importance of circumcision, human papillomavirus and smoking in in situ and invasive disease. Int J Cancer. 2005;116:606–16. https://doi.org/10.1002/ijc.21009. [DOI] [PubMed] [Google Scholar][Ref list].

7. Cooblal AS, Rampersad B. About the foreskin: parents' perceptions and misconceptions. West Indian Med J. 2015;63(5):484–9. https://doi.org/10.7727/wimj.2012.251. PMCID: PMC4655674 PMID: 25781287. Available from: https://pmc.ncbi.nlm.nih.gov/articles/PMC4655674/.

8. Puppo V. Embryology and anatomy of the vulva: the female orgasm and women's sexual health. Eur J Obstet Gynecol Reprod Biol. 2011;154:3. Available from: https://www.sciencedirect.com/topics/medicine-and-dentistry/vaginal-vestibule.

9. Fawcett RS, Linford S, Stulberg DL. Nail abnormalities: clues to systemic disease. Am Fam Physician. 2004;69(6):1417–24. Available from: https://www.aafp.org/pubs/afp/issues/2004/0315/p1417.html.

10. Taylor SC, Angela Kyei A. Chapter 2: Defining skin of color. In: Taylor and Kelly's dermatology for skin of color, 2e. Available from: https://accessmedicine.mhmedical.com/content.aspx?bookid=2585&sectionid=211763356#:~:text=.

Erythrasma

Symptoms

A 60-year-old woman presented with pruritic rashes on the neck, the elbows, and under the breasts. The onset of the rashes was gradual and she noticed them 1–2 days after a feeling of slight itching on the affected parts. The rashes were on for about 2 weeks as at the time she complained to the doctor. The itching was slight and so the discomfort from itching was not a bother to her. She described the rashes as not only slightly itchy but also caused a darkening of the affected parts. Reporting the skin condition to the doctor was really out of a concern about the skin darkening on the affected parts. The skin on the neck felt dry and she had a sensation of squeezing of the skin there; there was a similar sensation at the elbows but much less. She had a hard time avoiding scratching the affected parts and substituted the urge to scratch with rubbing the affected areas. The rashes were extending and she felt that there was a need to report. She also noticed that itching was a little more with the rashes in-between the skin folds of both breasts. It was inconvenient to wear a brazier, and she used it only when she had to go outdoors. She resorted to using clothes that could cover the elbows and

muffler (scarf, scarph, shawl) around her neck when she had cause to go to church or attend other social events. She had not applied any medication prior to consultation. She is hypertensive, with the blood pressure under control using Valsartan (an angiotensin receptor blocker) and Hydrochlorothiazide (a thiazide diuretic) in a combination tablet. She is not diabetic and does not have any manifestation of allergy on the skin or in any other part of the body.

Signs

Physical examination of both sides of this patient's neck and the flexural surfaces of both elbows showed hyperpigmented macular rashes with irregular margins. Figure 2.1 demonstrates the smallness and thinness of the lesions on the left side of the neck. There is mild hyperpigmentation when compared with unaffected skin; other parts of the lesions show that the lesions are almost of the same pigmentation as normal skin. Figure 2.2 shows the scaliness of the macules and wrinkling of the skin. Further features that are demonstrable in this Figure are extension of the rashes to the skin over the right mandible (this part looks similar to the patient's unaffected skin) and hyperpigmentation of the macules over her right trapezius (posteriorly—and in the image, top left, and close to the hair at the back). The anterior part of the middle portion of Fig. 2.2 shows skin that is in-

Supplementary Information The online version contains supplementary material available at https://doi.org/10.1007/978-3-031-97503-5_2.

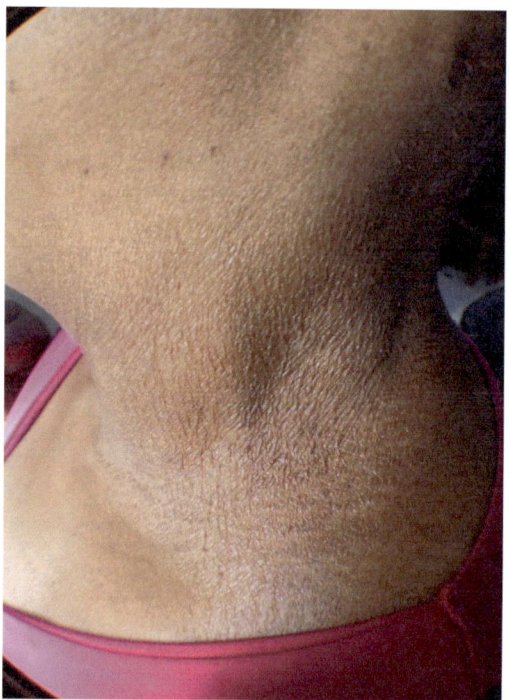

Fig. 2.1 Rashes on the left side of the neck of an adult patient

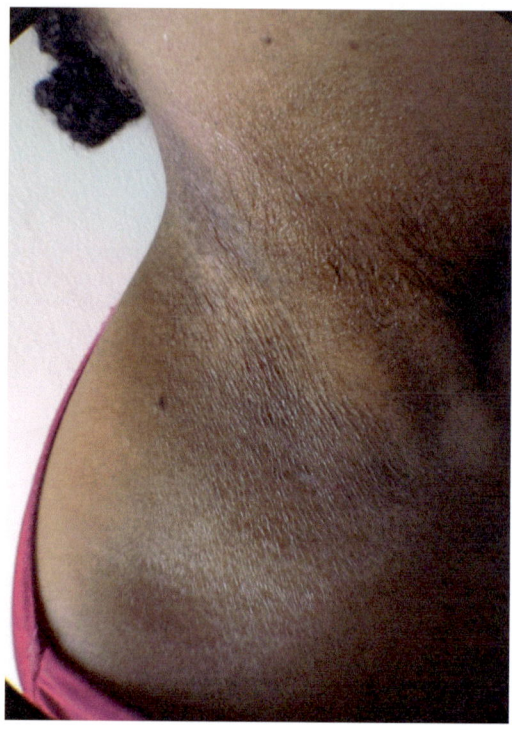

Fig. 2.2 Rashes on the right side of the neck of the same patient in Fig. 2.1

between normal pigmentation and hypopigmentation; this is especially the portion of the rash that affects the skin over the clavicular head of the right sternocleidomastoid muscle. Inspecting the skin posteriorly, the patient also has a single, ovoid, hyperpigmented (virtually black) papular rash at the border between the lateral end of the macular rashes and her normal skin. This is acquired melanocytic nevus. The lower portion of the affected area of the right side of her neck is the skin over the right supraclavicular fossa. The lesions here are more uniform in pigmentation as they are hyperpigmented. In this Figure, there is a gradual transition from the hyperpigmented rashes to unaffected normal skin, and in some areas (the supraclavicular rashes), there is a sharp demarcation. The rashes are slightly scaly and the affected skin appears wrinkled. Figure 2.3 is an enlargement which shows greater detail of the rashes in Fig. 2.2.

Figure 2.4 is the image of the same patient showing the rashes on her right elbow. The rashes are small macules which appear of normal pigmentation (and even hypopigmentation). The

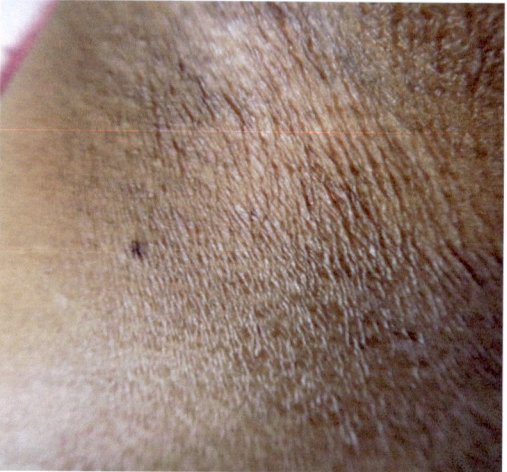

Fig. 2.3 An enlarged image of Fig. 2.2, showing greater details of the rashes

medial aspect of the right elbow (distal arm and proximal forearm) shows a clear demarcation between the hyperpigmented portion of the rashes and normal skin. Figure 2.5 shows the same area as Fig. 2.4. While the photograph for Fig. 2.5 was taken with a flash, the one for Fig. 2.4 was without

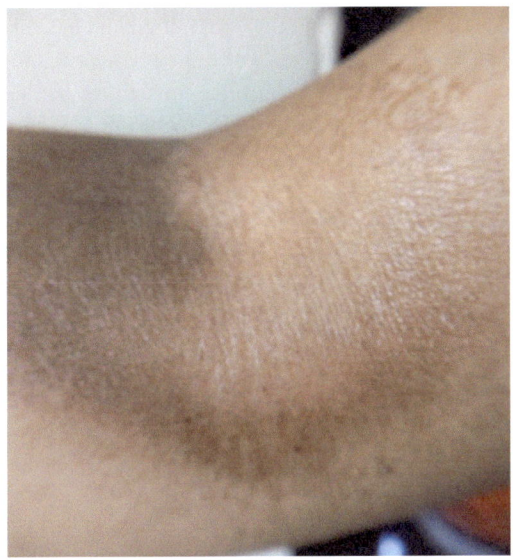

Fig. 2.4 The right elbow of the same patient in Figs. 2.1, 2.2, and 2.3

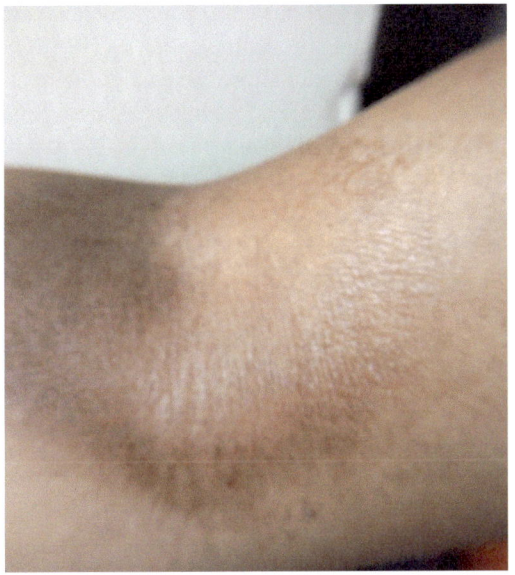

Fig. 2.5 The right elbow of the same patient in all previous figures on erythrasma

a flash. When preparing to create images of clinical conditions for documentation in a book or a journal, it is important to take many images using natural light without flash and using a flash. The author should choose the images that provide the clearest representation of the clinical condition in its natural state. Compared with Fig. 2.4, Fig. 2.5

does not demonstrate hyperpigmentation convincingly. The reader should note that this patient's two elbows were affected by this superficial bacterial infection of the skin although only the right elbow is used for this documentation.

Regarding the rashes on the elbows, there was no involvement of the extensor surfaces of the elbows and there were no scratch marks.

Etiology

Erythrasma is a superficial bacterial skin infection caused by a group of Gram-positive diphtheroids, prominently exemplified by *Corynebacterium minutissimum*. Moisture and heat encourage the proliferation of these organisms that are found normally on skin.

Usual Clinical Features

Erythrasma is an intertriginous macular eruption. The rash is hyperpigmented with more pigmentation at the periphery than the center (which may demonstrate clearing). There is usually a clear demarcation with the unaffected skin.

Investigations

When scales from skin scrapings from the lesion of erythrasma are examined under Wood's light, they fluoresce coral red, sometimes described as coral pink. Microscopic examination of skin scrapings from the lesions in potassium hydroxide (KOH) preparation does not demonstrate the positive findings in the following fungal infections: yeast infection (by *Candida albicans*), dermatophyte infections (by *Trichophyton*, *Microsporum*, or *Epidermophyton*), or pityriasis versicolor.

Treatment

Initial treatment of erythrasma consists of topical antibiotics, e.g., clindamycin 2% cream, fusidic acid 2% cream, or mupirocin 2% cream. Another topical agent that is effective for treating patients with erythrasma is Whitfield's ointment (12% benzoic acid and 6% salicylic acid). When it becomes necessary, second-line treatment is systemic therapy using the tetracyclines, e.g., tetracycline or doxycycline; good alternatives are the macrolides, e.g., clarithromycin or erythromycin—while clarithromycin 1 g single oral dose may clear the lesions, erythromycin needs to be taken 6-hourly for about 14 days. Drug adherence seems to be better with topical treatment than systemic treatment, perhaps due to less side effects with the former.

Follow-Up/Review

Follow-up consultation with the doctor would preferably be 1 week (or less) after commencement of therapy for erythrasma. During this consultation, the patient tells the doctor their observations regarding the symptoms and signs while the doctor re-examines the patient's skin. In practices that are not very busy and the condition is the only one or one of the few that presented within that period, the doctor is able to determine whether the patient's condition is better than before or the lesions have almost cleared. Sometimes, the doctor's assessment is a corroboration of the patient's observations and experiences, while at other times, the patient may be enthusiastic about a total resolution of the lesions and state that there is little or no improvement. During the follow-up care, the doctor is able to discuss the case in greater detail with the patient and include preventive measures.

Prognosis

The prognosis of erythrasma is good.

Discussion

The causative agent of erythrasma is the diphtheroid, *Corynebacterium minutissimum* [1]. In some patients, the superficial bacterial infection may run a chronic course.

The patient's skin looks wrinkled and has fine scales. The macular rashes have a predilection for where there are skin folds like the axillae, medial aspects of the thighs, inframammary folds (submammary area), inguinal folds, genitocrural folds, and interdigital webs of the lower extremities [2]. In this patient, the condition was very prominent on the neck; if it was only on the neck, irritant contact dermatitis would be considered as a differential diagnosis—the patient, however, hardly used necklace as part of her adornment.

In the Black skin, the rashes appear brown and occasionally slightly hyperpigmented.

The differential diagnoses of erythrasma include candidiasis, pityriasis versicolor, infections with dermatophytes (tinea axillaris, tinea corporis, tinea cruris), and terra firma-forme dermatosis [3, 4].

Mupirocin 2% cream is one of the effective medications for treatment of patients with erythrasma [5]. Due to the cost of mupirocin cream in low- and medium-income countries (LMICs), some patients cannot afford the cost of the treatment if they do not start the treatment early, and the condition spreads at one site or there are multiple sites with the rashes on each covering a reasonable area of the skin. It is, therefore, important to advise patients to report this (and other skin conditions) to the doctor soon after onset of symptoms.

Furuncle

Symptoms

The lady, in her early 60s, noticed slight discomfort in a circumscribed part of the right side of her abdomen. When she looked at the spot, she observed a tiny rash that was raised above the skin. Within 24 hours, she observed slight pain at the site; she also noticed that there was a red area that surrounded the rash in the initial stages. The pain was followed by an increase in both the size of the rash and the amount of pain that she had at the site of the rash. The pain was bearable and the pain score that she ascribed to the rash was either two or three. The rash was the only one at the

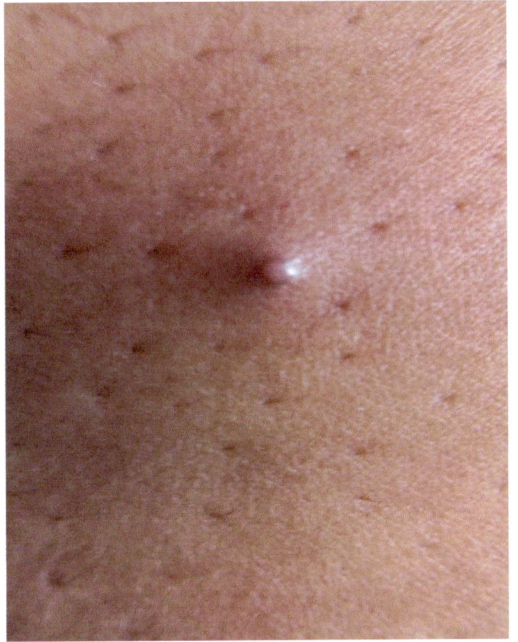

Fig. 2.6 An enlargement of a "boil" on the abdominal wall

time although she infrequently had similar ones. Just like in this episode, the rash was usually one and could be in any part of the body. She could not link the onset of the rash with anything as it seemed to "come out of nowhere" any time it occurred. She was curious as to the cause and observed that the appearance of this type of rash was unpredictable. Sometimes the rash would subside without any form of treatment, but this one showed no sign of regressing, 5 days after its onset. Rather than regressing, she was convinced that it was progressing for the surface had changed to yellowish—she believed that it contained pus. In the past, a doctor had told her that she should not scratch, squeeze, or open up that type of rash; what she did in this case was to rub it gently when she noticed pain. She had also taken about two doses of paracetamol before making the complaint about this rash.

She was not diagnosed with diabetes mellitus and she was unaware of anybody in her direct family who was diabetic. Her uncle's wife had diabetes mellitus and died some years previously and her male cousin (the aunt's only son) also had diabetes mellitus. This was, however, not a

direct family relationship. She is a known patient who is undergoing management of hypertension. Her blood pressure readings have been within the normal range after her doctor advised her to commence drug treatment about 4 years earlier. She sweated, although the degree of perspiration was normal compared to her husband who perspired excessively but had no similar skin condition. She did not sweat much and hardly engaged in physical exercises. She was glad that in this episode of the skin rash, the involvement was a part of her body that clothes covered, unlike previous instances when it could be on her face or another conspicuous spot. She not only desired to have adequate treatment for the condition but wanted to get information from the doctor during this consultation about how to stop the recurrence of the rash.

Signs

On examination, the patient was not in pain. When she exposed the rash, she did not, however, want the rash or the area to be touched, and the physician assured her that there would not be a need to touch it as most aspects of the examination did not require touching it. The rash was a single ovoid pustule that was about 4 × 2 mm, with the axis in the transverse plane. The surface was yellowish. The rash was raised from the skin, and there was a clear demarcation between it and the surrounding normal skin—there was no halo of hyperemia. The surrounding skin was smooth, and there was no evidence of scratching. The rest of the skin showed evidence of good care.

Diagnosis

The diagnosis of this condition is furuncle.

Treatment

Treatment of furuncle may be nonpharmacological, pharmacological, and surgical. Nonpharmacological management constitutes application of warm moist compresses which encourage drainage of the pus that is formed. Pharmacological management involves use of antibiotics (topically when warm compresses do not suffice, and oral antibiotics later if required). The antibiotics should be anti-staphylococcal. At the stage of this patient's furuncle, incision and drainage is a simple surgical procedure that satisfactorily treats it. In some patients, a furuncle undergoes self-drainage just like in some patients a furuncle undergoes resolution without any treatment.

Discussion

The sites that furuncles are expected to form are the neck, back, axillae, gluteal skin (buttocks), groin, and thighs [6]. They do occur in other sites, like in the patient whose case is discussed above. Furuncles are not preceded with or accompanied by fever—if there is fever, it is due to an associated illness and not primarily by the furuncle.

The usual clinical presentation of furuncles consist of an initially painful nodule that demonstrates local warmth over the furuncle and the immediate surrounding skin. In the Black skin, there is no evidence of surrounding inflammation (a redness) although in patients with light skin tone of Black skin the redness may be demonstrable. If the patient permits palpation, the papule causes tenderness. Eventually, the central part of the furuncle forms pus, converting the papule into a pustule. If it is left untreated, the pustular lesion becomes fluctuant and discharges its central part of the formed pus accompanied by some exudate [6, 7]. Depending on the immune status of the patient, there may or may not be healing with scar formation at the site of the infection.

Prognosis

The prognosis of a furuncle is good. If, however, a patient has frequent episodes of furuncle, especially when there are multiple furuncles in various parts of the body, it is important for the patient to have a detailed evaluation as there may

be diabetes mellitus, human immunodeficiency virus infection, or another cause of immune suppression.

Follow-Up Care

For a patient who has just one furuncle that resolves on its own or responds satisfactorily to topical or oral antibiotic treatment, there may be no need to visit the hospital again for follow-up care.

Hansen's Disease: Madarosis and Toe Resorption

Symptoms

The middle-aged male whose face is shown in Fig. 2.7 was a patient with leprosy undergoing treatment. He did not come to the hospital to complain about the loss of eyebrow hairs but for other health concerns. The treatment he received was from a hospital managed by the same faith-based organization that operated the hospital the author worked in. Enquiry revealed that the loss of hair on the affected part was not sudden but gradual. He did not engage in nose picking or picking eyebrow hair. There was no scar over the affected part. He was not on treatment for any

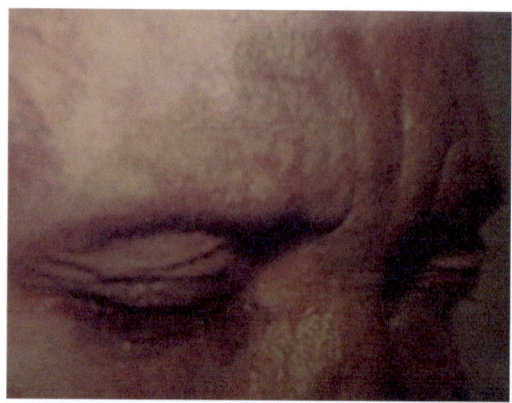

Fig. 2.7 Madarosis in a patient with leprosy. (Source: Reproduced with permission from *A Companion to Medical Students and Doctors*)

chronic illness. There were no eye signs suggestive of hyperthyroidism.

Signs

On examination, there was total hair loss on the eyebrows and this was bilateral. Figure 2.7 concentrated on the right eyebrow. The left eyebrow is shown only in part (the medial aspect). The patient had bilateral superciliary madarosis [8]. The skin of the eyebrows had uniform normal pigmentation. There was no scar as evidence of significant past trauma to either eyebrow. Movement of the eyebrows was normal. The eyelashes were intact.

Symptoms

Figure 2.8 is a photograph of the left foot of another male patient with leprosy. He was in his early 50s. He walked into the consulting room barefoot. He was one of the regular patients that came for consultation in the general outpatient clinic. The author was interested and, in addition to attending to the patient's immediate medical challenges, asked him questions about the deformity on his lower extremities. He had been a patient diagnosed with leprosy many years earlier. He said that he developed gradual reduction in the length of the ends of his toes. He eventually

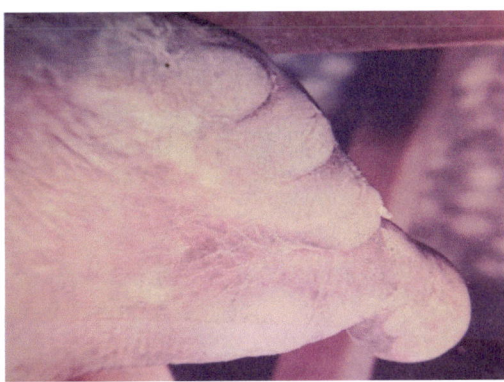

Fig. 2.8 Shortened toes in a patient with Hansen's disease. (Source: Reproduced with permission from *A Companion to Medical Students and Doctors*)

lost the fifth toe while the second to the fourth toes were stumps and the big toe was twisted.

Signs

On examination, the skin was husky and was dirty. The skin was also rough and thickened. It was difficult to determine if there was dyspigmentation of the skin (hyperpigmentation, hypopigmentation, or a mixture at portions of the feet). The distal part of the left big toe was deviated medially. The second, third, and fourth toes showed almost obliterated distal ends. The fifth toe was missing.

Etiology

Hansen's disease is a chronic infection caused by *Mycobacterium leprae*. It is one of the causes of madarosis. Madarosis may result from acute bacterial infection that targets the hair follicles on the eyebrows or eyelids. Madarosis occurs in some patients who undergo chemotherapy. Madarosis also occurs in trichotillomania patients. Bone resorption is one of the complications of leprosy. Bilateral madarosis is one of the features of lepromatous leprosy [8, 9].

Usual Clinical Presentation

Hansen's disease presents in many ways and affects various parts of the body including the skin, bone, eyes, and the nervous system. Madarosis is one of the skin presentations while bone toe resorption involves the skin and bone. This patient presented with superciliary (eyebrow) madarosis; madarosis may be ciliary (of the eyelashes).

In bone resorption, the toes are usually affected and so the patient presents with distal atrophy. Other features of leprosy pertaining to the feet, bone, and joint involvement are metatarsophalangeal osteoarthritis, chronic periostitis and osteitis, osteoporosis, ulceration and infection, pyogenic osteomyelitis, leprosy granuloma in bone, joint contracture, fibrous nodule in bone, and leprous periostitis [10].

Investigations

Investigations are not required to make the diagnosis of madarosis or foot resorption as they are obvious clinically; however, investigations may be required to identify the underlying cause if the patient is not a diagnosed leprotic patient. Blood tests should be performed to rule out hypothyroidism, hyperthyroidism, and autoimmune disease. Plain radiographs of the foot demonstrate lost or deformed terminal phalanges.

Treatment

When caused by an acute bacterial infection, madarosis should be treated with antibiotics. Topical minoxidil is useful for treating alopecia areata that affects the eyebrows. Prosthetic eyebrows and prosthetic eyelashes are available. Cosmetics can also be used to mask the condition. Eyebrow hair follicular transplantation is treated for patients with severe superciliary madarosis.

Prognosis

Prognosis of madarosis depends on the cause; when treatment restores or replaces the lost hair, prognosis is good. The prognosis of bone resorption and skin changes is not good as the deformity is severe enough to affect the patient's psyche.

Figures 2.9 and 2.10 show the face and upper chest of a man in his early 40s. He had lepromatous leprosy. The major feature in the photograph is multiple nodules and papules on the face and upper chest with fewer on the neck. The nodules are of various shapes and sizes and some of them are hyperpigmented.

Being a bacillus, *Mycobacterium leprae* is rod-shaped; it is characteristically described as an acid-fast bacillus. It is also an obligate intra-

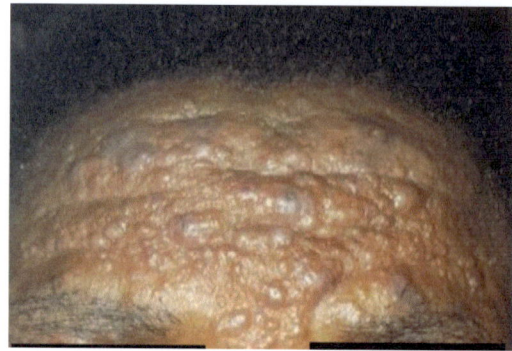

Fig. 2.9 The forehead of another patient with leprosy

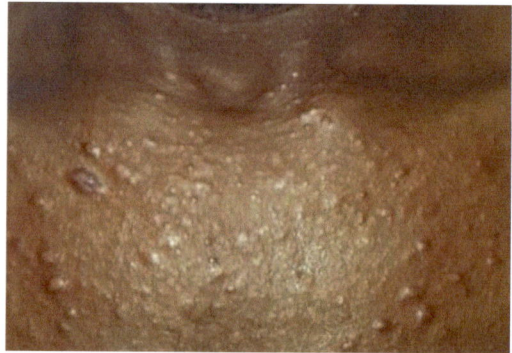

Fig. 2.10 The upper chest of a man in his early 40s

cellular bacterium. This bacterium prefers cool parts of the body. The incubation period may be as long as 30–50 years has been reported, but it is usually about 5 years. *Mycobacterium leprae* was identified in Norway by Armauer Hansen.

Subtypes or forms of Hansen's disease are five, viz.: TT, BT, BB, BL, and LL. Leprosy is more common in developing countries than in developed countries. A patient with good cellular immunity presents with TT disease. In leprosy, transition towards the TT disease pole is upgrading; downgrading is transition towards LL. The prognosis of LL form of the disease is poor.

In patients with lepromatous leprosy (LL disease), a bacillary index of 5 or 6 is expected. Lepromin test is strongly positive in the TT form of leprosy but negative in LL subtype. Cutaneous nerve enlargement is common in TT disease. Erythema nodosum leprosum (ENL) reaction is a common finding in LL form. When there are rashes with loss of sensation, the patient most likely has TT disease; in TT disease, there are macular rashes which are anesthetic, especially centrally. The rashes are scaly and of various sizes and shapes but may not be many.

With respect to skin biopsy histological findings, the following are correct: (a) normal epidermis is a feature in lepromatous leprosy; (b) in TT leprosy, there are on-caseating granulomas; (c) in LL leprosy, numerous acid-fast bacilli are present in histiocytes and nerves whereas in tuberculoid leprosy acid-fast bacilli are absent in histiocytes and nerves; (d) in TT leprosy, there is loss of hair follicles and sweat glands; and (e) destruction of nerves in the dermis occurs in tuberculoid leprosy.

The following are features that are expected in patients with lepromatous leprosy:

(a) Resorption of toe digits—It is one of the results of acute peripheral nerve damage in ENL reaction.
(b) Claw deformity of the hands. Another example is foot drop.
(c) There is a predilection of leprosy nodules for the face as seen in the patient whose photograph is shown in Fig. 2.9. The nose and lips are also affected and there is thickening of facial skin.
(d) Collapse of nasal cartilage—There is also nasal septum collapse, hoarseness of voice, and nasal speech. Anesthetic skin patches occur in patients with tuberculoid leprosy.

In this book, some dermatological conditions are described as presentations of systemic diseases. Leprosy is readily recognized as a disease affecting the skin and peripheral nerves. In a patient with leprosy, it is expedient to examine other parts of the body. With regards to the eye, the following are features of eye disease from leprosy: (a) Superciliary and ciliary madarosis—this loss of eyebrow and eyelash hairs makes the patient have leonine facies; (b) beading of corneal nerves; (c) reduced corneal sensation; (d) conjunctival hyperemia; (e) pannus; (f) avascular keratitis; and g) interstitial keratitis.

Based on the clinical presentation of the patient, appropriate investigations in leprosy may include the following:

- Skin lesion smears
- X-rays of hands and/or feet
- Skin biopsy
- Lepromin test
- Polymerase chain reaction

Medications that are efficacious in the treatment of patients with leprosy include rifampicin which is in the ansamycin class of macrolides; diamino diphenyl sulfone, i.e., dapsone; clofazimine, i.e., Lamprene which, for patients who are smear-positive, is added to rifampicin and dapsone and administered for twice the duration of treatment in these patients when compared to smear-negatives who are treated for 1 year; and chloroquine, steroids, non-steroidal anti-inflammatory drugs (NSAIDs), and salicylates which are useful in treating leprosy patients with reactions to treatment using the standard antileprotics.

Multiple-Choice Questions

1. Erythrasma: Which of the statements below is correct?
   A. It is a papular lesion.
   B. The lesions are aggravated by a cold environment.
   C. It may coexist with candidal intertrigo.
   D. A Gram-negative organism causes it, *Corynebacterium minutissimum*.
2. Which of the following associations pertaining to erythrasma is correct?
   A. Healthy lifestyle—No beneficial effect.
   B. Anhidrosis—Predisposing factor.
   C. Oral antibiotics—First-line treatment.
   D. Cutaneous candidiasis—Differential diagnosis.
3. Which of the following statements about furuncle is correct?
   A. It involves subcutaneous tissue.
   B. Pus arises from multiple openings.
   C. Palms and soles are common sites.
   D. It is synonymous with superficial folliculitis.

4. Which of the following statements about leprosy is incorrect?
   A. The causative organism is a Gram-positive acid-fast bacillus.
   B. Its incubation period may exceed 5 years.
   C. The hypopigmented macules in indeterminate leprosy may have normal sensation.
   D. Patients with tuberculoid leprosy have nodules and a negative lepromin test.

5. Which of the following statements about leprosy is correct?
   A. Etiology is a group of mycobacteria.
   B. The pathogen grows in Dubos-Lowenstein-Jensen culture medium and thyroxin sodium.
   C. The presentation is the same in every patient.
   D. Poor, minimal, cellular immune response by the host characterizes tuberculoid leprosy.

References

1. Martínez-Ortega JI, Franco González S. Erythrasma: pathogenesis and diagnostic challenges. Cureus. 2024;16(8):e68308. [QxMD MEDLINE Link]. [Full Text].
2. Kibbi A-G. Erythrasma. In: Dermatology. Medscape; 2024. Available from: https://emedicine.medscape.com/article/1052532-overview.
3. Forouzan P, Cohen PR. Erythrasma revisited: diagnosis, differential diagnoses, and comprehensive review of treatment. Cureus. 2020;12(9):e10733. https://doi.org/10.7759/cureus.10733. PMC7599055 PMID: 33145138. Available from: https://pmc.ncbi.nlm.nih.gov/articles/PMC7599055/.
4. Cohen PR. Terra firma-forme dermatosis of the inguinal fold: Duncan's dirty dermatosis mimicking groin dermatoses. Open J Clin Med Case Rep. 2015;1:1022. http://jclinmedcasereports.com/articles/OJCMCR-1022.pdf. [Google Scholar].
5. Greywal T, Cohen PR. Erythrasma: a report of nine men successfully managed with mupirocin 2% ointment monotherapy. Dermatol Online J. 2017;23:13030. [PubMed] [Google Scholar]. Available from: https://www.ncbi.nlm.nih.gov/pubmed/28537862.
6. Medecins sans frontiers (MSF). Clinical guidelines – diagnosis and treatment manual. Available from: https://medicalguidelines.msf.org/en/viewport/CG/english/furuncles-and-carbuncles-16689669.html.
7. Rehmus WE. Furuncles and carbuncles. In: MSD manual. Professional version; 2023. Available from: https://www.msdmanuals.com/professional/dermatologic-disorders/bacterial-skin-infections/furuncles-and-carbuncles.
8. Krishnan A, Kar S. Bilateral madarosis as the solitary presenting feature of multibacillary leprosy. Int J Trichol. 2012;4(3):179–80. https://doi.org/10.4103/0974-7753.100092. PMCID: PMC3500062 PMID: 23180932. Available from: https://pmc.ncbi.nlm.nih.gov/articles/PMC3500062/.
9. Palaniappan V, Karthikeyan K. Leonine facies and madarosis in lepromatous leprosy. Available from: https://watermark.silverchair.com/postgradmedj-98-e36.pdf?
10. Skinsnes OK, Sakurai I, Aquina TI. Pathogenesis of extremity deformity in leprosy – a pathologic study on large sections of amputated extremities in relation to radiological appearance. Int J Lepr. 1972;40(4). Available from: http://ila.ilsl.br/pdfs/v40n4a04.pdf.

Dandruff

Symptoms

This 13-year-old girl complained of a severely itchy scalp that had become worse over the years. She could not state precisely when the itching started. There was accompanying production of numerous tiny flakes from her scalp skin when she combed the hair or responded to the itching by scratching any part of the scalp. When she was younger, her mother had encouraged her to maintain a low hair cut, but now that she considered herself grown, she did not want to look different especially when she considered her hair longer and nicer than that of her age mates who maintained their hair and made different hairstyles according to their desire. Unfortunately, she noticed that she could not wash her hair frequently like when she maintained a "low cut," and the washing was principally when she undid the hair, washed, and dried it, before asking for a fresh hairstyle to be made for her. The two main symptoms of itching with concomitant scalp scratching and flaking on the skin of the scalp were matters of concern to her. She was not happy that her friends noticed her scratching her scalp and occasionally teased her by asking if she had lice in her long hair; she, however,

did not find any evidence of lice no matter how intensely and how carefully she combed her hair and looked out for lice. She feared that this condition may be lifelong as she did not intend to look different now or in the future, since in her culture a woman should look like a woman and not a man—it is men that either maintain a low cut or shaved their scalp although recently young men were maintaining long hair as it "happens abroad." This patient had high expectations that she would receive treatment that would solve the skin condition.

Signs

Figures 3.1 and 3.2 are photographs of the head of a teenage female with plaited hair. The spaces between the done hair expose her scalp.

On examination, the scalp showed a covering of what could be described as "debris" making normal scalp skin unrecognizable. Figure 3.1 shows a significant portion of her scalp demonstrating both the plaited hair and the gaps between them. Figure 3.2 is a close-up photograph of a part of the scalp showing recently scratched scalp in-between braided hair. This portion demonstrates flakes of skin on the space and the squames extending to cover surrounding scalp hair.

Supplementary Information The online version contains supplementary material available at https://doi.org/10.1007/978-3-031-97503-5_3.

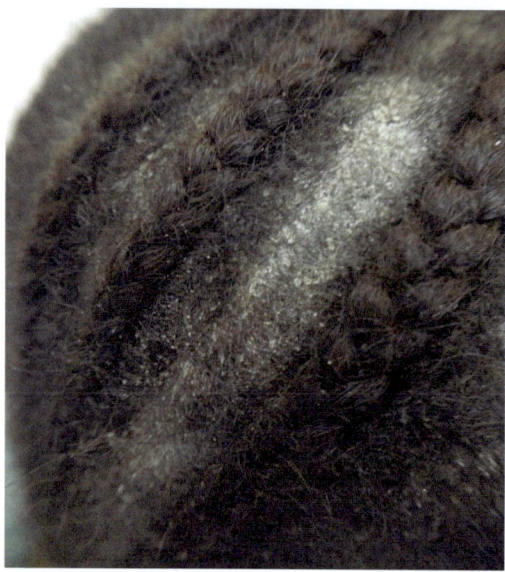

Fig. 3.1 The head of a teenage female with plaited hair

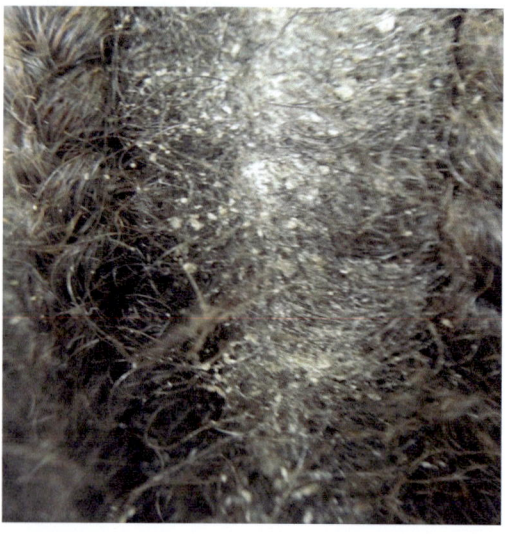

Fig. 3.2 The scalp of the same teenage female with plaited hair

Diagnosis

Dandruff

Etiology

Dandruff is seborrheic dermatitis that is limited to the scalp [1]. The etiological agent is *Malassezia furfur*, a yeast, the overgrowth of which is linked with the condition. Abundance of sebum on the patient's scalp is also a factor. It is not one of the.

Treatment

For this patient, the prescription was selenium sulfide 2.5% shampoo [2]. The author convinced the patient to have her hair cut to become significantly short but not for her scalp to be shorn. The explanation was that the shampoo in the practice area is expensive (when available) and small in volume compared to regular shampoos. The shampoo need to make satisfactory contact with the scalp skin for effectiveness; if she maintained the long hair, undid the hairstyle, washed it, and applied the shampoo, she would simply waste the shampoo as it would be applied mostly to the long and thick hair rather than the scalp. She was to apply the shampoo two to three times weekly and each time, allowing it to contact the scalp for 5–10 minutes, before washing it off. The mother figure who brought her to the clinic was encouraged to have patience with her as the treatment would necessarily entail her spending a longer time in the bathroom especially on the days she had to wash the hair and apply the shampoo.

Reservoirs of the etiological yeast may be significantly reduced by applying shampoos that contain selenium sulfide 2.5%; selenium sulfide 1% shampoo is available, but the 2.5% is the preferred concentration for management of dandruff. Other shampoos are effective and contain ketoconazole or ciclopirox [2].

Prognosis

For good prognosis, patients with dandruff should be informed that they should use the prescribed shampoo regularly; this is particularly important for female teenagers and adults who maintain long hair as the target of shampooing in dandruff is the scalp and not the hair. Achieving a good prognosis may, therefore, require assigning a reasonable budget of funds for the shampoo and time for shampooing. For patients who cannot cope with the demands of effective treatment, they should be advised to maintain low hair length.

Follow-Up Care

Using selenium sulfide 2.5% that was prescribed for the treatment of this patient as an example, the principle would be that the patient do more of a personal care of the hair as enunciated earlier but to maintain the therapy—which after a successful clearance of the rashes may require weekly application of the shampoo for months and years. The patient should be made aware of the fact that dandruff is as a result of the peculiarities of the scalp skin that encourages *Malassezia furfur* to proliferate. The patient should also return to the clinic for evaluation by the doctor or the specialist. Further check-up visits may be longer than the initial one(s) when the patient would have taken active participation in the management of this usually chronic scalp skin condition.

Discussion

Usual clinical features There is pruritus of the scalp which is sometimes severe enough to make the patient scratch; scratching releases flakes of the skin from the scalp in various amounts depending on the severity of scaling in the disease.

Investigations Investigations are usually not required as it is essentially a clinical diagnosis. When investigations are deemed necessary, histological examination of affected skin shows the features of seborrheic dermatitis; these include the classical finding called "shoulder" parakeratosis in which follicular openings are surrounded with parakeratosis in the acute phase [3]. In parakeratosis, maturation of epidermal keratocytes is incomplete—the outermost layer of the epidermis, the stratum corneum, still demonstrates nuclei in its cells.

Pityriasis Versicolor

The following photographs are to demonstrate how late some patients with pityriasis versicolor tend to go to the hospital to seek for a solution to the skin condition and how extensive the skin disease can be.

Symptoms

The symptoms of the patient in Fig. 3.3 consisted of whitish rashes on the trunk and the limbs. The rashes had been present for at least 5 years. The rashes, apart from being whitish, were only slightly itchy—and the itching occurred only when the patient worked for long periods outside the house and sweated. The patient first noticed the rashes on the upper chest, followed by the face. The patient did not feel concerned at the time but started worrying when a close relative observed that the rashes were plenty on the patient's back. Apparently, the rashes may have started at the same time as the ones on the anterior chest wall. Over the years, the rashes had spread to anterior and posterior surfaces of the upper limbs. The patient was a poor patient and did not see the need to commit scarce funds to go to the hospital on transport, registration and consultation, and purchase of drugs or to use the time considered as precious for petty trading and subsistence farming to be on the queues characteris-

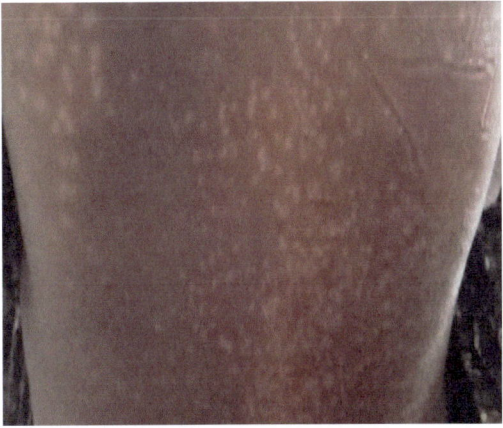

Fig. 3.3 The back of a patient with multiple rashes

tic of hospitals—even the ones closest to this patient. The patient was considering getting married and the looks of their skin was embarrassing. This patient feared that having such extensive rashes that changed the normal pigmentation of their skin would not augur well for the marital relationship. The patient's expectation was a cure as soon as possible.

Signs

Figures 3.3 and 3.4 On examination, the patient's posterior trunk was about 75% covered by the hypopigmented macules [4]. Although they could be hyperpigmented or hypopigmented in other skin types, these rashes are hypopigmented in the Black skin. Some of the macular rashes were discrete and irregular in shape, some formed islands, and others were coalescent. Figure 3.4 rashes demonstrate coalescence and marked irregularity in their outline.

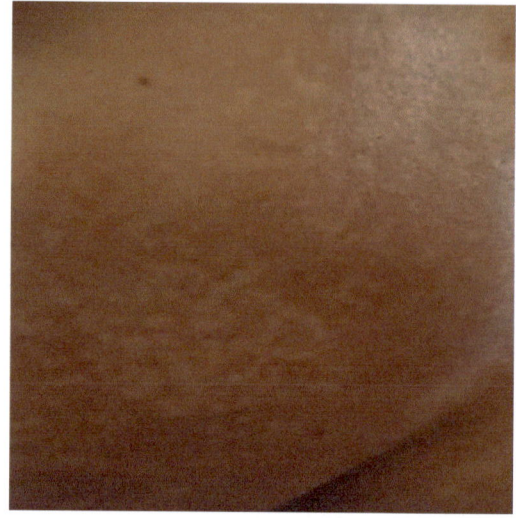

Fig. 3.4 The left side of the lower abdomen of the patient

Figure 3.5 This photograph of another patient's left upper back and the posterior surface of the left arm demonstrate the multiple lesions that characterize late presentation of this dermatological condition. With regards to the back, many patients are not aware that the rashes are on their back too—this has been highlighted in the history of the first patient (Figs. 3.3 and 3.4). The features are almost the same as documented for the first patient although those features are more readily appreciated in this enlarged image showing only a part of the back, compared with Fig. 3.3 that showed most of the back

Figures 3.6 and 3.7 show the rashes on a third patient. This patient was a 17-year-old girl. The macular eruption affected her upper extremities and both anterior and posterior aspects of the trunk.

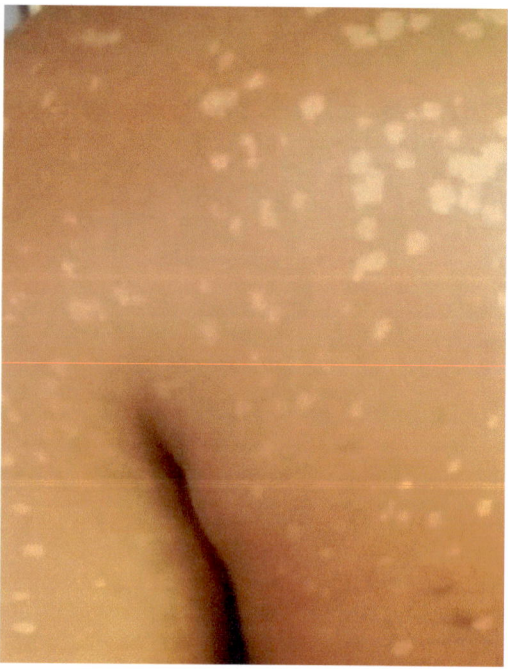

Fig. 3.5 Rashes on the left upper back

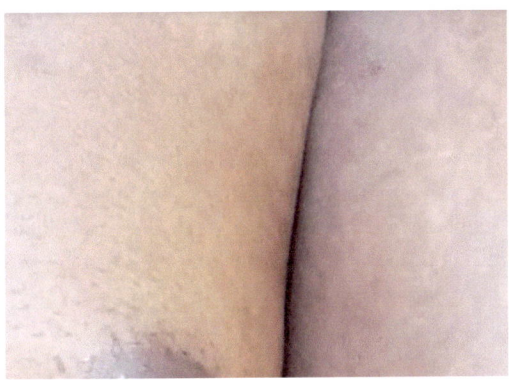

Fig. 3.6 Pityriasis versicolor affecting the left upper chest and the left arm

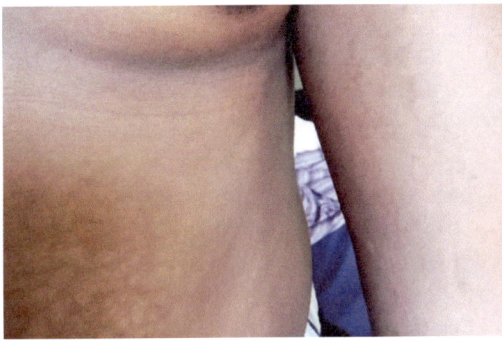

Fig. 3.7 Rashes on the left side of the patient's abdomen and the left arm

Diagnosis

Pityriasis versicolor

Etiology

Pityriasis versicolor is a superficial dermatological condition that is caused by the organism *Pityrosporum orbiculare*—the yeast form of *Malassezia furfur*.

Treatment

These three patients had extensive infection and required systemic treatment with oral antifungal creams.

Prognosis

Prognosis is good when the patient presents early (at the initial stages) of pityriasis versicolor when the macular eruptions are few and respond satisfactorily to topical application of antifungal agents. With extensive coverage of the body, the treatment may take slightly longer and the patient may require a further 6 weeks for the pigmentation of the skin to become normal. It is usually safe to ask the patient to take the oral medications until the lesions clear and to continue for a further minimum period of 2 weeks to ensure that the dimorphic yeasts are eliminated from the stratum corneum.

Follow-Up Care

Follow-up care helps both the physician and the patient in the sense that in some practice settings (like the one from which these clinical cases were obtained) the patients may not take their medications as prescribed, may not have enough money to buy the medications when prescribed, and therefore may not commence treatment until much later. In such cases (or when the doctor suspects that they could occur), the patient should be informed to return for a review in 2 weeks to "see how the medication is working." When the patient returns and the physician compares the status of the skin rashes with that of the initial or previous visit, an assessment of whether there was commencement of treatment or adherence to treatment would be made. It is better to counsel the patient at this visit that the treatment results are based not only on the prescribed medication but also on the commitment of the patient to treatment. For patients who have had the condition for years, it is imperative that the physician clearly communicates the fact that the treatment duration may be longer than they expect and encourages them to be on treatment. Financial considerations are not the only parameters that dictate patients' adherence to treatment as some patients who are covered by health insurance still do not go through the treatment course; they get tired and give up especially as pityriasis versicolor is a benign condition. Female patients tend to bother about the looks of their skin more than male patients.

Discussion

The etiological agents of pityriasis versicolor are dimorphic yeasts. They belong to the genus Malassezia. The causative organism also goes by the name *Pityrosporum orbiculare.*

The parts of the body that are usually affected are the trunk (initially upper), neck, face, and upper limbs.

The lesions are commoner during the warm seasons (summer) in temperate region, but in the tropical countries, the weather is warm most times; there may not be a specific season with a higher prevalence of pityriasis versicolor.

The diagnosis may be made clinically, but it is better to subject scrapings of affected skin to potassium hydroxide preparation and thereby confirm the diagnosis. When these are examined under the microscope, they show fungal elements. The fungal elements have both spaghetti appearance and meatballs appearance; these are indicators of the yeast and short hyphae [5, 6]. Other investigations that may be required are Gram staining, culture of specimen, and skin biopsy.

It is important to state that in people who are dark-skinned, pityriasis versicolor does not significantly present as hypopigmented macular eruptions [7]; in people with Black skin (especially of the deep tone), they are hypopigmented rashes.

Treatment of pityriasis versicolor may be by topical preparations like shampoos containing selenium sulfide 2.5%, ketoconazole shampoo, or zinc pyrithione shampoo—zinc pyrithione is fungistatic (it is also bacteriostatic). These and creams of azole antifungal medications provide effective treatment for pityriasis versicolor, but they are usually on the expensive side when this infection involves a large area of the body. For patients who have multiple relapses, they may require prophylactic treatment in addition to repeated therapy.

Tinea Capitis

Symptoms

The photographs are of the scalp of a 2-year-old boy. The mother complained that the multiple scalp rashes started about 3 weeks earlier. The rashes were few at the beginning but had increased in number to five. The rashes that appeared first had also increased slightly in size. The rashes were itchy as the patient had been scratching the scalp, particularly the affected parts. This was the first episode. The child did not have similar rashes in any other parts of the body. The mother said that the lesions were so pruritic that she assisted the patient to scratch it using a brush rather than letting the son continue scratching with his fingernails; using a brush alleviated the intensity of the rashes, especially initially. As it is common among the patients that we treat, perhaps because many drugs are available for purchase without prescription, the mother reported that she had been applying the following with some improvement: an antiseptic agent in undiluted form (the active ingredient is chloroxylenol), an alcohol-based cleaning agent, and an antifungal shampoo (with active ingredient ketoconazole). She brought the son because the response to her treatment was not satisfactory. When asked, she said that the only other person in the household with a similar eruption was the nanny. To mask the lesions, the mother took the son to a barber's shop to obtain a low haircut.

Signs

The image in Fig. 3.8 shows the patient bending to make the selected macular rash on the scalp very visible for the photograph to the taken. The boy's occiput is at the top while the neck is towards the top right of the image; his face is not visible in the image as he was pointing towards the floor. On examination, there were multiple irregularly shaped relatively hairless patches. Figure 3.8 shows the rash on the first day of consultation (a close examination shows two small macules lateral and inferior to the large one—on the image they are to

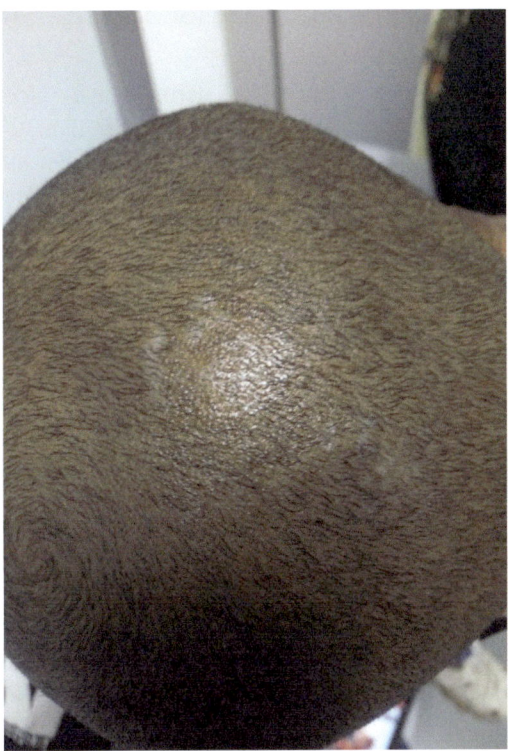

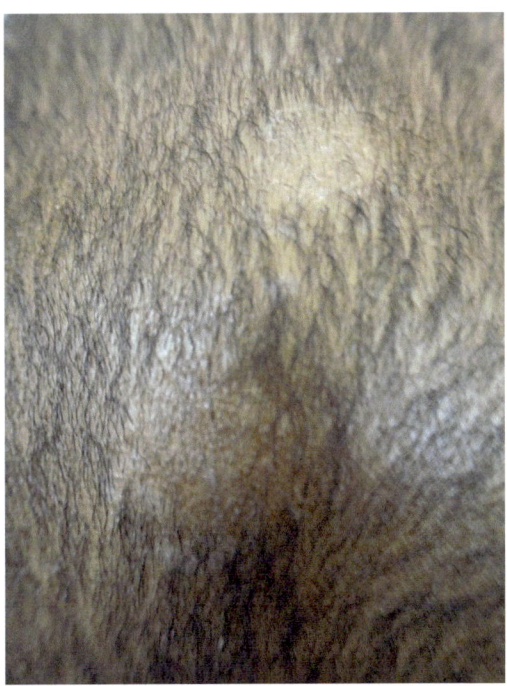

Fig. 3.9 Scalp skin rashes in the same child at 2-week follow-up consultation

Fig. 3.8 Macular rashes on the scalp skin of a 2-year-old boy

the right and slightly lower than the one of interest). This large rash (and the other two small ones) is on the left parieto-occipital scalp skin. The child's hair, having been cut, was almost at skin level, and the appearance of the rashes is demonstrated. The macular eruptions were of various sizes ranging from approximately 1–3 cm at the widest diameters. On close examination, there was a distinct demarcation between each macule and normal skin, despite the low haircut; there were no vesicles at the borders of any rash. There was no difference in pigmentation between the macules and surrounding unaffected skin—the large macular rash on Fig. 3.8 exemplifies the features of the others.

There were no scratch marks and no scar formation. Figures 3.9 and 3.10 show the same patient when he was brought back for review 2 weeks later. The two rashes in Fig. 3.9 are very distinct due to hair growth on normal skin during the 2-week interval between the two consultations.

Unfortunately, the parents had continued applying what they were applying and had neither obtained nor started applying the prescribed cream on the rashes.

N.B. Figure 3.9 is an enlargement of the rash in Fig. 3.8, and Fig. 3.10 is a further enlargement of the original macule of interest in Fig. 3.8 2 weeks after the first consultation. During this consultation, the author was interested in knowing why the rashes were larger and not regressed, only to extract the unfortunate information that the parents were yet to buy the medication that the author prescribed and therefore had not started using it on the child.

Figure 3.10 is a close-up image of the largest of the rashes in the field of the photograph. Central clearing is expected in tinea capitis, but in this patient, there is an elevation in the center from healing of a recent injury resulting from the child scratching the rash.

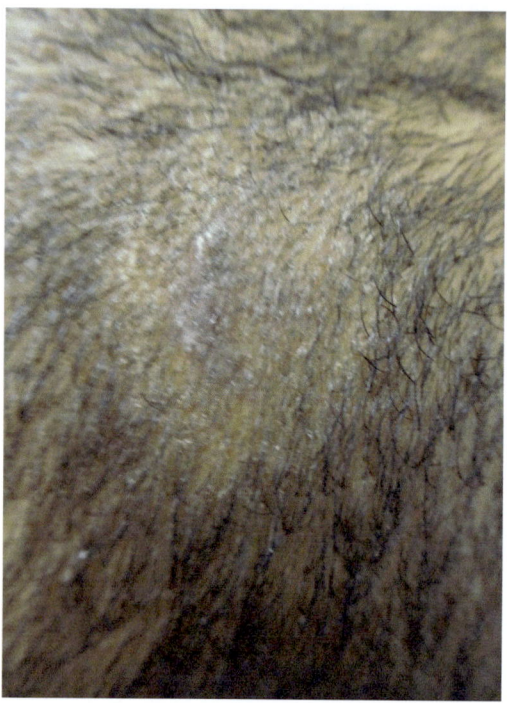

Fig. 3.10 Tinea capitis in the same child. The purpose of this image is to demonstrate two features: (a) magnification of the image in Fig. 3.8. Using a magnifying glass is useful in examining some clinical conditions in dermatology; this image replicates the features of that practice. (b) To show scalp hair loss that tinea capitis caused in that portion (parieto-occipital) of the scalp

Diagnosis

Tinea capitis

Treatment

Any antifungal from the groups that are efficacious for a dermatophytosis may be used. This patient was placed on ketoconazole cream as the not so many lesions did not require oral medication. The mother was advised to purchase the prescribed cream and continue applying the cream for 10–14 days after the rashes had cleared; this was to ensure effective treatment.

N.B. The nanny of this boy was the teenage girl whose scalp showed dandruff. She was also given a prescription of oral antifungal medication for her scalp lesions.

Etiology

Tinea capitis is one of the dermatophyte infections. The etiological agents are the dermatophytes *Trichophyton*, *Microsporum*, and *Epidermophyton*. This superficial skin infection affects the scalp.

Prognosis

Though tinea capitis may be a chronic fungal infection, this course is easily broken if the population from which the patients come are made aware of the importance of affected persons to consult doctors for prompt and adequate treatment. Spread is stemmed when contacts are identified and treated. Sometimes the infection is acquired in school or in the neighborhood. Among adults sharing combs, towels, headgear, etc. or having close bodily contact as may occur in certain overcrowded living conditions like internally displaced people's camps and some prisons may facilitate spread of the infection; therefore, attending to these conditions prevents the spread and improves prognosis.

This case was chosen as it is an atypical presentation of tinea capitis having been tampered with, thus causing an alteration from the clinical features that are usual at 3 weeks.

Discussion

Tinea capitis is a superficial dermatosis; it affects patients of all ages but principally children. When adults are affected, there may be risk factors that contributed to it, such as poverty, overcrowding in their living circumstances, or any cause of immunological depression. The macular lesions affect the scalp, eyebrows, and eyelashes [8].

Usual clinical features Untreated, this fungal infection runs a chronic course. The patient is usually a young child, but it could affect teenagers, young adults, and older adults. The rashes are macules usually starting small and increasing in size; they are also few at the outset but increase in number over time. The macules are in the form of irregularly shaped rings and the alternative name of the skin condition is scalp ringworm. As a macule increases in size, the active growing borders may develop papules or vesicles while the central portion of the rash demonstrates clearing due to healing. There may or may not be hypopigmentation or hyperpigmentation when compared with surrounding normal skin.

Investigations Tinea capitis is usually a clinical diagnosis based on a detailed history and proper physical examination of the lesion(s). However, in some patients the doctor may deem it expedient to request fungal studies on skin scrapings obtained from the lesions. Microscopic examination of the preparation demonstrates fungal elements of the causative dermatophytes.

Follow-Up Care

Regarding the index case and the patient with the condition, follow-up has been briefly discussed above. This is important as the observations by the physician (even if it is not the same doctor who attended the case in an earlier visit or previous consultations) are useful in assessing response to treatment and giving additional advice to the patient or parents of a minor. The information shared with them may be correction, commendation, or encouragement regarding playing their own part. Sometimes, other family or financial considerations may impinge upon a successful follow-up care.

Tinea Corporis, Dyschromia, and Striae Distensae

Symptoms

This patient was a middle-aged woman who came to the hospital and complained of a worsening abnormal skin color changes consisting of lightening and darkening, many initially itchy rashes that were extending in size and increasing in number despite recently becoming less pruritic, and many stretch marks that made her look older than her age, causing her frustration and embarrassment.

During further history, this woman said that she had used cosmetics for at least 3 years with the sole purpose of achieving skin lightening.

During consultation by a dermatologist following referral by a medical officer, detailed history, including drug history, showed that this patient used steroid creams, mercury-containing creams, antifungal creams, and local herbs.

Signs

She was a middle-aged woman with a combination of abnormal skin color changes consisting of hypopigmentation and hyperpigmentation, scaly multiple and extensive irregularly shaped macular rashes, and many stretch marks that belied her age.

Figure 3.11 shows oblique/longitudinal stretch marks on the anterolateral part of the upper and mid portions of the left thigh; describing from their top and back, these hyperpigmented stretch marks run anteroinferiorly. The marks were raised from the skin, but on palpation, there was a feeling of thinning of the stretch mark skin giving the sensation that the affected parts were slightly depressed.

With respect to the right thigh, there are multiple scars on the anterior surface of that thigh. The scars are variegated with mostly hyperpigmentation but some showing hypopigmented portions within the hyperpigmented scars. There were similar scars on the lateral and medical aspects of the right thigh, but the photograph is only one and thus does not show the full clinical picture like some other conditions shown in this book. The skin of the thighs also shows areas that are hypopigmented relative to other parts of the skin and multiple scars.

The medial aspects of the upper part of the two thighs show marked hyperpigmentation. From this photograph, it cannot be determined whether the affected skin is just uniformly hyperpigmented or there are hyperpigmented macular eruptions superimposed; the patient was not willing to expose that portion for examination.

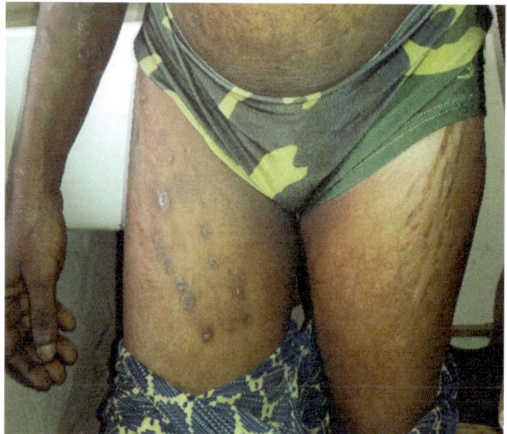

Fig. 3.11 Anterior thighs, lower abdomen, and lateral surface of the right forearm and hand

Figure 3.12 is the photograph of the upper limb of the patient with the triple conditions. The image shows multiple and extensive rashes. The lesions are a potpourri of macules, plaques, and scars. The lesions are not only of various shapes but also of diverse sizes. The shapes may be summarized as irregular as none has a regular shape like round, ovoid, or crescentic. Some lesions are discrete while others are coalescent. The right upper limb shows some hyperpigmented scars and many areas of hypopigmentation—this mixture may easily be described as dyspigmentation.

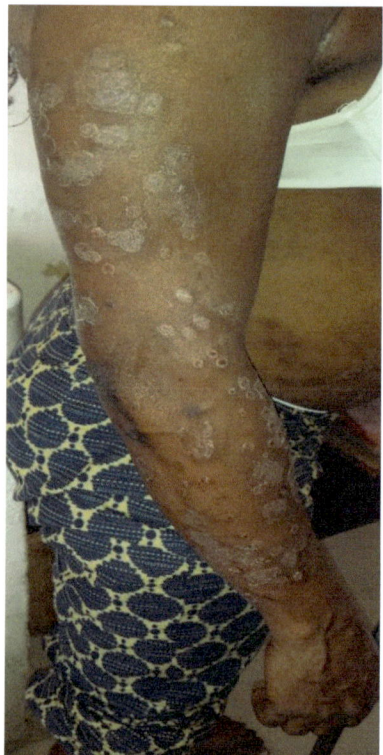

Fig. 3.12 The lateral aspect of the right arm, posterolateral aspect of the right forearm, and dorsum of the right hand

Diagnoses

Tinea corporis, Dyschromia, and Striae distensae

Treatment

The treatment approach for this woman was complicated. There was a major psychological component mixed with the physical and financial. Regarding the psychological, she was unhappy, frustrated, and embarrassed that at her age she had such "terrible skin." This was worse when she was informed that her use of cosmetics over the years to achieve the desire to look fair like fair women whom she admired had conspired against

her and contributed principally to the dyschromia and stretch marks. It was difficult for her to accept this as some people who used the same or related products did not have the kind of skin condition she presented with. It also took time to make her not dwell on self-blame when she finally accepted that she had spent her money to cause the multiple skin conditions that developed. The physical part was the realization that it would take a long time for her skin to recover somewhat, but perhaps not return to the status quo ante; she was to stop all the cosmetics she was using (and she used a combination even currently—and had used countless body creams over the years). She was encouraged to use simple creams and stick to the simple ones whether they were expensive or not. If she desired to make any modifications to her body cream or lotion, she should look at the small print on the container regarding the constituents and ensure that there was no hydroquinone and no mercury—and these sometimes had alternative fanciful names that many users do not recognize as the injurious products. The financial aspect of the treatment was that she needed the care of a specialist (dermatologist). Only dermatologists would be able to monitor the treatment. Finally, she would need multiple follow-up visits to the dermatological clinics for a long time. She attended the dermatological clinics.

Prognosis

Prognosis of tinea corporis is good but recurrence could occur in patients who do not protect themselves from reinfection by autoinfection. At other times, infection or reinfection could be secondary to exposure to fomites like sharing towels and various forms of clothing. Prognosis of dyschromia and striae distensae (stretch marks) is not good compared to that of tinea corporis. In dyschromia, dyspigmentation may be hyperpigmentation or hypopigmentation; either way it unleashes significant psychological trauma on patients with darker skin [9]. This is more especially on patients with Black skin. It takes considerable time to cause damage to skin structure and function to have the result as dyschromia and stretch marks. It also takes a long time to correct the changes in Black skin, and the cooperation and understanding of the patient are more pertinent during management by the specialist.

Follow-Up Care

This was done by the dermatologists. The author believes that the patient would get better with time as she overcame the initial discouragement, particularly when she was informed of the cause.

Discussion

In some patients, there may be more than one dermatological condition. The conditions may be similar but occur in different sites e.g., tinea cru-ris and onychomycosis or dissimilar in etiology but present with similar symptomatology e.g., scabies and tungiasis with severe pruritus. The patient whose photographs are used for this triple topic had a combination of tinea corporis, stretch marks, and dyschromia.

Tinea Corporis

Tinea infection affects various parts of the body. It is caused by the dermatophytes *Trichophyton*, *Epidermophyton*, and *Microsporum*. The commonest cause of tinea corporis, worldwide, is *Trichophyton rubrum*—being implicated in more than 40% of cases. Tinea corporis is a dermatophytosis affecting non-glabrous (hair-bearing) skin. This means that infection affecting the palms and soles, face, lips, and ears that do not bear hair (glabrous) are excluded. Tinea infection that affects glabrous skin bears specific names ending with faciei (face), manuum (for palms), and pedis (for feet), respectively. Some parts of the body that grow hair have names for tinea infection occurring there, e.g., tinea capitis for the scalp. In children, tinea corporis may be secondary to tinea capitis. Tinea corporis may take the form of tinea incognito in patients undergoing corticosteroid therapy, while HIV-positive patients may have disseminated form of the fungal infection.

Clinical presentation Tinea corporis is initially erythematous (which may not show classically in the dark-skinned) and takes various forms and thus may be plaques, papules, pustules, vesicles, or scaly and assume various shapes. The peripheral part of the rash is more active, and the increase in proliferation of epithelial cells results in scaling; the central portion shows healing, new, and healthy skin.

Investigations Results of laboratory investigations are, viz., microscopic examination of KOH wet mount of skin scraping shows fungal elements; histological examination of punch biopsy specimen stained with hematoxylin and eosin shows spongiosis, parakeratosis, and superficial inflammatory infiltrate; periodic acid-Schiff staining may show septate branching hyphae in the stratum corneum.

Treatment Treatment of tinea capitis is with the use of drugs effective for other dermatophyte infections, i.e., topical, or oral use of azoles or allylamines. The determinant of what the doctor prescribes may be the patient's age, extent of the skin covered by the infection, pregnancy, or lactation.

Dyschromia

Treatment for post-inflammatory hyperpigmentation may consist of the following:

- Azelaic acid
- Corticosteroids
- Hydroquinone
- Tretinoin
- Mandelic acid
- Trichloroacetic acid
- Vitamin C with a full-face iontophoresis

Skin-lightening agents have a place clinically in the management of hyperpigmentation disorders, e.g., post-inflammatory hyperpigmentation and melasma. The challenge is when there is uncontrolled and nonprescription use of these agents, the decision to use them being principally that of the females and some males who use them; this situation is likely in some parts of Africa, the Caribbean, and India.

For outside clinical use, persons who use skin-lightening creams do so because they have dark spots on exposed parts of their bodies or because they are not satisfied with their natural complexion—preferring a tone or complexion lighter than the natural. The problem with the latter is that when they opt for topical application there is a tendency for such patients to apply the medication/cosmetic agent over the entire body or a significant part of exposed skin and use the product(s) over a protracted period lasting months or years—in summary, they purchase and use these products as cosmetics. Skin lightening agents are found in many outlets in some countries where regulatory controls are lax. These drugs may contain mercury and are cheap and affordable for many people. Unfortunately, many users of these products are either lowly educated or do not bother to read the product labels to know the ingredients. Mercury may not be written exactly, as it may be stated as quicksilver, cinnabaris, calomel, or hydrargyri oxydum rubrum. Non-mercury skin-lightening agents include hydroquinones, steroids, and arsenic. Both mercury and hydroquinones inhibit melanin synthesis. Examples of steroids are clobetasol propionate and betamethasone. In some of the products, the concentration of mercury, hydroquinones, or arsenic may be higher than the upper levels allowed for cosmetics. Some cosmetics contain more than one active ingredient.

The skin of the patient whose photographs, Figs. 3.11 and 3.12, are shown above demonstrates some of the adverse effects of use of steroids and skin-lightening preparations. Many dermatological preparations are a combination of steroid-antifungal-antibiotic agents. Whether used singly or in combination, corticosteroids applied over a protracted period may result in recalcitrant dermatophyte infections. Irrational and uncontrolled use of topical corticosteroids cause skin atrophy (thinning of the skin), hypopigmentation, depigmentation, or dyspigmentation.

Striae distensae (Stretch Marks)

When stretch marks become mature, the striae that they form are white bands. These bands have irregular shape and are depressed; their long axes are parallel to the lines of skin tension [10]. Stretch marks are also results of this inappropriate use of steroids. Prolonged use of potent corticosteroids over a wide skin area may lead to renal hypertension. Similar use of high- or low-dose mercury-containing cosmetic preparations may result in renal toxicity.

Tinea Cruris

Tinea cruris is one of the dermatophytoses. It is, therefore, a superficial mycosis.

Though the infection is found in all regions and all races, it is commoner in males than females and is more prevalent in warm, hot, humid regions.

Symptoms

This patient, in his late 20s, presented in the hospital with the complaint of itching, rashes, and discoloration of his scrotal skin and the inner upper thighs for more than 2 months. The itching was severe and became more prevalent in the night. He used to wear tight underwear, but the rashes, over time, prevented him from wearing them as the tightness did not allow him to scratch or rub with ease; he had to be struggling to get there, and the frequency of scratching or rubbing to assuage the itching was too much for him. It was now easier for him to get some relief since the underwear gave him adequate space; this was his first time having the rash. He wore the same pant for at least 3 days, and although his work was mainly physical with consequent sweating, he could not change his underwear as frequently as he knew that he ought to; due to insufficiency of water in the community where he lived, he preferred to wash all his clothes for the week during the weekends.

The patient did not have a similar rash in any other part of the body. He was not a patient with obesity, diabetes mellitus, or hypertension. He lived alone, was unmarried, currently had no girlfriend, and did not share clothes or towels with anybody.

When he went to a "chemist shop" recently, he was given a cream that the shop operator (not a pharmacist) told him has more than one medicine inside it. He noticed some reduction in itching, but the rash was there and seemed to be increasing in size and the skin darkening was not lessened.

He feared that this rash was becoming a long-lasting condition, and he was not happy with the fact that he had to be cautious not to scratch "through clothes" in the presence of people. He wanted to know the cause, especially as he wanted to know what he could do to stop it and prevent it in the future. He believed that having come to the teaching hospital, he would receive the best treatment. He was willing to spend money to treat the condition for he had spent

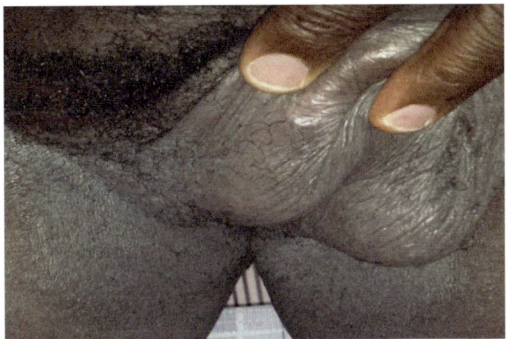

Fig. 3.13 Hyperpigmented macular eruption on scrotal and genitocrural skin

money since the onset of the rash without obtaining the desired relief.

Signs

Figure 3.13 shows the groin of an adult male with an extensive bilateral macular rash with ill-defined borders which are not readily identifiable. The rashes consisted of a large, continuous, well demarcated, and macerated patch on the scrotum and inner thighs. Satellite lesions which are seen in candidal skin infection are not obvious in this image. In this man with scrotal involvement and the near absence of scrotal hair, such absence is due to depilation occasioned by scratching and pulling the hairs.

Diagnosis

Tinea cruris

Etiology

Tinea cruris is caused by *Trichophyton*, followed by *Epidermophyton*. Of the trichophytons, the commonest specie that causes it is *Trichophyton rubrum*. Other trichophytons are *Trichophyton tonsurans*, *Trichophyton mentagrophytes*, and *Trichophyton verrucosum*. *Epidermophyton floccosum* also causes this infection.

Treatment

The patient was placed on miconazole powder to be applied twice daily until 2 weeks after the rashes cleared. The additional medication was a second-generation antihistamine, levocetirizine 5 mg, to be taken orally daily for 2 weeks. The patient was informed that the pruritus would end before the rashes would disappear. He was encouraged to use the medications as prescribed. He was encouraged to maintain his weight for his body mass index was normal, and he should ensure that he should adopt a lifestyle that would prevent the development of diabetes mellitus. He was also advised to continue wearing underwear that was not tight but should either wash them more frequently; alternatively, he could procure more underwear if he could not dispense with the habit of bulk laundry.

Prognosis

Prognosis is good when the patient is inquisitive and willing to apply the information on the risk factors, adherence to treatment, and prevention of tinea cruris.

Follow-Up Care

Every patient should be advised to return to the clinic at the agreed time; the first follow-up visit is particularly important as the physician is able to assess the patient's level of cooperation with the treatment. Further appointments may be based on the availability of both the patient and the doctor (especially if a dermatologist). Even this aspect of care should be discussed with the patient and, preferably, be patient centered. If the timing of the appointment is highly restrictive, some patients may not keep the appointment or some appointments.

Discussion

Usual clinical presentation History taking should place emphasis on onset, duration of initial symptoms and recurrence, additional symptoms, and extension of the initial lesion. Ask the patient if there are similar or other skin conditions in other parts of the body, e.g., the hands, feet, under the breasts, nails, etc. Other information that should be sought for include practices that encourage acquiring the infection and its recurrence. Practices like wearing tight-fitting clothing, especially underwear, for extended periods or sharing laundry, e.g., towels, underwear, and bedding with persons who have dermatophytosis, can lead to acquiring the infection which is also spread by fomites. In parts of the world where many drugs can be procured over the counter, it is important to ask the patient what medications have been ingested or applied to the rashes—application of steroidal creams (or steroid-containing) may provide a temporary respite, especially to the pruritus, but they cause the spread of the skin infection. Obesity, diabetes mellitus, and excessive sweating also predispose people to acquiring tinea cruris.

Initial symptoms are a rash (or rashes) with pruritus. The area of involvement is primarily the groin, but the surrounding skin, e.g., pubic area, lower abdomen, and upper thighs, may be affected.

The rash is macular and may be of any shape. The rash has borders that are usually clearly demarcated from normal skin or gradually fade into normal skin. There may be coalescence or confluence of rashes creating irregular shapes. The center of a rash heals over time while the borders spread. The healing part may become hyperpigmented to various degrees. There is a tendency for patients to respond to intense pruritus by scratching; this may lead to excoriation and superimposed bacterial and candidal infection. Chronicity may show as dryness, scaling, lichenification, and hyperpigmentation at the genitocrural folds and upper thighs.

Differential diagnoses of tinea corporis include erythrasma, allergic contact dermatitis, candidal intertrigo, irritant contact dermatitis, seborrheic dermatitis, etc. History taking may assist in ruling out some of the above skin diseases. A known diabetic patient with genitocrural rash may well be having candidal intertrigo especially if the rash is grayish-white with satellite lesions at the borders. A patient with atopy and exposure to or use of synthetic, tight-fitting clothing may be having allergic contact dermatitis. For another patient, there may be occupational exposure to an irritant either by touch or use that may cause irritant contact dermatitis. Erythrasma is equally a macular skin disease and may affect other intertriginous parts of the body, but is drier, and produces tiny skin flakes.

Investigations In patients with the provisional diagnosis of tinea cruris, investigations include skin scraping and microscopic examination of the scales in potassium hydroxide wet mount. The result is positive for tinea cruris, but it could be negative. After repeat tests, the result may be positive—and so more than one test may be done. Scale culture identifies the precise fungus causing the tinea cruris. Other tests are examination of the rash under Wood's lamp (which produces ultraviolet radiation) in a dark room—which shows coral red fluorescence in erythrasma. Punch biopsy may be useful also. In tinea corporis, histopathological examination of appropriately stained tissue sections shows characteristic presence of neutrophils in the stratum corneum, perivascular inflammation in the epidermis, and the presence of spores and branching hyphae.

Treatment The treatment of tinea cruris, like other dermatophytosis, may be challenging because patients sometimes try the treatment by self-prescription and suggestion from relatives, friends, or colleagues before consulting a doctor. At other times, they are impatient to use prescribed medications for the period recommended, especially after they notice satisfactory improvement or clearing of the skin lesions. Moreover, some patients find it difficult to break habits that tend to perpetuate the infection or to encourage its recurrence. It is, therefore, important to do the following:

- Give patients enough information to enable them to see the importance of avoiding direct or indirect contact between other fungal-infected parts of the body and the groin, e.g., hands and feet. With hands, the contact is usually direct and with feet it is indirect. They should wear socks before putting on underwear.

- Treat all dermatophyte-infected sites in the body concurrently.
- Encourage weight loss by patients who are overweight or obese.
- Work together with diabetic patients to achieve and maintain glycemic control.
- Avoid dampness of the groin by drying the area well and use loose, non-tight-fitting underwear.

Effective topical and oral antifungals for treatment belong to the allylamine and azole classes.

Tinea Pedis Interdigitalis

Symptoms

The patient whose feet were photographed is a 61-year-old retiree. He complained of a recalcitrant itchy rash in-between his right fourth and little toes with a duration of more than 1 year. During

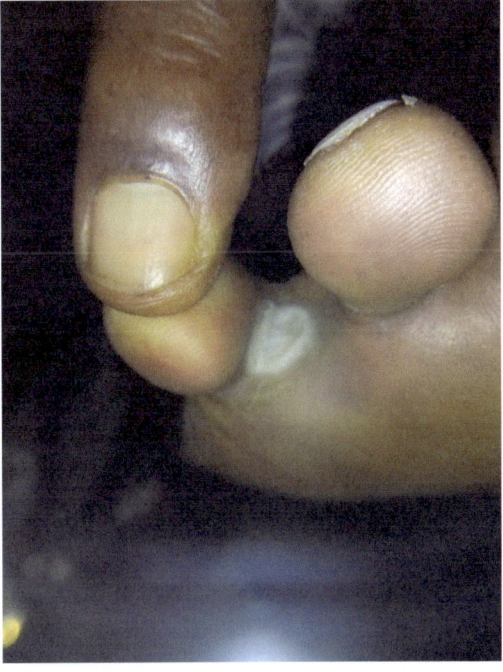

Fig. 3.14 Rash in-between the right fourth and little toes

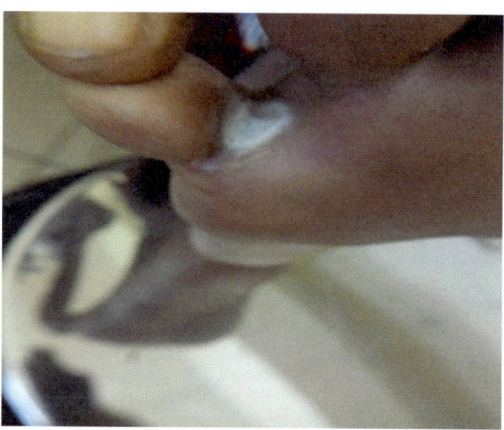

Fig. 3.15 Rash in-between the patient's right fourth and little toes

this period, he has used a myriad of creams and sprays with no significant relief. Apart from the itching, he feels discomfort and occasionally pain in the affected foot. For some months, he has found free toed footwear more comfortable to wear and he came to the clinic wearing a pair.

Further history showed that the patient had the rash in only that location. He did not have a positive history of a similar rash earlier in his life. He has not been in a profession that requires wearing covered shoes or boots for protracted periods. He was a highly placed official in his church, but he was not required to officiate regularly. He was not a diabetic patient and has not had cause to use antibiotics for prolonged periods or irrationally.

According to this patient, he was upset when he went to a private hospital and the young doctors refused to refer him to a specialist when he made the request. He brought the empty packet of the antibiotic that he purchased based on the prescription; he had exhausted it without any improvement. He also brought evidence of other drugs he had taken recently including an unexhausted canister of a spray he was asked to spray on the rash.

Signs

For adequate examination, the patient was asked to use his hands to separate distal ends (tips) of the right fourth and fifth toes as far as he could

without causing himself additional pain. On examination, he had a whitish plaque only in the fourth/fifth interdigital cleft of the right foot. Although it was mainly in the cleft, the rash was shifted laterally keeping the medial border of the rash away from the lateral surface of the fourth toe; rather the rash affected the medial border of the fifth toe in addition to the fourth interdigital cleft. The surface of the rash was clean, and there was a clear demarcation between the rash and unaffected skin. The rash was slightly tender but the patient was able to move all toes of the right foot. There was no involvement of the nails, and all toenails were normal in shape and color. However, the surrounding plantar skin was slightly erythematous.

Diagnosis

On clinical grounds, a putative diagnosis of tinea pedis interdigitalis may be made. This is subject to appropriate investigations and their results to confirm the diagnosis.

Etiology

Tinea pedis interdigitalis is the result of infection by the dermatophyte *Trichophyton rubrum*.

Treatment

As indicated above, treatment should be commenced early in the course of this infection. Antifungals from various classes are used: imidazoles, allylamines, benzylamines, and pyridones. These are effective for topical administration when applied early and for satisfactory length of time. It is good practice to advise the patient that even when the lesion has cleared the antifungal should be used for a further approximately 2 weeks and that adherence to use any of the drugs is important. Antimycotics may need to be taken orally especially when the infection is chronic.

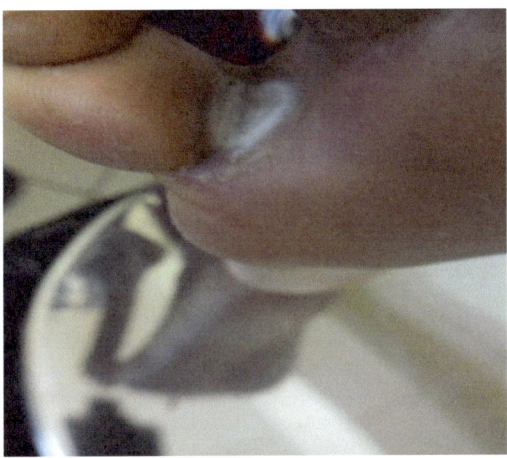

Fig. 3.16 Rash in-between the patient's right fourth and fifth toes

Prognosis

When the patient understands the cause of the disease, its chronicity, and tendency towards recurrence, the prognosis is good. This is because the patient will not treat it as a simple bacterial infection that frequently responds to 5–7 days' treatment; will pay attention to proper foot care, proper use, and care of footwear; will make life-style modifications to ensure weight control, will prevent diabetes mellitus and HIV infection, and will ensure control of diabetes mellitus if a patient is already with diabetes mellitus.

Follow-Up Care

The care for a patient who has tinea pedis inter-digitalis follows the same principle for other der-matophyte infections of the skin; the major addition is that the patient should be adequately educated on the need to avoid autoinfection which may be responsible for reinfections. Secondly, the patient should be informed that the disease runs a chronic course and so the treatment should be strictly adhered to, to ensure that the infection is eliminated. Preventive measures like foot care should be reemphasized during follow-up care as many patients do not document in writing (or any other means) what the doctor said. For a busy

practice that attends to only dermatological condi-tions or general conditions but inclusive of skin diseases, it may save time to print simple and brief guidance and give to appropriate patients.

Discussion

Usual clinical features This dermatophyte infection is a disease that runs a chronic course; it is also called chronic intertriginous tinea pedis. It is better to prevent it or, at least, treat it satisfac-torily as early as possible.

It is an intertriginous fungal skin infection of the spaces between the toes. There seems to be a predilection for the smallest interdigital space and that is between the fourth and fifth toes. The infec-tion, like other intertriginous infections that affect skin folds, involve spaces that are warm and moist. The rash is white or grayish-white. It is pruritic. It may be painful when there is fissuring.

Investigations The diagnosis can be made from the history, but since there are differential diagno-ses and there could also be superinfection, it is important to carry out some investigations. Investigations include skin scrapings for fungal studies using potassium hydroxide (KOH) prepa-ration and microscopic examination; this differen-tiates between *Candida albicans* infection which demonstrates the yeast and this dermatophyte infection that shows *Trichophyton rubrum*. Wood's lamp differentiates it from erythrasma. Diabetic patients are prone to developing this infection, and it may be the pointer that the patient with this skin infection is diabetic and should commence treatment; blood and urine tests are sufficient to make this diagnosis or rule it out.

Multiple-Choice Questions

1. Pityriasis versicolor: Which of the statements below is correct?
   A. It rarely affects the upper part of the trunk.
   B. Lesions are hypopigmented, non-scaly macules.

C. Lesions are usually non-pruritic and coalescent.

D. It responds to treatment with erythromycin.

2. Tinea capitis: Which of the statements below is correct?

   A. It has a predilection for newborn babies.

   B. Candida species are the etiological organisms.

   C. It is characterized by broken hairs and scaly areas of the scalp.

   D. It does not respond to treatment with ketoconazole.

3. An 11-year-old girl is brought to your clinic on account of a second rash on the body. The rashes are almost round and pruritic. Which of the following would best enable you sustain a tentative diagnosis of tinea corporis?

   A. Close bodily contact with a cousin on recent visit having similar rashes.

   B. Positive history of carbuncle 1 month earlier.

   C. Skin scrapings demonstrating superficial dermatophyte.

   D. Blood culture to rule out bacterial secondary infection.

4. A 39-year-old factory supervisor with a 9-month history of interdigital rash between the most lateral two toes presents to the clinic with a 6-week complaint of itchy rashes in the groin area. Which of the following is a correct association?

   A. Infection by self-inoculation is unlikely.

   B. Infection at the two sites is most likely occupation-related.

   C. Treatment should terminate on disappearance of the rashes.

   D. The etiological agent is unlikely to be a yeast.

5. With respect to tinea cruris, which of the following associations is correct?

   A. Etiology—Same as for moniliasis.

B. Pathophysiology—Fungal invasion of dermal layer.

C. Clinical feature—Grayish-white plaque.

D. Preventive measure—Use of appropriate fitting cotton underwear (undergarment).

References

1. Borda LJ, Wikramanayake TC. Seborrheic dermatitis and dandruff: a comprehensive review. J Clin Investig Dermatol. 2015;3(2):10.13188/2373-1044.1000019. https://doi.org/10.13188/2373-1044.1000019. PMCID: PMC4852869 NIHMSID: NIHMS754376 PMID: 27148560. Available from: https://pmc.ncbi.nlm.nih.gov/articles/PMC4852869/.

2. Handler MZ. Seborrheic dermatitis treatment & management. In: Dermatology. Medscape; 2023. Available from: https://emedicine.medscape.com/article/1108312-treatment.

3. Tucker D, Masood S. Seborrheic dermatitis. In: StatPearls [Internet]; 2024. Available from: https://www.ncbi.nlm.nih.gov/books/NBK551707/.

4. Łabędź N, Navarrete-Dechent C, Kubisiak-Rzepczyk H, Bowszyc-Dmochowska M, Pogorzelska-Antkowiak A, Pietkiewicz P. Pityriasis versicolor—a narrative review on the diagnosis and management. Life (Basel). 2023;13(10):2097. https://doi.org/10.3390/life13102097. PMCID: PMC10608716 PMID: 37895478. Available from: https://pmc.ncbi.nlm.nih.gov/articles/PMC10608716/.

5. Swick BL. Pityriasis versicolor. BMJ Best Practice; 2024. Available from: https://bestpractice.bmj.com/topics/en-gb/861.

6. Schwartz RA. Superficial fungal infections. Lancet. 2004;364(9440):1173–82.

7. Aljabre SH, Alzayir AA, Abdulghani M, et al. Pigmentary changes of tinea versicolor in dark-skinned patients. Int J Dermatol. 2001;40(4):273–5.

8. Handler MZ. Tinea capitis. In: Dermatology. Medscape; 2024. Available from: https://emedicine.medscape.com/article/1091351-overview.

9. Halder RM, Richards GM. Management of dyschromias in ethnic skin. Dermatol Ther. 2004;17(2):151–7. https://doi.org/10.1111/j.1396-0296.2004.04015.x. PMID: 15113282. Available from: https://pubmed.ncbi.nlm.nih.gov/15113282/.

10. Alaiti S. Striae distensae (stretch marks) clinical presentation. In: Dermatology. Medscape; 2022. Available from: https://emedicine.medscape.com/article/1074868-clinical.

Herpes Zoster

Symptoms

The 40-year-old female patient complained of rashes on the left thigh for 1 week. The rashes erupted at the site of discomfort, "heat," and itching which started about 3 days prior to the first rashes. The rashes were just about three at the outset but have increased in number. The rashes congregated on only the affected part. She had an imprecise pain which she said was more of "mild fiery pain." The pain was tolerable and the pain score was just about 2 of 10. She did not have any other local symptoms, neither did she have constitutional symptoms like fever, malaise, weakness, or nausea preceding the symptoms or as at when she made the presenting complaints in the clinic.

The patient said that she had a similar set of rashes some 9 months earlier, but that episode was on another part of the body. She was not a patient with HIV or AIDS, hypertension, diabetes mellitus, or obesity. She was an employee of a company, was satisfactorily remunerated, and had access to medical treatment sponsored by the company.

She had not taken any medication and had ensured that despite the itching she did not scratch the rashes or break them—even if she were to succumb to the desire, she constantly

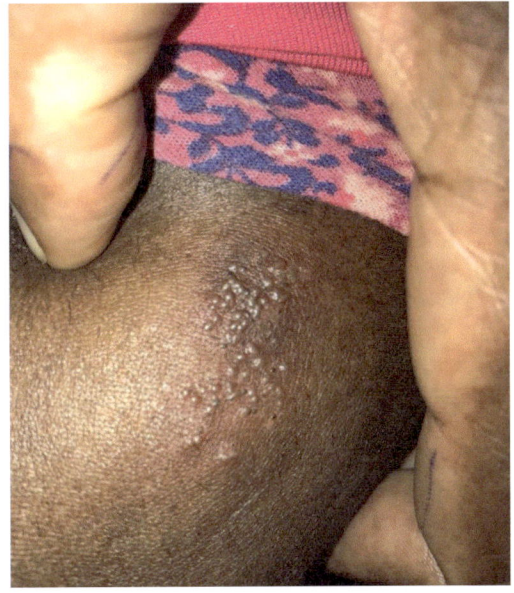

Fig. 4.1 Rashes on the thigh of an adult female patient

remembered the pain would become aggravated; what she did was to rub it with her fingers.

Although she was not certain of what it was, she was worried that this was the second time she was having it; she desired to know what it was and to have a solution to this episode and prevention of a recurrence.

Supplementary Information The online version contains supplementary material available at https://doi.org/10.1007/978-3-031-97503-5_4.

Signs

Examination of the skin condition showed that the rashes were on the lateral surface of the proximal part of the left thigh. The rashes were grouped vesicular eruptions that roughly formed an oval shape. In terms of size, each was "pin head," but the conglomerate lesion was about 6 × 3.5 cm at the longitudinal and transverse planes, respectively. The vesicles were slightly tender, and although many appeared to congregate with virtually no space, they still appeared discrete and there was not convincing coalescence. Each vesicle was more-or-less circular, had a smooth surface, and did not discharge their contents. The pigmentation of the affected part was the same as unaffected skin; her skin tone was moderate for Black skin.

Diagnosis

Herpes zoster

Etiology

Varicella-zoster virus (a reactivation of the virus infection) [1].

Treatment

Although this patient did not access treatment soon after the onset of the rashes, she was placed on acyclovir cream. She was to apply it at least four times on the days she went to work and six times daily on weekends. She was to ensure that the cream was no longer discernible on the skin before allowing her dress to tough the affected part. (In this practice setting, acyclovir is the most readily available and affordable of the effective antiviral creams; others [valaciclovir and famciclovir] are either too expensive for the average patient or unavailable.)

She was encouraged to continue with avoidance of any other measures to the affected part, just the way she had done before coming to the clinic. She was placed on levocetirizine 5 mg daily for 10 days. She was also placed on prednisolone 10 mg three times daily for 3 days, 5 mg daily for 3 days, and finally 5 mg daily for 3 days. She was requested to keep a follow-up appointment 1 week later. She was not in significant pain and was placed on a combination tablet comprising acetaminophen and caffeine. Some patients would need warm compress and calamine lotion. This patient did not require such treatment and she actually visited the clinic from work.

Prognosis

The prognosis of herpes zoster is good, except for patients who are malnourished, generally of poor health, or with reduced immunity from HIV infection, diabetes mellitus, or on chemotherapy.

Follow-Up Care

When she came for follow-up, there was regression of the lesions as seen in Fig. 4.2. She was informed again that herpes zoster is a viral infection that affects nerves. In a healthy patient like

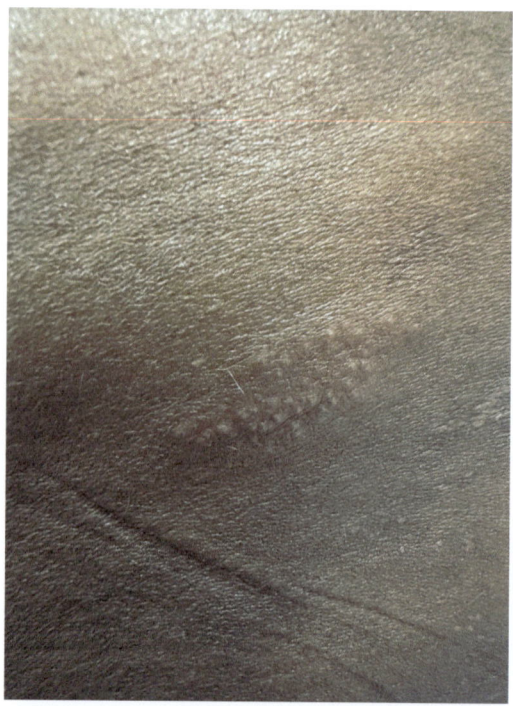

Fig. 4.2 The rashes about 1 week of taking the prescribed treatment

her without HIV infection, obesity, hypertension, or diabetes mellitus but running a very busy schedule in her office and at home, it would help if she could reduce her stress level—as this could minimize her risk of recurrence of the lesions from reactivation of the etiological agent.

Discussion

Herpes zoster is a vesicular eruption that is the result of a reactivation of the Varicella zoster virus. The patient would have had chicken pox, and the causative virus remained dormant, only to be reactivated to cause herpes zoster (shingles) later in life. Spread of the infection does not happen by close contact with the patient with the eruptions unless the contact never had chicken pox or has never been vaccinated against chicken pox.

Prevention of herpes zoster is by vaccination with *two* doses of recombinant zoster vaccine (RZV) also called Shingrix. This is efficacious for individuals who are aged 50 years or above. For individuals who are 19 years and older and are concomitantly at risk of the infection due to depressed immunity, the vaccine is also recommended [2] to prevent shingles and related complications in adults 50 years and older.

Genital Molluscum Contagiosum

Symptoms

This male patient, aged 22 years, presented with penile rashes he observed within the past 4 months. The rashes were neither painful nor pruritic. He did not have rashes in any other part of the body. The rashes became causes of concern to him only because they were increasing in number. He was sexually active but said that he did not practice unprotected sex. He was HIV negative. He was currently on isotretinoin tablets for treatment of severe acne that was unresponsive to other drugs; when asked why he did not mention anything about the genital rashes although he had been attending the clinic for severe acne, his

response was that he felt that the lesions would resolve on their own.

Signs

Figure 4.3 On examination, he had multiple, discrete, essentially round, less than 5 mm papular rashes some of which were umbilicated. They were the same in pigmentation with the surrounding skin. The rashes concentrated on the dorsal part and sides of the shaft of the penis, sparing the glans. There was no tenderness and there were no scratch marks on the surrounding skin. None of the popular eruptions appeared traumatized.

Etiology

The disease is viral and the causative agent is the DNA poxvirus, molluscum contagiosum.

Risk factors for genital molluscum contagiosum include being sexually active, immune depression, and living in warm areas that are equally humid in addition to the first two just listed [3]. Risk factors for molluscum contagiosum at other body sites include warmth, humidity, and atopic dermatitis. Since it is a direct person-to-person bodily contact infection and a nosocomial infection, good hand hygiene and good personal hygiene are preventive measures against acquiring or transmitting the disease.

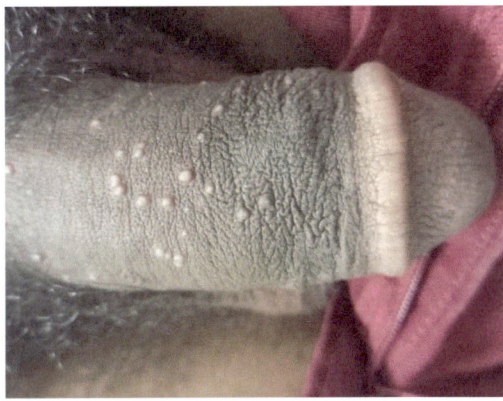

Fig. 4.3 Penile rashes

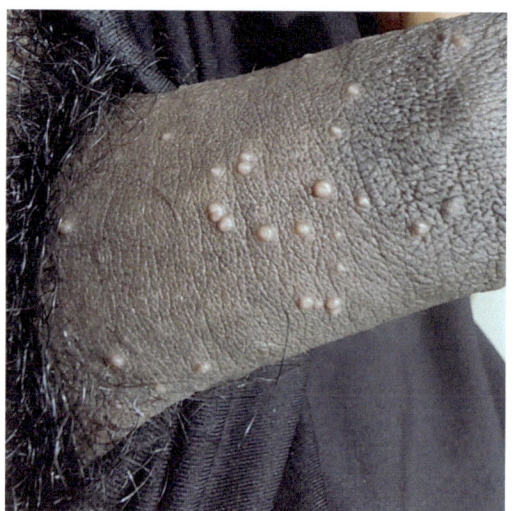

Fig. 4.4 Penile rashes, enlarged

These skin lesions are limited to the epidermal layer of skin.

Diagnosis

Genital molluscum contagiosum

Treatment

In this patient, treatment was a necessity as its location made it imperative for the patient to receive immediate treatment by the dermatologist. The dermatologist was to determine which method of treatment.

For most other sites of this viral skin infection, it should be communicated to the patient that it is self-limiting; though the condition is self-limiting in some patients, in others it may require treatment especially if the site presents an aesthetic embarrassment like facial lesions, or if their presence gives an almost constant foreign body sensation, e.g., the fornix of the eyelid.

When treatment is required, it may consist of cryotherapy using liquid nitrogen, curettage, electrocautery under topical anesthesia, or application of laser.

Oral therapy with cimetidine is principally used in children.

Topical treatment consists of podophyllin, tretinoin, iodine and salicylic acid, imiquimod, or cantharidin. The challenge is that a topical agent is applied to lesions individually, and the procedure could be burdensome in patients with multiple lesions and those who have them in sites that they cannot apply these topical agents with precision or their hands do not reach—in which case they need another person to help them do the application on the rashes.

Intralesional interferon is effective for treating extensive facial lesions in immunocompromised patients. This mode of treatment gives better results in those with intact immunity.

Follow-Up Care

For this patient, it was left for the dermatologist. The principle would be the same as for (or similar to) many dermatological conditions as described in this book.

Prognosis

Prognosis is good but the patient should know that there may be further episodes of infection if they are re-exposed by sexual contact or physical contact with another person with the lesions. Moreover, the patient should be informed that an episode may last for weeks, up to a few months, or a few years, but they hardly continue beyond about 5 years. When treated with curettage, there may be scarring at the site of some of the lesions.

Discussion

Usual clinical features The rashes in molluscum contagiosum are usually small discrete dome-shaped papules which are under 6 mm. These papules are umbilicated for they demonstrate a central indentation or pitting [4]—the umbilicated area contains a caseous plug. They have the same color as normal skin—see Fig. 4.5. Usually, they are neither painful nor pruritic, but pricking, scratching, or traumatizing them in

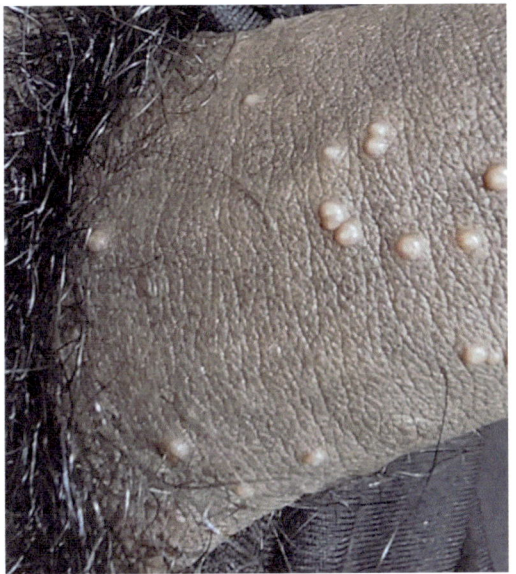

Fig. 4.5 A close-up photograph of the fine features of the lesion; these should be looked out for in the patient

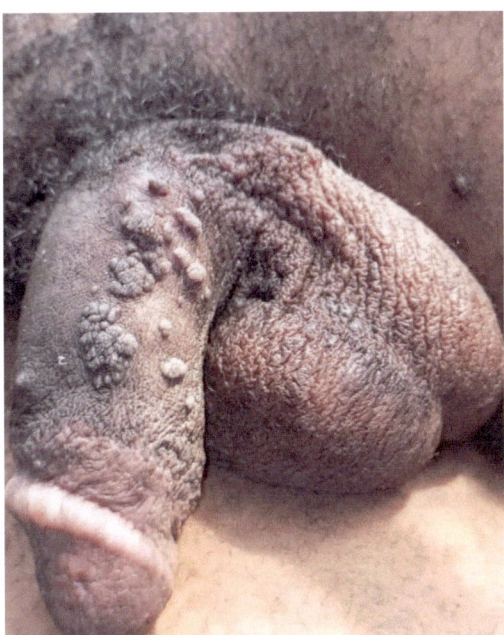

Fig. 4.6 Penile growths in warts

another form may lead to superimposed bacterial infection and associated pain. They could be few or many. Mollusca may appear in any part of the body, but commoner sites include the trunk, groin, posterior surface of knees, axillae, and anterior elbow.

The lesions may be genital as in the case presented here; in such cases they may be in the anal area of the penis, vulva, or vagina. Genital molluscum contagiosum, although it may be alarming to the patient, is a benign viral infection [4].

Molluscum contagiosum does not affect the palms and soles.

The patient who has relatively large lesions that are in parts of the body they can examine clearly, they may find the fluid within. Attempts at removing the fluid or the lesion may not only cause superimposed bacterial infection but spreading of the rashes by autoinoculation.

Molluscum contagiosum in patients with severe HIV infection presents as extensive facial mollusca; such patients almost predictably have low CD4 cell counts.

Investigations In healthy individuals, investigations may not be required as the diagnosis can be made clinically following a good history and physical examination. In patients with genital Mollusca, it is necessary to investigate to rule out coexisting sexually transmitted infections or conditions that are associated with immune suppression, especially HIV infection. In lesions with uncertain diagnosis, biopsy should be done, and histopathological examination shows Henderson-Paterson bodies also called molluscum bodies; they are intracytoplasmic inclusion bodies. Polymerase chain reaction (PCR) is also useful as it detects the causative virus.

Penile Warts

Symptoms

This patient in his late 20s reported multiple growths on the penis. The duration was under 1 year. The onset of the lesions was gradual, but the course was progressive and relentless. The growths were not associated with pain but were occasionally pruritic. There was no similar growth in or around the anus. He did not have a bleed from the urethra and had no discomfort or pain associated with urination. He practiced only vaginal sex, did not know whether any of his sexual partners had vaginal lesions, but was certain that there was none with obvious vulval lesions. He was unaware of his HIV status. This was the first time he had noticed this kind of growth on any part of his body. The major concern of the patient lay in the fact that these lesions were increasing in number and in size; the other issue was the appearance of his penis which he considered unsightly. He did not know why he had them, could not figure out the result of the progressive nature of the lesions, and desired to have a permanent solution to the medical condition.

Signs

On examination, there were multiple growths on the penile shaft; they affected every part of the shaft (the dorsum, sides mainly, and the ventral surface least), but the glans penis and the coronal sulcus were spared. Ventrally, the median raphe of the penis (genital median raphe) had no growth, but the few growths were on either side of this skin line. The growths were of various sizes—the smaller ones were solitary but the large ones were cauliflower shaped and seemed

to be a conglomeration of small ones. They were of various sizes but between 2 mm and 2 cm. Only the smallest ones were papular; the others were irregularly shaped and the larger ones formed whorls with ridges, but there was no fissuring or bleeding. They were firm in consistency, non-tender, and attached to the skin and had the same color as the immediate surrounding unaffected skin. Despite a thorough examination, there were no growths on the scrotum—not even small ones.

He did not have similar growths in the perianal area. There was no evidence of bleeding per urethram.

Diagnosis

Penile warts

Etiology

The etiological agents of genital warts are epidermotropic human papillomaviruses (HPVs), especially HPV-6 and HPV-11. Genital warts are low-risk benign human papillomavirus lesions. The viruses that are in this classification have a lower impact as carcinogenic agents;

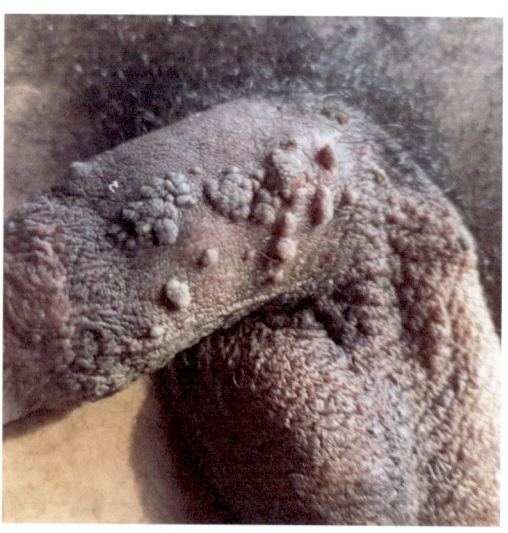

Fig. 4.7 Penile growths in warts

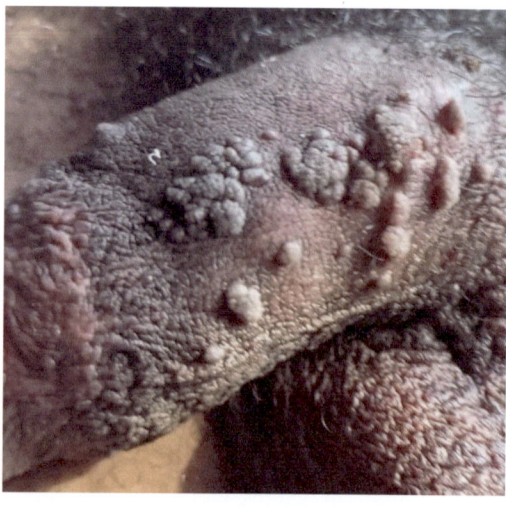

Fig. 4.8 A close-up photograph of the penile growths

this is why they are called low-risk HPV (lrHPV) [5].

This close-up photograph of penile warts is to give the reader fine details to include when documenting a case of penile warts pre-referral or presurgery.

Treatment

In mild early cases, the patient may be prescribed topicals to apply, e.g., Podofilox (podophyllotoxin) solution or gel, 5-fluorouracil, catechins ointment, or imiquimod cream. The physician should select the patient based on, among other things, the small size, visibility, and easy reach by the patient; the patient should also understand the instructions on application and have good vision and steady hands.

When it is necessary for the doctor to apply the treatment, it may be done in the clinic using trichloroacetic acid or bichloroacetic acid solution applications or interferon injections.

Extensive cases, like in the male patient, discussed in this topic may require surgical excision, electrodessication, and curettage, electrocautery, carbon dioxide laser therapy, cryotherapy, and infrared coagulation are modalities of treatment, but surgical excision tends to yield the best success rate and least recurrence rate.

Prognosis

The prognosis for genital warts is variable as the lesions can regress spontaneously within 1 year, become static, or recur after treatment. Treatment does not ensure eradication of HPV infectivity.

Follow-Up Care

Figure 4.9 shows one of the benefits of follow-up care. In this patient, it was gratifying to both the patient and dermatologist that the extensive lesions had regressed satisfactorily. Having experienced the course of this disease and the treatment process, the patient was convinced that it

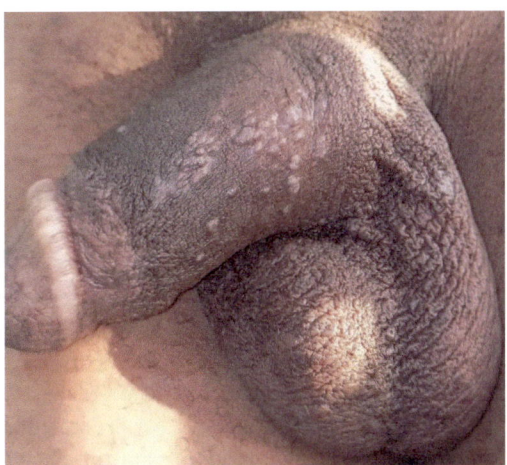

Fig. 4.9 The result of treatment using electrocautery

was good judgement to cultivate and maintain safe sexual practices as the patient had now become aware of the possibility of reinfection.

Discussion

Human papillomavirus (HPV) is non-enveloped and double-stranded. In addition, it is a circular DNA virus. The virus is the etiological agent of multiple epithelial lesions and cancers [6]. Human papillomavirus subtypes 6 and 11 are low risk or non-oncogenic; these viruses cause condylomata and low-grade precancerous lesions [7]. Concomitant infections by different types of HPV can occur [8].

Usual clinical presentation Genital warts (also known as condyloma acuminatum [single] or condylomata acuminata [plural]) are viral skin infections affecting both male and female external genitalia. The lesions may be papular, filiform, lobulated, cauliflower shaped, pearly, or fungating. They are firm and irregular in surface and borders. Common sites are the penile shaft and the glans penis in males and vulva, vagina, and cervix in females. Depending on the patient's sexual practice preference, there may be perianal lesions, oral, or pharyngeal lesions also. There may or may not be color change in the lesions; when there is color change, it is usually hyperpigmentation. When present, pruritus may be variable in intensity.

Vulval Warts

Symptoms

The patient with the image shown in Fig. 4.10 presented in the general outpatient clinic with the complaint of a growth in her "private part." She said that the growth had quickly increased in size over the nearly 1 year preceding her presentation in the clinic. She had a positive history of unprotected sexual intercourse with her boyfriend, and she tested HIV-positive.

She sought treatment in a peripheral public hospital where she was treated with podophyllin 15% for a few weeks. She was not satisfied and decided to travel to the teaching hospital in the State and abandon the treatment as she had not noticed any satisfactory improvement. She was attended to in the general outpatient clinic of a Teaching Hospital and referred to the dermatolo-

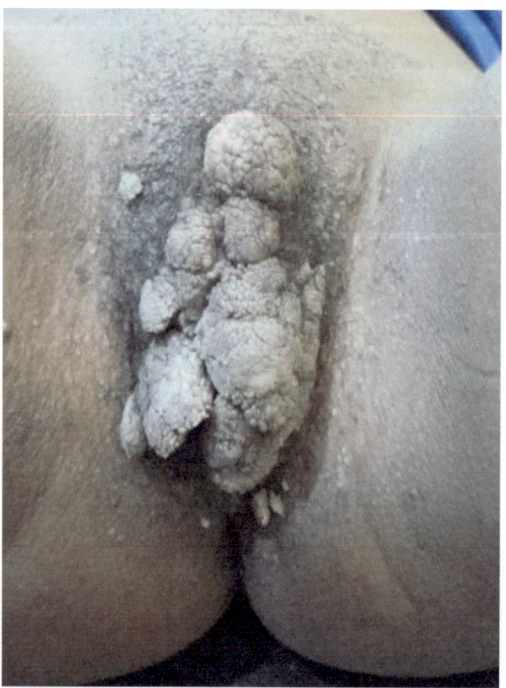

Fig. 4.10 The perineum of an 18-year-old patient

gist from whom she received treatment with good results.

Signs

Figure 4.10 is the photograph taken during pretreatment. Podophyllin may have smeared the inner thighs repeatedly, giving the appearance of concomitant candidal infection (this is not evident in this image although it was obvious during physical examination).

This pretreatment photograph shows obliteration of the view of the vulva by multiple growths. The growths are of various sizes with the major one clustered over the introitus and arising from the labia. The larger growths are cauliflower-shaped and are either overlapping at the edges or almost so.

A close examination also shows that there are smaller growths on the right genitocrural fold and the inner aspect of the proximal part of the right thigh and an isolated, round lesion on the right thigh close to the mid-point of the left extreme of Fig. 4.10. There are also lesions on the hairy part of the vulva lateral to the anatomical location of the right labium majus—a prominent one is located towards the anterior part (upper portion of the image). On the corresponding part of the left side, there are multiple tiny growths that give the left genitocrural fold a "rough" appearance.

Other lesions are between the posterior end of the visually obliterated vulva and the anus—three are on the left side and one on the right side; these have the appearance of hanging lesions or small pedunculated versions of the massive growths.

Diagnosis

Vulval (vulvar) warts

Etiology

Of the many epidermotropic human papillomaviruses (HPVs), HPV-6 and HPV-11 are the most frequent types incriminated in the etiology of genital warts.

Risk factors for acquiring this infectious growth include early commencement of sexual activity, use of oral contraceptives, smoking, and maintaining multiple sexual partners.

Figure 4.11 shows the patient's vulva with just vestiges of the warts, dyspigmentation of the skin, and irregularity of the margins of the labia majora.

Treatment

Treatment can be by any of the following modalities:

- Surgical excision.
- Cryotherapy.
- Infrared coagulation.
- Carbon dioxide laser therapy.
- Electro-dissection and curettage.
- A combination of these modes of therapy may be used.

The size and recurrence of the lesions are some of the considerations for choice of mode of

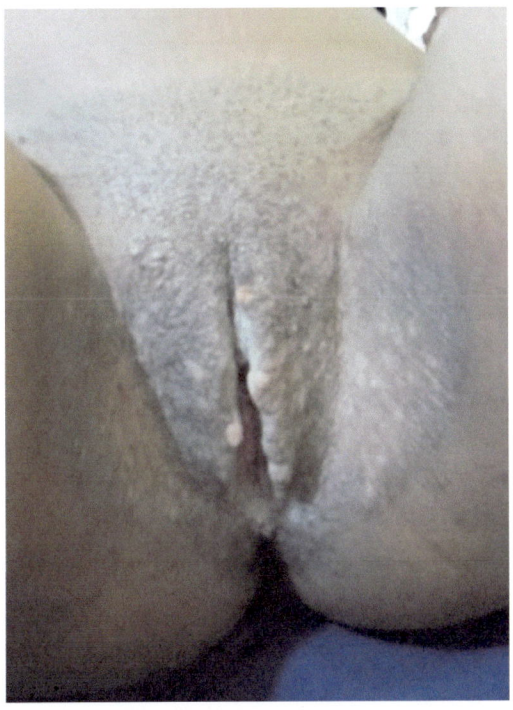

Fig. 4.11 The photograph taken posttreatment

treatment. The massive size in this young woman necessitated electro-dissection and curettage.

Drugs are also useful, and these come as injections or topical application as gels, creams, and solutions. Examples of topical drugs are trichloroacetic acid, podophyllin, 5-fluorouracil, and imiquimod. An example of injections is interferon.

It is recommended that sexual partners be evaluated and treated.

Discussion

Genital warts (condyloma acuminata) are growths that arise in the genital area of both males and females. It is associated with sexual exposure to a partner or partners who are infected with the human papillomavirus (HPV).

In females, the vulval (vulvar) lesions are as shown in the photographs above, but they could be smaller or more extensive. There may be discharge when mucous membranes of the urethra, vagina, or cervix are affected [9]. Pregnancy may cause latent lesions to become active. Activation of latent lesions or aggravation of currently active lesions may occur in immunosuppressive states. Examination should entail speculum examination in women for likely vaginal or cervical lesions. Hairy portions of the patient's perineum should be examined as hair may obstruct the presence of some lesions there. The lesions may be transmitted to sexual partners, may grow in some patients to the point of disfigurement, and in a few patients may undergo malignant transformation. There may also be recurrence of the lesions post-therapy.

Sites In females, genital warts could be in the labia, vaginal walls, or cervix. (In males, it may be found on the glans penis, penile shaft, or the scrotum.) In both sexes, the growths may be found on the skin of the perianal area, the rectal walls, mouth, or throat. The mouth and throat locations are susceptible in people who practice oral sex.

Presentation The lesions are irregularly shaped, firm, and generally not painful. They may be pruritic. They could bleed during sexual intercourse.

As exemplified in the above photographs, genital warts could be small, discrete, extensive, and clustered. Other presentations are papules, plaques, pearly, or fungating growths. Some of them are flat and some may be too small to be readily identified as warts. Examination of patients should involve searching for evidence of other STIs, e.g., discharge, ulcerations, etc. Passage through the birth canal may lead to respiratory tract infection in a neonate, while presentation in small children should arouse the suspicion of sexual abuse. The growths caused by the common HPV-6 and HPV-11 are benign, and they hardly undergo transformation into a carcinoma. Large vulvar lesions as the type shown may get larger during pregnancy and interfere with parturition or cause urethral meatal trauma with likely acute urethral obstruction and consequent urinary obstruction. The disfigurement from large vulvar growths may present a psychological burden on some patients.

Clinical course Following a 3–40-week latency period, the virus infects host cells with a predilection for the basal layer of the epidermis. Latent infection may be activated by immunosuppression and pregnancy. If left, untreated genital warts may increase in size, number, or both—they may also regress spontaneously or remain static.

Differential diagnoses Differential diagnoses of genital warts include condyloma lata, herpes simplex, keratosis follicularis, vulvar neoplasia, nevi, and vulvar neurofibromatosis.

Investigations Investigations should aim at identifying concomitant sexually transmitted infections like chlamydia, gonorrhea, HIV, and lues. In some patients, additional investigations may be required, e.g., polymerase chain reaction for typing of the HPV or histopathological examination of biopsy specimens in recurrent cases or in patients that there is suspicion of malignant transformation of the lesions. Some lesions undergo spontaneous remission.

Investigations should not be limited to the ones for genital warts but should include the ones for concomitant STIs, e.g., HIV, gonorrhea, syphilis, and chlamydia. Cytological analysis of Pap smear samples, colposcopy, or polymerase chain reaction may be required. Biopsy specimens may be taken for examination in patients with recurrence or suspected transformation to a cancer.

Prevention Vaccination plays an important role, and the nonavalent vaccine, 9vHPV, covers HPV subtypes 6, 11, and 7 others: HPV types 16, 18, 31, 33, 45, 52, and 58 [10]. Children and young female adolescents aged 15 and below need two doses of the vaccine, while adolescents and older individuals aged 15–45 require three doses within 6 months.

Prognosis

When patients do not respond adequately to treatment, there is actual treatment failure, or recurrence. The possibility of immunosuppression exists and should be investigated if it was not done earlier. Tissue biopsy with histopathological examination is required in such cases also.

Follow-Up Care

This patient was followed-up by the dermatologist and members of the team she was allocated to. The author obtained satisfactory details of the management of this case from the dermatologist in charge of the management of the patient for the purpose of documentation of this case.

Multiple-Choice Questions

1. In herpes zoster which of the following is correct?
   A. There is predilection for males.
   B. The lesions follow the distribution of a peripheral nerve.
   C. Pain is not a prominent feature.
   D. The lesions are usually bilateral.

2. With respect to herpes zoster (shingles), which of the following associations is correct?
   A. Etiology—Herpes simplex virus (HSV).
   B. Disease progression—Vesicles, papules, then macules.
   C. Site of predilection—Abdominal dermatome.
   D. Population requiring treatment—Immunocompromised.

3. Warts: Which of the statements below is correct?
   A. They are caused by flaviviruses.
   B. They are common in the elderly.
   C. They demonstrate hyperkeratosis.
   D. Those of the venereal variety are always acquired by sexual contact.

4. A 26-year-old sexually active female presents to you with genital rashes and fever. Which of the following would make you consider herpes genitalis as the diagnosis?
   A. Cauliflower growth in the genitals.
   B. Painless vulval ulcer.
   C. Bilateral painful genital vesicles.
   D. Intense pruritus vulvae.

5. With respect to genital warts, which of the following statements is correct?
   A. The specific etiological agent is human papillomavirus-6 (HPV-6).
   B. Meatal warts frequently cause urinary retention.
   C. Multiple warts are a rarity.
   D. Painless, pruritic growths are characteristic.

References

1. Nair PA, Patel BC. Herpes zoster. In: StatPearls [Internet]; 2023. Available from: https://www.ncbi.nlm.nih.gov/books/NBK441824/.
2. CDC. About shingles (herpes zoster). Available from: https://www.cdc.gov/shingles/about/index.html.
3. American Academy of Dermatology Association (AAD). Molluscum contagiosum: who gets and causes. Available from: https://www.aad.org/public/diseases/a-z/molluscum-contagiosum-causes.
4. Bhatia AC. Molluscum contagiosum. In: Dermatology. Medscape; 2024. Available from: https://emedicine.medscape.com/article/910570-overview.
5. Egawa N, Doorbar J. The low-risk papillomaviruses. Virus Res. 2017;231:119–27. https://doi.org/10.1016/j.virusres.2016.12.017. Available from: https://www.sciencedirect.com/science/article/pii/S0168170216307146.
6. Luria L, Cardoza-Favarato G. Human papillomavirus. In: StatPearls [Internet]; 2023. Available from: https://www.ncbi.nlm.nih.gov/books/NBK448132/.
7. Leslie SW, Sajjad H, Kumar S. Genital warts. In: StatPearls [Internet]; 2023. Available from: https://www.ncbi.nlm.nih.gov/books/NBK441884/.
8. Sendagorta-Cudós E, Burgos-Cibrián J, Rodríguez-Iglesias M. Genital infections due to the human papillomavirus. Enferm Infecc Microbiol Clin (Engl Ed). 2019;37(5):324–34. [PubMed] [Reference list].
9. Ghadishah D. Genital warts clinical presentation. In: Emergency medicine. Medscape; 2018. Available from: https://emedicine.medscape.com/article/763014-clinical.
10. National Cancer Institute. Recombinant human papillomavirus (HPV) nonavalent vaccine. Available from: https://www.cancer.gov/about-cancer/treatment/drugs/recombinant-hpv-nonavalent-vaccine#:~:text=.

Scabies

Symptoms

At the time of consultation, the female patient whose back is shown in Fig. 5.1 was aged 54 years. She complained of having itchy rashes on her lower back. The rashes also affected her armpits and under the breasts [1]. Having had no similar rashes previously, she strongly believed that they were associated with her sharing her bedding and clothing with a long-time friend who visited her [2]. This belief was predicated on the fact that the friend had similar rashes, and when her visitor scratching her body, she enquired and the response she received was that some of the pupils she taught had similar rashes. The friend's visit was 3 months earlier, and the visit was for 2 weeks. She noticed itching 3 weeks after her friend's visit ended, and this was soon followed by the rashes. Initially, the rashes were few, but they had become many and intensely pruritic. On enquiry, she could not associate greater intensity of pruritus during nighttime despite the specificity of the question. She was definite that there was no aggravation or relief from bathing with water and her normal soap. She said that since the onset of the rashes there has been none on her face. She did not have any on the webs of her fingers or toes. She felt very inconvenienced by the rashes. She indicated that she had used a couple of drugs including benzyl

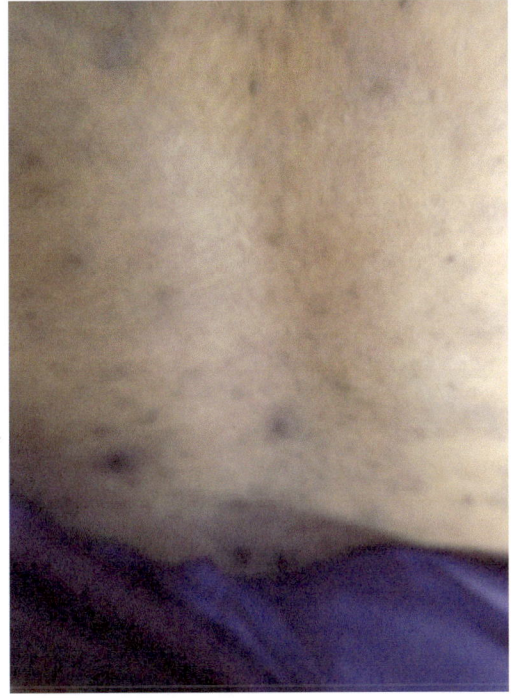

Fig. 5.1 A close-up photo of the skin showing hyperpigmented scars on the patient's back

benzoate that was suggested to her to apply, but there was improvement.

Signs

On examination of the part of the back which was the part of the body she was willing to expose for examination, there were multiple hyperpigmented

Supplementary Information The online version contains supplementary material available at https://doi.org/10.1007/978-3-031-97503-5_5.

papules on the lower back; these were associated with scars—more in the midline of the lower back and the left half lateral to the midline at the waistline [1]. There were no obvious scratch marks despite her indication of scratching from the severe pruritus (this was perhaps due to masking by cream she applied prior to coming to the hospital).

Diagnosis

Scabies

In this patient, the diagnosis was made primarily from the characteristic history, including noninvolvement of the face [3].

Symptoms in Pediatric Patients

Regarding the second patient, an infant, the mother complained of itchy rashes on both hands of the child. The rashes affected other parts of the body, but the hands were affected most. The itching was said to be all day long but most severe at night, preventing the child and her from sleeping well. The child scratched the hands and other affected parts. The child was said to be very irritable. There was a positive history of similar rashes in the patient's older siblings.

Signs in Pediatric Patients

Figures 5.2 and 5.3 show the palm and dorsum of the left hand of a 7-month-old female.

On examination, the hand is swollen, and the photograph of the palmar surface of the hand shows the skin at the sides of the fingers to be bulbous over the joints. The fingers, interdigital spaces, dorsum, and palm of both hands show multiple papules, some pustules, and a few ulcers. There are scratch marks (on close scrutiny) on the skin just distal to the dorsal surface of the metacarpophalangeal joint of the index finger—

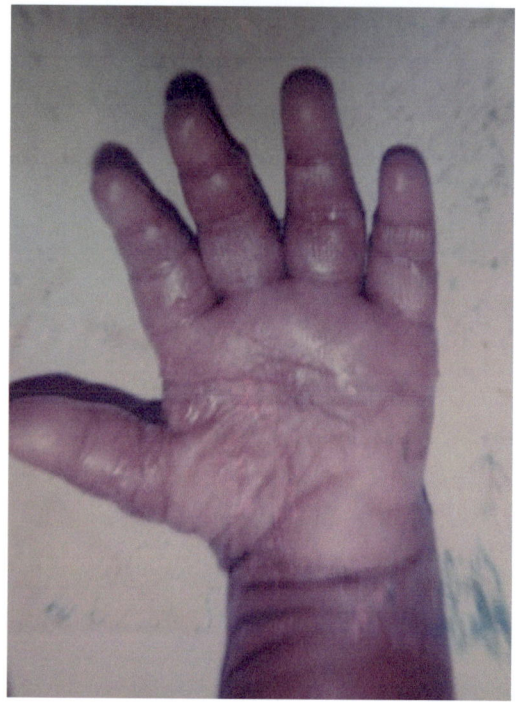

Fig. 5.2 Bulbous left palm and fingers of a baby with vesicles

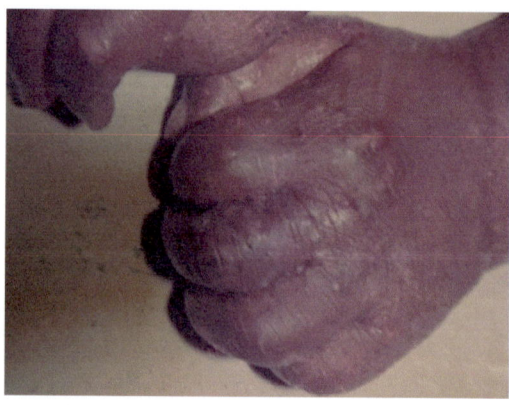

Fig. 5.3 The dorsum of the hand and fingers of the child in Fig. 5.2. showing the same lesions

the scratch marks terminate just before the hyperpigmented circular superficial ulcer.

Diagnosis

Scabies

Treatment

Treatment of scabies in children and adults is usually by topical application of any of the following agents to the entire body to save the face—to protect the eyes. The drugs (scabicides) are as follows:

- Benzyl benzoate emulsion 10–25%
- Permethrin cream 5%
- Malathion 0.5% in aqueous base
- Sulfur ointment 5–10%

In adults (excluding pregnant women), Ivermectin is an effective oral alternative for treating patients with scabies. Children who weigh >15 kg may also take Ivermectin.

All close contacts of the patient should be treated as they may be infested before becoming symptomatic.

Etiology

The etiological agent of scabies is the mite, *Sarcoptes scabiei var hominis* [4].

Discussion

The pathophysiology is a delayed type IV hypersensitivity reaction of the patient's skin to *Sarcoptes scabiei var hominis*, its feces, and eggs [5].

Usual clinical features in scabies The principal features of scabies are papular eruptions that are so pruritic that they induce scratching; the pruritus predominates in the night [5]. The nocturnal severity of these rashes sometimes disturbs sleep. Scratching could lead to trauma to the papule and secondary bacterial infection manifesting as pustules, e.g., impetigo. Scratching also causes excoriation of the surrounding skin, and in some patients, there may be scratch marks. Scabies affects children mainly, but people of any age can acquire this infection. Overcrowding is an important predisposing factor as it encourages close bodily contact; in such settings, open or covert sharing of clothing and other items like bedding is feasible.

In school-age children, scabies has the propensity to cause stigma (when the classmates, schoolmates, and teachers are not knowledgeable about the disease and when it occurs in a child from a poor family background); the pediatric patient may therefore have the consistent disturbed sleep at night being extended to school hours with manifestation as sleepiness during classes, or frank absenteeism during the illness [6, 7]. Scratching and wounding of the skin from severe pruritus in these pediatric patients, and others, may result in impetigo from superimposed infection by *Streptococcus pyogenes* or *Staphylococcus aureus*. Thus, it is important for the general medical practitioner to note that a child could, from untreated or poorly treated scabies, develop acute rheumatic fever, glomerulonephritis, or sepsis [8]. The parents, at least, should be adequately educated.

Investigations Scabies can usually be diagnosed clinically from a thorough history taking and physical examination of the rashes, noting the parts of the body affected. Since the mite burrows into the skin to lay eggs, skin scraping of burrows when examined under the microscope demonstrates the mites and their eggs. Dermoscopy is another means of investigation for diagnosing scabies. As just stated, scabies is principally a clinical diagnosis.

Prognosis

Prognosis is good when the patient is given adequate information of the disease, e.g., the risk factor in family, school, residential, and other settings, and so the patient or relevant/responsible authorities prevent overcrowding and thus limit close bodily contact. The other information is that treatment should be repeated to eliminate newly hatched mites as the eggs are not killed by the drugs. Thirdly, clothing, bedding, and similar items of the patient should be put in boiling water before washing, washed with a washing machine and using a hot dryer cycle afterwards, or dry cleaned. Clothes should be dried under direct sunlight by hanging on a line not spreading them on grass.

Follow-Up Care

Follow-up care is to ensure that the patient is responding appropriately to the treatment. The treatment may be changed if the patient (or patient's parent) complains of a side effect that may prove to be a stumbling block to successful treatment; the reviewing physician must consider any such impediment. The follow-up consultation is occasionally an appropriate occasion for reevaluating the patient's grasp of the information that was given regarding prevention of recurrence of scabies—and their desire to implement the suggested measures.

There are patients who need encouragement to eradicate this skin infestation, especially poor patients (or patients from poor families like the infant whose elder siblings currently had the skin disease and whose symptoms and signs commenced before the onset in the child). Regarding this child, the additional cost of treating the entire family was reduced by prescribing benzyl benzoate 25% emulsion for the siblings at home as insisting on their being brought to the hospital for consultation would have been too costly and too inconvenient for the family—especially the mother who, culturally, was the one to take care of such matters pertaining to children. It was also more encouraging for the mother to embark on treating the older children when she had evidence of the efficacy of the treatment in the youngest child (the index patient); the treatment of the older ones would be less challenging than that for this infant whose hands had to be covered with socks up to, and slightly beyond, the wrists to ensure that the baby did not suck the hands to

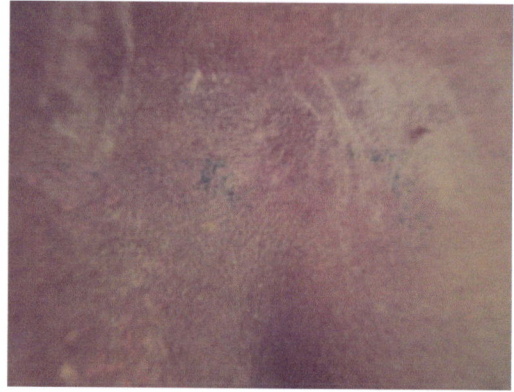

Fig. 5.4 The lower back of a patient with superficial scratch marks. (Source: Reproduced with permission from *A Companion to Medical Students and Doctors*)

which the medication had been applied. New socks that fit the hands must be bought for this purpose unless there are fitting socks that must be washed, dried, and ironed prior to use for this treatment.

Onchodermatitis

Symptoms

This adult in the mid-30s complained of having itchy rashes for about 1 year. The rashes affected the lower back, buttocks, and thigh up to the legs, bilaterally. The itching was intense, exhibited no increased intensity during nighttime, and involved the skin of the affected parts, not limited to the rashes. He was concerned that his skin was no longer normal when compared with before his institutionalization in an overcrowded correctional center; he had not developed the rashes. Then, he was not the only one with the rashes.

Signs

On examination, he had multiple macules with indistinct borders. There were multiple scratch marks [9]; these were on both sides of the lower back, just superior to the natal cleft, but there was no rash between the gluteal folds. Scratch marks and similar macules were on the thighs.

The skin had irregularly shaped patches of hyperpigmentation and hypopigmentation. Palpation of the skin showed thickening. There was no fissuring and there were no papules, pustules, or small scars.

Diagnosis

Onchodermatitis

This diagnosis was made following skin snip microscopy that was positive for *Onchocerca volvulus*. This patient was attended to in a peripheral secondary care hospital that, at the time, did not have the more modern facilities for investigation for this parasitic skin infection.

Treatment

Ivermectin was available in this practice setting, and a single 150 µg/kg body weight dose of Ivermectin sufficed to eliminate microfilariae from the patient's skin for many months.

Etiology

Onchodermatitis is the skin manifestation of onchocerciasis, river blindness, and a chronic disease that affects many body systems and is caused by the nematode, *Onchocerca volvulus*.

Discussion

Usual clinical features Patients with onchodermatitis present with maculopapular rashes on any part of the skin. The rashes may cluster or may be scattered; they appear at unpredictable times. There is usually no pain, and there may be no itching in some patients at a certain point in the course of the disease. However, in most patients, the pruritus is mild, moderate, or severe. There is usually corresponding scratching, and this could be severe in patients with severe pruritus; such patients show evidence of scratch marks. Over time, the skin becomes thickened (lichenified), and changes in pigmentation occur showing patches of hyperpigmentation and others with various degrees of hypopigmentation (depigmentation [partial pigment loss] or leopard skin [total pigment loss])—in either case the hair follicles are surrounded by normal pigmentation. Skin atrophy is another feature of onchodermatitis. There may be skin ulceration and bleeding from scratching; secondary bacterial infection of the skin may result. Apart from the dermatitis just described, onchocerciasis causes skin conditions like onchocercomas (onchocercomata) with subcutaneous nodules, hanging groin in males or females with atrophy and inelasticity skin in the groin—it may be bilateral or unilateral.

Investigations Microscopic examination of skin snips of the patient's skin was carried out, and it revealed the presence of multiple microfilariae. Obtaining skin snips is invasive and more modern methods are preferred.

Enzyme-linked immunoassay (ELISA) requires finger stick samples of blood and is therefore less invasive than microscopic examination that requires taking skin snip specimens. ELISA uses antigens of microfilariae, and being an immunological test, it is also more sensitive than skin snip microscopy; the downside is that it does not differentiate between a previous and a current infection. People in endemic areas may therefore show a positive result without having a current infection.

Polymerase chain reaction (PCR) may be done using skin snip or skin scratch specimens; the latter is less invasive but yields result with equal accuracy. In resource poor areas, the high cost is a limitation. PCR is a more sensitive test than skin snip microscopy in patients with low levels of infection. Unfortunately, patients who require the test are frequently impecunious.

Treatment A single 150 µg/kg body weight dose of Ivermectin suffices to eliminate microfilariae from skin for many months. The drug does not kill adult worms but minimizes the release of microfilariae by the adult nematode.

Ivermectin is derived from *Streptomyces avermitilis*. The drug paralyses the nematode at the neuromuscular junction.

Moxidectin at 8 mg/kg body weight has shown the potential to reduce the rate of transmission of the infection during the interval(s) between rounds of treatment than Ivermectin does. Elimination of the parasite in patients is expected to be more rapid with this newer drug. It is related structurally to Ivermectin. The drug is recommended for use by patients who are at least 12 years old.

Prognosis

Onchodermatitis is a chronic dermatological infection, and the prognosis is linked to the time of presentation of the disease in the hospital, promptness of treatment, and prevention of a reinfection.

Follow-Up Care

Drug treatment may need to be repeated. One of the challenges in the practice setting is refusal or inability of patients to return to receive care. This may be because of the great inconvenience involved in the to-and-fro journeys for accessing medical care in hospitals and the long waiting times in overcrowded general outpatient clinics; after the long wait, the patient is referred to a dermatology clinic for diagnosis and commencement of treatment. In some hospitals, these clinics do not run every day as a tertiary hospital may have no dermatologist, one dermatologist, or at most two. The other reason is inability to bear the cost of treatment when they present late in the course of the disease—like this patient. The recommendation of the World Health Organization (WHO) for treating onchocerciasis with Ivermectin is a least once yearly for 10–15 years [10]. The cost of treatment is not necessarily financial when it pertains to the medications, as this should be (and is frequently) free; the cost is linked to the what has just been described—the cost of

patients making themselves available for treatment. The best situation is the population-based mass drug administration that takes the treatment to the population and can provide treatment for asymptomatic patients or those who have undiagnosed onchocerciasis in the earliest stage of the disease.

Multiple-Choice Questions

1. Which of the following statements about onchocerciasis of the skin is correct?
   A. Leopard skin is involvement of skin of the back
   B. Pruritic papular rashes are features
   C. Skin snip microscopy is the gold standard for early disease
   D. Enzyme-linked immunosorbent assay is less sensitive than skin snip microscopy

2. A 40-year-old resident of an area known to be endemic with onchocerciasis is almost blind and presents in the clinic with skin manifestations of the disease. Which of the following findings is in tandem with lichenified onchodermatitis?
   A. Confluent, excoriated, hyperpigmented papulonodular plaques
   B. Multiple, solid papules each with dimension >1 mm
   C. Palpable, movable, nodule over a bony prominence
   D. Wrinkling and dryness of the skin

3. In a 5-year-old patient with scabies, which of the following statements is correct?
   A. The causative organism is a tick
   B. Pruritus may be severe enough to result in sleepiness during classes at school
   C. Vesico-pustular eruption affect the face
   D. Eruption of large blisters causes ulceration with excruciating pain

4. A 27-year-old otherwise unemployed commercial sex worker positive for HIV presents with features suggestive of scabies. Which of the following statements is correct in this patient?
   A. Limitation of rashes to facial and palmar sites is typical

B. Extensive pruritic and eczematous rashes is usual
C. Severe pruritus is one of the complaints
D. Concomitant fungal infection is unlikely
5. With respect to the treatment of scabies, which of the following is a correct association?
A. Ivermectin—Repeated course 21 days later
B. Permethrin—Mandatory two courses
C. Topical corticosteroids—Useful in severe pruritus
D. Crotamiton—The best treatment modality

References

1. Mayo Clinic. Scabies. Available from: https://www.mayoclinic.org/diseases-conditions/scabies/symptoms-causes/syc-20377378.
2. Murray RL, Crane JS. Scabies. In: StatPearls [Internet]; 2023. Available from: https://www.ncbi.nlm.nih.gov/books/NBK544306/#:~:text=.
3. Dinulos JGH. Classic scabies. In: MSD manual. Professional version. https://www.msdmanuals.com/professional/dermatologic-disorders/parasitic-skin-infections/scabies.
4. World Health Organization (WHO). Scabies. Available from: https://www.who.int/news-room/fact-sheets/detail/scabies.
5. Tidman ASM, Tidman MJ. Intense nocturnal itching should raise suspicion of scabies. Case Rep Pract. 2013;257(1761):23–7, 2. PMID: 23808128. Available from: https://pubmed.ncbi.nlm.nih.gov/23808128/.
6. Swe P, Reynolds S, Fischer K. Parasitic scabies mites and associated bacteria joining forces against host complement defence. Parasite Immunol. 2014;36(11):585–93. https://doi.org/10.1111/pim.12133. [DOI] [PubMed] [Google Scholar].
7. Jackson A, Heukelbach J, Filho A, Campelo Júnior EB, Feldmeier H. Clinical features and associated morbidity of scabies in a rural community in Alagoas, Brazil. Trop Med Int Health. 2007;12(4):493–502. [DOI] [PubMed] [Google Scholar].
8. Parks T, Smeesters PR, Steer AC. Streptococcal skin infection and rheumatic heart disease. Curr Opin Infect Dis. 2012;25(2):145–53. https://doi.org/10.1097/QCO.0b013e3283511d27. [DOI] [PubMed] [Google Scholar].
9. Medecins sans Frontiers (MSF). Onchocerciasis (river blindness). In: MSF medical guidelines. Available from: https://medicalguidelines.msf.org/en/viewport/CG/english/onchocerciasis-river-blindness-16689892.html#:~:text=.
10. World Health Organization (WHO). Onchocerciasis. https://www.who.int/news-room/fact-sheets/detail/onchocerciasis.

Alopecia of the Scalp

Alopecia

Symptoms

This young lady with little financial support from her direct parents or close family members noticed a gradual loss of her fairly long hair. Her preferred salon provides her with satisfactory hair grooming in the form of plaiting her natural hair for a reasonable amount, compared to the more expensive salons. She also observed that for some months (she keeps or "manages to maintain" the hair) for up to a month, and the hair style she chooses used to consist of many small and tightly packed finished hair many months back. Due to the loss of hair which she noticed as pronounced when she went to redo her hair, she opted for less tight styles, with the current one shown in the photograph as an example.

She came to the hospital to complain about this hair loss as the professional hairdressers did not give her any effective remedy.

Signs

Figure 6.1 shows the scalp of a young lady in her early 20s. The photograph shows extensive, irregular, and patchy hair loss with an island of apparently normal hair distribution on the frontal part of the scalp. The absence of hair is irregular and affects the top of the scalp posteriorly and the

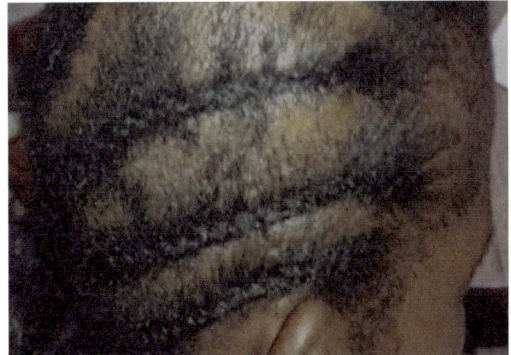

Fig. 6.1 The right side of the scalp and a part of the face of a patient with alopecia

parietotemporal scalp bilaterally. A close examination of the photograph shows that the patches of alopecia areata have the same degree of pigmentation as the patient's unaffected skin. Additionally, despite having alopecia, this patient maintained peripheral scalp hair and still presented with plaited hair in the hospital for the consultation; perhaps traction was an insignificant factor in the etiology of alopecia in this patient.

Figure 6.2 shows the "top" of the scalp of an infant with extensive loss of scalp hair involving the posterior end of the frontal scalp (left end of the image), parietal scalp of which the image shows mainly the left side (towards the lower portion of the image), and the occipital scalp (towards the right side of the image). The hair loss creates an irregular pattern of portions of exposed scalp.

I. Ukot, *Understanding Diseases in Skin of Color*, https://doi.org/10.1007/978-3-031-97503-5_6

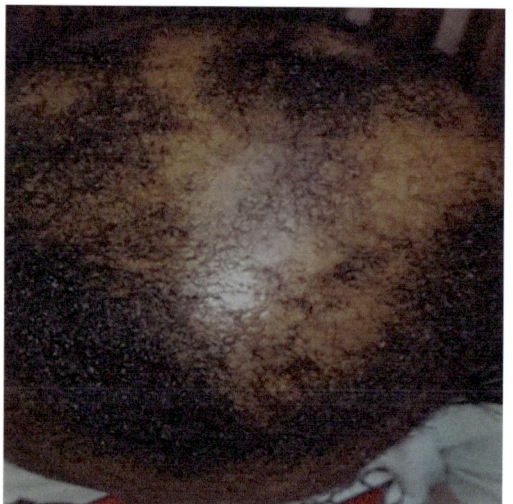

Fig. 6.2 The scalp of an infant

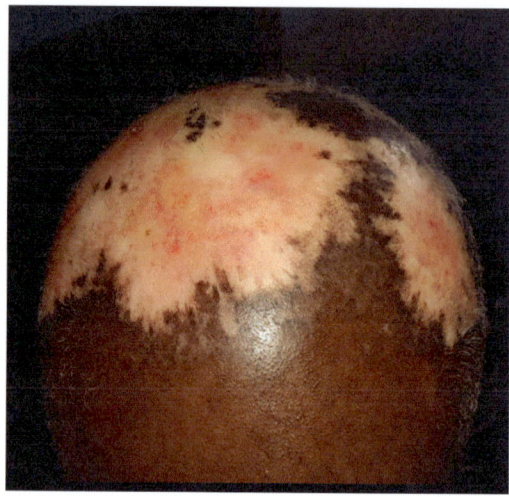

Fig. 6.3 The scalp of a middle-aged man with cicatrical alopecia

Diagnosis

Alopecia of the scalp

Etiology

Alopecia is classified as an autoimmune disorder. In alopecia, the patient may have a family member who has the condition or some other related diseases, e.g., vitiligo, autoimmune thyroiditis, etc. If genetic, it is polygenic. Apart from autoimmune disorder, chronic severe traction may cause alopecia.

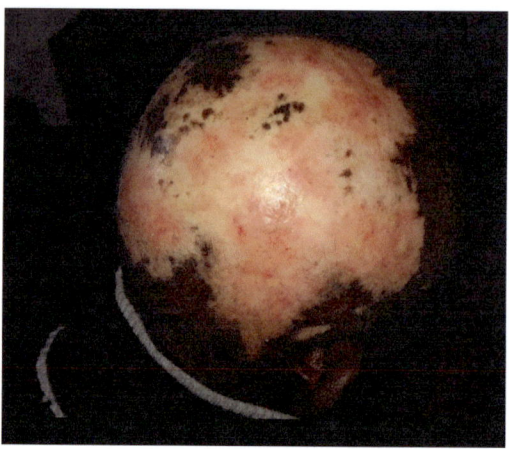

Fig. 6.4 The scalp of the same patient in Fig. 6.3

Symptoms

Regarding this third patient (whose scalp is shown in Figs. 6.3 and 6.4), he could not link the severe scalp hair loss with failure of hair regrowth to any particular action, activity, or event. He, however, knew that it was a slow process spanning many months, but the condition had become very embarrassing to him recently. He desired to obtain treatment from the specialist to whom he was promptly referred following this short documentation.

Signs

Figures 6.3 and 6.4 are photographs of the same patient; they demonstrate the scalp of a middle-aged male. They show extensive scalp involvement (temporal, parietal, and occipital scalp).

Figure 6.3 shows an irregularly shaped scarring of the scalp going posteriorly and laterally from the posterior part of the frontal scalp. There is a complete loss of hair on the affected portions. There are islands of normal scalp skin pigmentation. These islands are separated from one another by the affected part—on the right side of the image, the irregularly shaped strip of normal frontal scalp skin continues posteriorly nearly forming a T with another strip of normal skin from the left parietal scalp skin (towards the right of the image), but the full formation of the letter T is prevented by a bridge of affected skin that connects the larger affected right parietal scalp with the smaller left component. A close examination of the scalp beyond the peripheral part of the affected scalp shows some gray hairs on the unaffected portion at the left side, top, and right side of the photograph.

Figure 6.4 is a right-side view of his scalp showing his right ear. There are islands of normal scalp skin pigmentation—normal when compared with the patient's right ear which is in the lower part of the field of this image. Just as in Fig. 6.3, this image shows depigmentation of scalp skin with multiple areas of redness; this permanent redness cannot be described as hyperemia.

Diagnosis

The condition is scarring alopecia.

Etiology

Scarring (cicatrical) alopecia may be caused by conditions that present significant injury to scalp hair follicles. These include the following:

- Severe chemical burns
- Discoid lupus erythematosus (DLE)
- Systemic lupus erythematosus (SLE)
- Irradiation
- Kerion
- Dissecting folliculitis
- Central centrifugal cicatrical alopecia (CCCA)

Treatment

Treatment of alopecia is by injection of intralesional steroids (anti-inflammatory), cyclosporine (immunosuppressant), diphenylcyclopropenone, or squaric acid dibutylester.

Other nonsurgical methods of treatment include the following:

- Ketoconazole—an antifungal agent.
- Finasteride and dutasteride that block the enzymatic conversion of testosterone by 5-alpha-reductase to dihydrotestosterone thus reducing circulating serum testosterone and enhancing male scalp hair growth since testosterone does the opposite [1].
- Minoxidil, platelet-rich plasma, adenosine, and low-level laser light therapy inhibit scalp hair loss and stimulate growth of new hair.

In well-selected cases of alopecia, the patient may be offered follicular-unit grafting for hair transplantation [2].

Prognosis

The prognosis of alopecia is not good, especially when it is cicatrical alopecia. When it is due to traction, it is good, as it can be alleviated by stopping the offending activity. It is important to refer the patient to a dermatologist so that the cause of the alopecia is identified following appropriate investigations on the index patient.

Follow-Up Care

As in most dermatological conditions, follow-up care is required in patients with alopecia. The causes are varied, and depending on the cause of alopecia, the patient may need short-term or long-term follow-up care.

Brief Discussion

Alopecia is the absence of hair in parts of the body where hair normally grows. The scalp is where there is high density of hair. When the absence of scalp hair is partial, it is referred to as alopecia areata, but when there is total absence of hair on the scalp, the condition is alopecia totalis. The absence of hair on the entire body is alopecia universalis; it is a rare and extreme condition.

In a part of the world where girls, young women, and even the elderly ones prefer their normal, natural hair, alopecia of any degree other than the most minimal is a dermatological-cum-aesthetic concern for women.

In men, there is a high prevalence of hair loss from androgenetic alopecia (AGA) also referred to as male androgenetic alopecia; it is the commonest form of alopecia among men. Men suffer from the psychological burden of this condition which tends to reduce their quality of life. AGA is a type of alopecia that is found in men and occurs as early as age 30 in some individuals—the older a man is, the higher the possibility of developing this form of alopecia [3].

Detailed history with investigations by the specialist to rule out some of the differential diagnoses is essential in making the diagnosis.

When there remain a few hairs in progressive acute alopecia areata, examination of such hairs at the junction or border with normal skin shows them to have the "exclamation mark" in which the end of the hair that abuts with skin is thin and has a propensity to break [4].

The onset of alopecia is usually sudden. The affected part of the skin is neither pruritic nor painful. In some cases, there may be spontaneous regrowth of hair, but in others treatment is required though the result of treatment may not be satisfactory.

Chronic and severe traction to hair like in females who plait or braid their hair and the hair style or plaiting/braiding technique or method necessitates excessive pulling on the scalp hair up to its roots—and the condition of too much traction is maintained. Warning signs include scalp pain, folliculitis, and superficial ulceration of the scalp skin. Such hair loss may be reversed when the implicating practice is stopped, or the offending hairdo is undone promptly.

Hidradenitis Suppurativa

Symptoms

"Boils" in the left armpit for many years was the complaint in this 40-year old obese patient who is not a diabetic. The symptom started more than 15 years before presentation to the author. The history from the patient was that of recurrent "boils" that would appear, persist, discharge foul-smelling pus, resist treatment, and eventually heal only to recur after a few months. The patient had associated pain but there was no fever. She had gone to many hospitals without obtaining the desired relief and had recently become quite aware of the unwholesome odor of the discharge from her armpit. This was a deterrence to attending the general hospitals or other public hospitals where she would sit close to and beside other patients in the general outpatient clinics. She did not believe that using antiperspirant and perfumes masked the malodorous discharge satisfactorily. According to her, she would have respite following taking prescribed medications, but, sooner or later, the discharge would recur. She felt distraught and embarrassed and needed a permanent solution to the health challenge.

Signs

Hidradenitis suppurativa Figure 6.5 shows two carbuncles at the apex of the left axilla. The larger carbuncle which is close to the skin covering the posterior wall of the axilla is discharging purulent material, while the other that is anterior and medial to the larger one is not. The larger carbuncle measured 4 cm × 2 cm, while the smaller one measured 2 cm × 1 cm. On the skin in-between the anterior and posterior axillary walls and inferior to the carbuncles is a long nearly S-shaped scar where the patient had similar

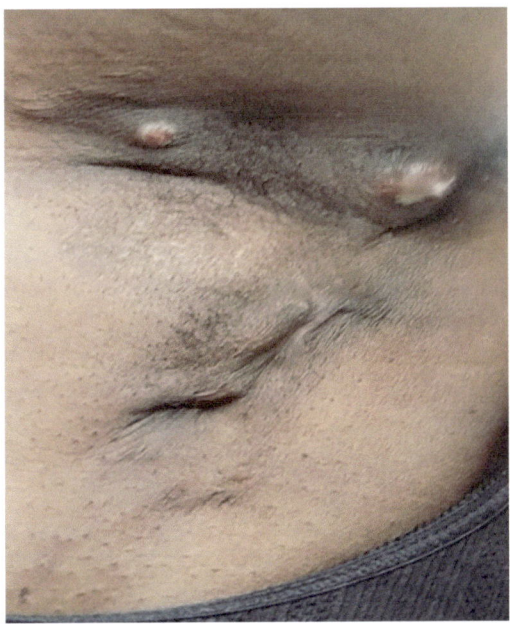

Fig. 6.5 The left axilla of a patient

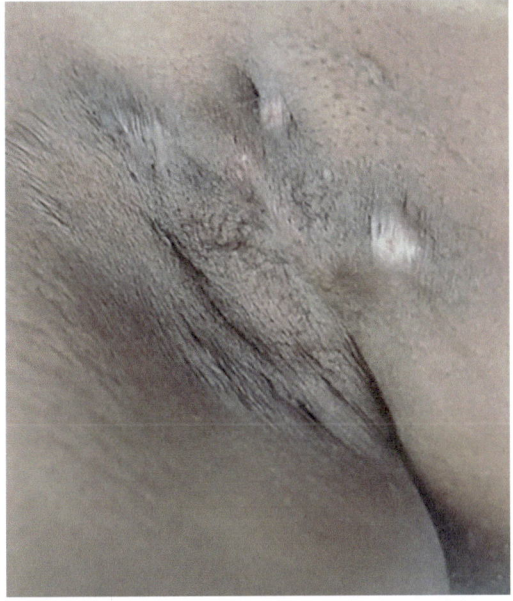

Fig. 6.6 Also showing the left axilla of the middle-aged female

lesions previously. This figure shows the left arm abducted and partly elevated to make the axillary lesions visible for physical examination and taking the photograph.

In Fig. 6.6, the lesions shown are after purulent discharge had subsided. The axillary skin where the scarred lesions are located demonstrate hyperpigmentation when compared to unaffected skin. The scars, particularly the two in the upper part of the image, show depression—this finding is a pointer to the deep-seated location of the nodules, abscesses, and tunnels in hidradenitis suppurativa [5].

Diagnosis

Hidradenitis suppurativa

Etiology

In hidradenitis suppurativa, there is an abnormality in the epithelium of terminal follicles in parts of the body that have apocrine sweat glands, e.g., axillae, sub-mammary area, and groin. Over time, there is bacterial infection repeatedly and eventual sinus formation and scarring at the affected part(s).

Treatment

Surgery provides relatively satisfactory results with acceptably low recurrence rate in locations other than sub-mammary where the rate could be up to 50%. Wide excisions are preferred as the recurrence rate is lower (<15%) [6].

The advice for patients with this condition should include the following:

- Weight reduction for those who are overweight or obese
- Wearing light clothing of non-synthetic material—which could help maintain coolness and encourage evaporation of perspiration
- Avoidance or cessation of smoking
- Using simple toilet soaps
- Applying warm compresses
- Maintaining general good personal hygiene

Discussion

Pathology Sweat glands are one of the exocrine glands. There are three types of exocrine glands, viz., holocrine glands, eccrine (merocrine) glands, and apocrine glands. Some sweat glands are apocrine glands just like mammary glands while others are eccrine glands. Hidradenitis suppurativa affects apocrine sweat glands. It is important to remember that apocrine sweat glands and sebaceous glands—with hair follicle—form a pilosebaceous unit. Apocrine sweat glands, unlike merocrine (eccrine) sweat glands that open directly onto skin, open into the upper (or terminal) part of hair follicles. This means that their milky and proteinaceous secretion (produced by the secretory portion of the gland and carried by its excretory duct outwards) opens into hair follicles just like sebaceous gland secretion does. Pathologically, obstruction of distal end of hair follicle is from plug formation found in hyperkeratosis of follicles with infundibulofolliculitis; there is also periductal folliculitis [7].

The patient is usually healthy-looking and could be obese. The onset is insidious and usually in adolescence and early adulthood. It is not expected in prepuberty as full development and function of apocrine sweat glands is from sex hormone stimulation starting at puberty. It runs a chronic course and could be debilitating. Complications may arise and include development of keloids, scars, contractures, and reduced mobility of the affected area from contractures. Hidradenitis suppurativa has an association with arthritis and metabolic syndrome [8]. There is a female preponderance of hidradenitis suppurativa. Hirsutism is common in patients with hidradenitis suppurativa. Hyperandrogenism appears to be a related factor in hidradenitis suppurativa. The following are considered risk factors or trigger factors in hidradenitis suppurativa: cigarette smoking; mechanical irritation, e.g., shaving and depilation; and chemical irritation, e.g., application of deodorants. Menstruation, stress, exposure to undue heat, and excessive sweating are considered as factors that aggravate hidradenitis suppurativa.

Presentation Primary lesions are painful papules that may be smaller or larger than 1 cm; they may also be nodules or abscesses which the patient describes as painful, and tenderness can be elicited on palpation; there may be double-ended comedones and dermal contractures which show as elevation or depression of the skin. These "primary lesions" are synonymous with "typical lesions." Presentation of hidradenitis suppurativa, therefore, has a wide range depending on when the patient presents for consultation; it could be papules, discharging papules, abscesses, sinuses, fistulae, or scars from cicatrization. In the advanced, third, stage, there is diffuse presentation or many sinus tracts or abscesses that are linked in the area involved. With two draining abscesses although without inflammatory nodules, this patient's case falls into moderate in the six-stage physician global assessment (PGA).

Investigation and Diagnosis Investigations could be useful, and these consist of laboratory and imaging. Blood tests include full blood count with differential white cell counts and platelet counts, erythrocyte sedimentation rate, and serum protein electrophoresis—which may show abnormalities; ultrasonography may show increased thickness of the skin in affected parts; since associated infection is polymicrobial, bacteriology may yield any bacteria, but the commonly encountered ones are *Staphylococcus aureus*, coagulase-negative staphylococci, and anaerobic bacteria like anaerobic streptococci and the *Bacteroides* species. Immunohistochemistry tests are also done in centers that provide the services; histology which shows similar findings between hidradenitis suppurativa and acne vulgaris, i.e., hyperkeratosis of the infundibulum—which gives rise to horny impactions reminiscent of comedones [7]. The *diagnosis* is essentially clinical, consisting of fitting history of location, onset, duration, progression, and physical findings.

Prognosis

Spontaneous resolution is rare, but relentless progression of the disease is common. Patients may experience frustration and despair and may subject themselves for surgical procedures much later in the course of the disease.

Follow-Up Care

Hidradenitis suppurativa is a chronic disease with a high tendency to recur, even after surgical intervention. It is important to familiarize patients with the characteristics of this disease; doing so increases the chances of their returning for follow-up care.

Subungual Hemorrhage

Symptoms

Figures 6.7, 6.8, and 6.9 are photographs of the right index finger of a middle-aged left-handed man who injured the finger by accidentally closing the car door on the hand a few weeks earlier. He had put a small bag on the back seat of the car, got distracted by his mind being occupied with family challenges that were ongoing at the time,

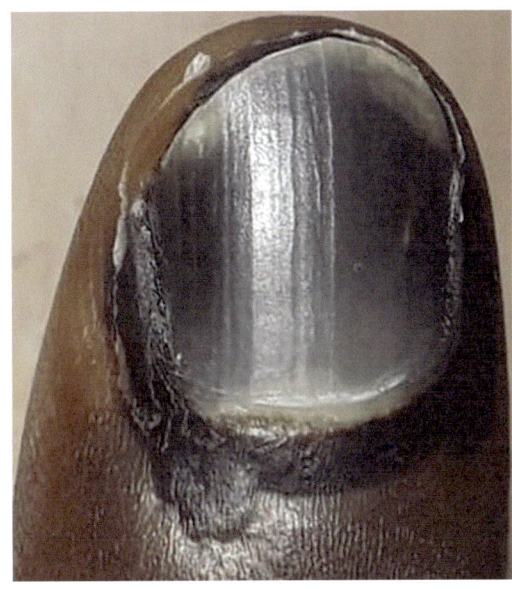

Fig. 6.8 Subungual hemorrhage on the day of trauma to the distal phalanx. (Source: Reproduced with permission from *Essentials for Practice of Medicine in the Frontline, Volume 2*)

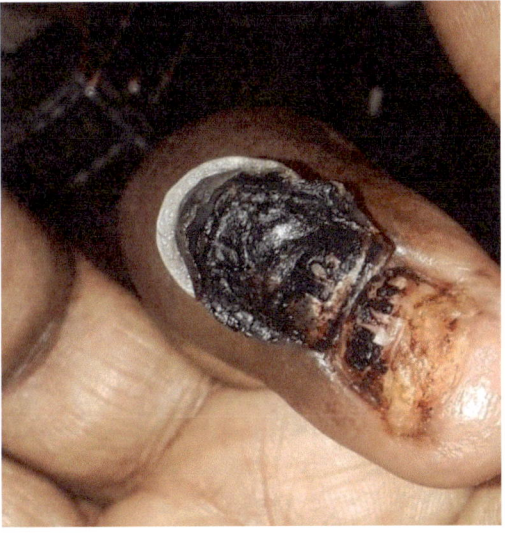

Fig. 6.9 Subungual hematoma many days after trauma to the distal phalanx. (Source: Reproduced with permission from *Essentials for Practice of Medicine in the Frontline, Volume 2*)

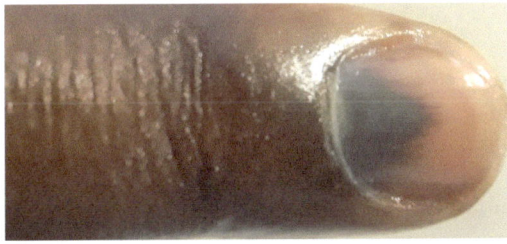

Fig. 6.7 Trauma to the distal phalanx of the right index finger. (Source: Reproduced with permission from *Essentials for Practice of Medicine in the Frontline, Volume 2*)

and slammed the door shut while not fully removing his right hand. Initially, and for about 1 week, the patient suffered from excruciating pain which was throbbing and continuous. The pain was severe enough to disturb sleep and hamper his activities of daily living and his regular work. It was impossible for him to use the computer in the workplace, and his physician, appreciating the amount of pain and distress, gave him a few days off work. At the time, and on the day of injury, his pain score was 8 of 10.

Signs

Figure 6.7: Soon after the injury, there was a collection of blood under the nail plate. The first part of the nail to lose its color to black was the lunule (lunula)—this was not the total as a close look shows an altered lunule but no obliteration. The original position of the lunule became the base of a triangle. The blood is tracked under the nail plate in a manner that showed the middle portion had a more rapid movement of the blood, as it formed the peak of the triangular area (reminiscent of a mountain lying on its side). This description is because of the orientation of the nail in the image. The base of the triangle appears uniform, but the remaining two sides of the triangle demonstrate spikes (spicules) of blood.

Figure 6.8: The blood collection was rapid and, on the same day, obliterated the normal color of the nail plate—save the resistant portion of the lunule which is still evident on close scrutiny of the mid-portion of the base of the triangle. There was marked tenderness over the nail plate, and the patient hardly allowed examination of the affected nail. Examination of all the skin folds (lateral, medial, and proximal nail folds) shows their involvement as they are black, and the difference between them and the immediate surrounding skin of the right index finger is clear. There was darkening of the skin on the dorsal surface of the affected finger proximal to the eponychium, but the image does not satisfactorily demonstrate this feature. Evidence of blunt trauma to the palmar skin of the distal phalanx of the neighboring right first finger (thumb) was in the form of slight swelling of that phalanx compared with the left and a darker hue of the skin of this patient with Black skin of intense dark tone. The right index finger and fingernail went through a series of changes until they got to this stage.

Figure 6.9: The photograph taken of the affected finger and nail more than 1 week after the accident occurred. At this stage, the nail had flipped off its base (nail bed) but was not detached from its finger. The hematoma associated with the now exposed inner surface of the nail plate is thicker and more extensive than that at the proximal part of the nail bed. At this point, the affected lateral and medial nail folds (which were initially bulbous from the trauma) had almost completely healed and looked normal.

Diagnosis

Subungual hemorrhage of the right index fingernail with subungual hematoma

Etiology

Subungual hemorrhage is the result of significant trauma to the nail plate and nail bed. In some cases of hand trauma that involves the fingers and fingernails, there may be nail avulsion; the latter is a surgical condition. Subungual hemorrhage may or may not be due to trauma, but even if it is posttraumatic, with significant amount of blood collecting under the nail plate, it may not require surgical intervention as trephining may reduce the severe pain by relieving the pressure under the nail plate.

Treatment

Treatment of traumatic subungual hemorrhage immediately following the injury consists of RICE—*r*est, *i*ce application, *c*ompression, and *e*levation of the affected part. Adequate doses of analgesia should be prescribed for the patient. Some patients may need benzodiazepines to enable them to sleep. When trephining is required, adequate precaution should be taken to avoid introducing infection into the nail bed via the surface opening.

Prognosis

Prognosis of subungual hemorrhage and resultant subungual hematoma is good. The patient witnesses the positive results of the treatment. The degree of pain and disturbance of normal function that are associated with this condition (especially when it is severe like in this patient) is enough to keep the patient cautious to avoid a repetition of the causative trauma. The patient feels gratified that although the nail was lost, another nail grows to replace it—and the new nail is usually normal.

Follow-Up Care

This patient was one of the best patients that this author has had in terms of cooperation for follow-up care. The images used for this case study are a few compared to what are available. The images are enough to tell the chronological story of subungual hemorrhage.

Brief Discussion

In subungual hemorrhage, blood usually shows on just a portion of the nail initially; blood continues to accumulate, and the entire nail becomes black if there is no intervention. The degree of trauma that causes subungual hematoma may eventually lead to loss of the nail plate that is virtually lifted off the nail bed.

When a patient has a traumatic injury to the fingers, they should be encouraged to seek proper and prompt medical attention and adhere to the treatment prescribed by a doctor. The patient should also be made to see the importance of keeping a follow-up consultation appointment. Since prevention is better, it is necessary to educate patients and parents of young children on prevention of trauma to the hands and fingers. Most people do not appreciate the importance of their fingers and hands until they have conditions that affect this part of the body.

Subungual hematoma due to trauma is not a primarily dermatological condition but a surgical condition that has significant aesthetic implications associated with a skin appendage, the nail. For patients who are highly self-aware and are particular about their appearance, the duration of this health condition may not only be a period of bearing the pronounced initial pain (which gradually reduces over time with taking analgesics that are appropriate with the level of pain that the patient experiences) but also an interference with their psyche. The patient who requires support and care in this respect should be availed with them.

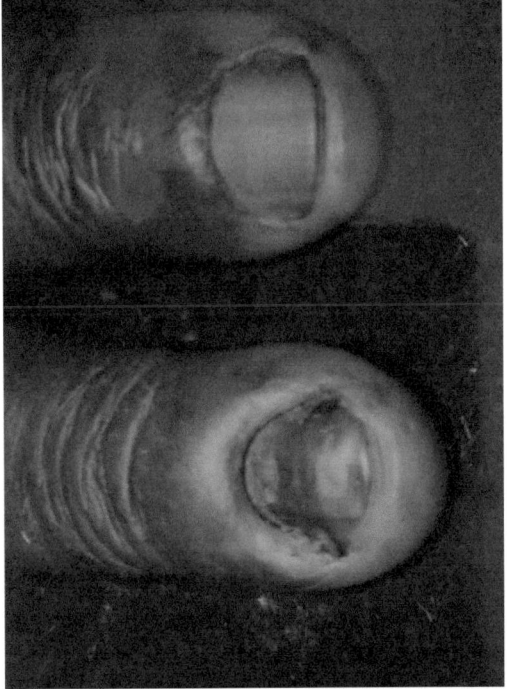

Fig. 6.10 Discoloration and disfigurement of the right middle fingernail

Onychomycosis

Symptoms

The patient with this condition complained of discoloration and disfigurement of his right middle fingernail. He had only mild pain which was on the skin surrounding the nail (nail folds) rather than the deformed nail. He did not have a similar change in any other fingernail or toenail. He did not have a similar nail condition in the past and did not have anyone in his family with something close to it. He was a farmer and was not involved directly or primarily with wet work that would involve his hands spending significant work time in water or other liquids. The symptoms were insidious, and he could not state categorically when the changes started, but it was at least 7 months prior. He came to the hospital as he was concerned about the situation not improving, rather getting worse, and he did not have any idea what might have caused it. He expected to obtain answers during the consultation and hoped that there would be a quick resolution to the condition.

Signs

On examination of the affected hand, the nails of the right thumb, index finger, ring finger, and the little finger were clipped level with the fingertips except the ring fingernail that receded beyond the fingertip. The nails were consistent with expectation from one who worked the land manually. The dorsi and palms were rough with no evidence of application of oil or cream before the patient's coming to the clinic. The hands were, however, clean and dry.

Examination of the right middle finger and its nail showed a flattened, brownish-black nail. The nail plate was intact. It was difficult to clearly define the lunule. There was bulbous swelling of the nail folds laterally, medially, and proximally. The ulnar border of the distal part of the finger showed an area of nailfold excoriation; the swollen nailfold and the excoriated area were tender.

There was no discharge. The proximal and medial nail folds, though swollen, were dry and non-tender.

Etiology

Etiological agents of onychomycosis are mainly dermatophytes especially *Trichophyton rubrum* and *Trichophyton mentagrophytes* contribute to 90% of cases with the former making up 70%, but non-dermatophyte molds and *Candida* (yeast) also cause onychomycosis.

Etiology of paronychia is usually bacterial agents in acute cases and fungi in chronic paronychia.

Treatment

Onychomycosis treatment with drugs may be with topical drugs like ciclopirox and efinaconazole; systemic drugs such as terbinafine, itraconazole, and fluconazole; or a combination of topicals and oral. In some patients, there may be nondrug treatment additionally, e.g., surgical, chemical (using urea), laser, or photodynamic therapy.

Treatment of acute paronychia is with antibiotics, and for chronic paronychia, antifungals are required. These drugs are effective as topical preparations. Warm soaks thrice or four times daily may suffice in the early stages of acute paronychia.

Prognosis

Patients with onychomycosis should be informed of, and made to accept, the fact that drug therapy takes weeks to months to be effective as the sole form of treatment and that the stage of the infection at which they seek treatment may be a determinant of duration of therapy and necessity or otherwise of additional or adjunctive treatment. After full treatment, topical drugs may be needed to prevent recurrence of this infection.

Follow-Up Care

This patient was "lost to follow-up care" in the sense that he could not cope with repeated visits to the busy Christian mission hospital in the rural area where the author worked at the time. This was a common experience with patients who were mostly farmers and had to travel long distances to come to the hospital. In doing so they would sacrifice the entire day, leaving home early in the morning and spending significant time on the queue for their turn to be attended to by extremely busy general practitioners, only to return home late in the evening.

The more detailed attention that this patient received was because the author was particularly interested in the dermatological condition he presented with—and he did not come to the hospital solely because of this condition but had other immediate health concerns. Although this patient was interested in obtaining a solution to the nail condition, his mien showed that he was not prepared to return to the hospital for the first follow-up visit even when he was asked to request to be "posted to" this author on the day of the first follow-up visit (spaced conveniently, in the mind of the author, 6 weeks away). The patient did not return, or if he returned he may have misplaced the piece of paper on which the doctor's name was written.

It is of note that in this busy primary and secondary care setting in a rural area, there were always relatively few doctors who were willing to work in such a location for less pay than in government hospitals in towns and private hospitals in the cities. This was despite the perk of living in one of the bungalows "doctor's quarters" that the early Christian missionaries had built to encourage Nigerian doctors to take up employment with them. At the time that this author worked in this mission hospital, it was many decades after the establishment of the hospital, yet the incentive of a comfortable and "free" accommodation did not achieve the anticipated "pull effect" envisioned by the mission.

Finally, the author's experience was that posting of patients to the consulting rooms for them to be attended to by doctors was officially a random activity; this meant that even if the patient had brought and presented the piece of paper with the doctor's name on it, it would not have been of any import to any of the junior staff whose duty it was to do the allocation of patients to consulting rooms. No doctor had a defined consulting room, and a patient who had waited for a long time to consult with a doctor would not want to return to the back of the queue on realizing that the doctor they expected to see was not the one in the consulting room they were about to enter. This detail is provided in this particular follow-up care report to demonstrate the challenges in obtaining suitable cases for a detailed report from outpatients when mobile telephony was not available in the country.

Discussion

Usual clinical features The usual presentation of onychomycosis consists of discomfort, disfigurement with/without discoloration of the nails, and occasionally pain. In severe cases, onychomycosis may have an untoward effect on the patient's occupation, e.g., in occupations where wearing boots is mandatory or prolonged repetitive manual work involves the nails. In some patients, the appearance of the affected toenail(s) or fingernail(s) may impact negatively on their quality of life; this is especially when multiple nails are affected or both fingers and toes are involved.

There are five recognized types of onychomycosis, viz.:

- Proximal subungual onychomycosis
- Distal lateral subungual onychomycosis
- White superficial onychomycosis
- Endonyx onychomycosis
- Candidal onychomycosis

Paronychia is an infection of soft tissue around the nail(s) of toes or fingers. There is erythema of the affected part, swelling, and pain which are features of cellulitis; this may progress to pus formation (abscess). In chronic paronychia, there is usually bulbous non-fluctuant soft tissue that may be mildly painful or painless, and there may be no erythema.

Investigations Although tentative diagnosis of onychomycosis can be made on clinical grounds and treatment commenced, specifying the subtype of onychomycosis requires investigations. Such investigations may go beyond fungal studies using 20% potassium hydroxide (KOH) with dimethyl sulfoxide (DMSO) and microscopic examination of the nail specimen to curettage and examination of specimen of the nail bed, to removal of the nail plate to obtain specimen from the proximal part of the nail plate where the lunule is, to doing culture studies on nail specimens. Specimens may, therefore, be taken from the nail plate surface, ventral surface of the nail, proximal part of the nail, distal part of the nail, and lateral and medial parts of the nail.

Investigations in paronychia include Gram staining microscopy with culture and sensitivity studies on discharge or drained specimen from the swelling. Fungal studies using KOH and microscopy are useful in chronic paronychia. If herpetic whitlow is suspected, Tzanck smear is required. Blood sugar level should be checked in patients with repeated acute paronychia, and diabetic control should be investigated for in known diabetics.

Onychomadesia

Symptoms

Onychomadesia On 21 December 2024, 7 weeks prior to this documentation, the mother of this 6-year-old girl said that she was clipping the daughter's nails—a requirement by the school regarding the appearance of their pupils—when she noticed that one of the fingernails appeared to be coming off "the base" of that fingernail. She asked the daughter "Did you hit your nail somewhere?" and

the daughter responded in the negative. Apparently, the daughter had not even noticed any change in her nail. The mother felt worried because she remembered that about 4 months earlier, a doctor advised the daughter to take food that contains calcium "to strengthen her bones" when the mother reported that the daughter refused to take full cream milk or cow milk in any form; this was quite unlike many children of her age group. Despite the doctor's counsel, she had allowed the daughter to still have her way for about 3 months as she was eating other foods and taking snacks and sweet drinks that most children take at home, school, and at children's parties. It was only with great persuasion that the child started taking milk only about 3 weeks prior to the onset of the nail anomaly. The mother mentioned that 2 weeks prior to this discovery, the two children (the patient and the younger brother just over 1 year old) were ill with both having fever. When they went to the hospital that the mother's office uses, the pediatrician examined them and the findings on the patient were redness and swellings in the throat for which the pediatrician prescribed an antibiotic and a painkiller. Nothing happened in the intervening period during which she had recovered from the throat infection.

However, in the next 2–3 weeks after the finding in one of the right fingernails, the mother notices that there was a similar involvement of other nails in the right finger. There was brownish discoloration of some nails, and one of the nails assumed a yellow color, which was unusual and observed for the first time since the child was born. The mother was worried that the part of the nail that appears white was the first part that was affected by this condition, and it appeared eaten up leaving an irregular second end of the nail that should have only one free end at the tip. The nails of the finger fell off painlessly until all went through the same process. Each of them was lifted from the nail bed from the beginning portion of the nail and eventually loosened toward the front and dropped off when the nail plate was close to the free edge of the nail at the tip of the finger.

The left fingernails followed the pattern just described for the right hand, and four of the nails on the left that loosened and dropped off save the left thumb nail. The last set of nails to be affected were the toenails. The toenails of both toes eventually dropped off except the big toenails which were equally affected, but the process was slow and the nails were still attached to the nail bed as at the time of this documentation. The mother said that the child would sometimes wake up in the morning and find a nail on the bed sheet. There was no pain in either the hands or the feet other than occasional mild discomfort. Within 3 weeks of dropping off, new nails were already forming or had almost fully formed. The newly formed nails that replaced the lost ones were normal in shape and color.

Signs

Figure 6.11 shows the changes in the nails of the young girl; the changes consist of disruption in the integrity and continuity (index and middle fingernails) and alteration of color (ring and little fingernails).

Figure 6.12 shows the second (index) fingernail with an inverted V-shaped proximal portion of the fingernail. Just beyond the irregular margins of the V, there is a light yellow discoloration of the nail plate that affects almost half of the remaining nail. The color of the rest of the nail plate is normal. The skin of the finger (including the skin of the proximal, lateral, and medial nail folds) are normal in shape and color. The edge of the fingernail is also normal in color and curvature.

The yellow discoloration of a few of the nails on the right and left fingers are best demonstrated by the right middle fingernail plate in Fig. 6.13. Other features described for the index fingernail are present in the middle fingernail plate although not as marked.

From Fig. 6.14, the two hands show that the skin on the dorsi of the hands are normal in every respect. The only abnormalities are in the fingernails of both hands.

This case study is presented in a chronological order, making it slightly different from all other cases reported in this chapter and the book. It is to demonstrate how a case study is recorded for the reader to have a correct mental picture of the medi-

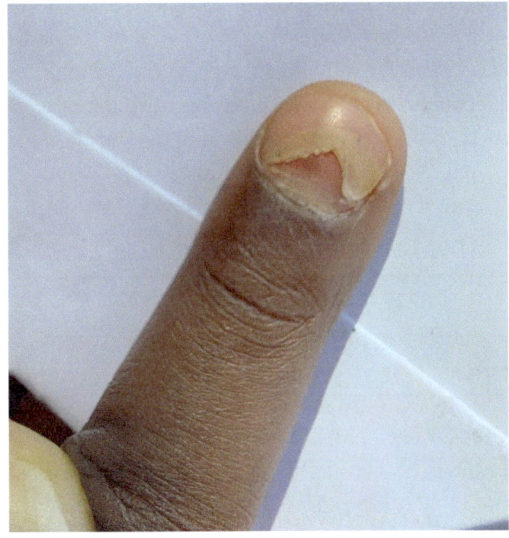

Fig. 6.12 The right second (index) fingernail

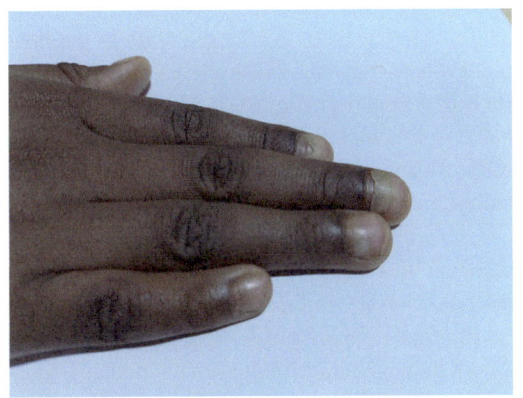

Fig. 6.11 Fingers of the right hand of a 6-year-old girl

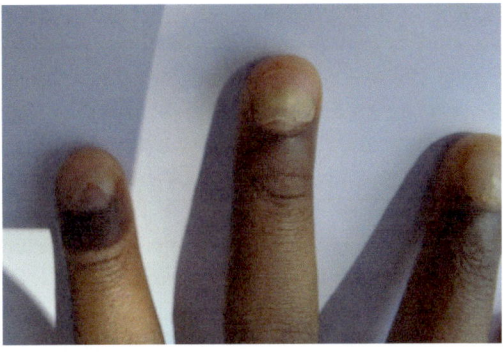

Fig. 6.13 The right index, middle, and ring fingers and fingernails

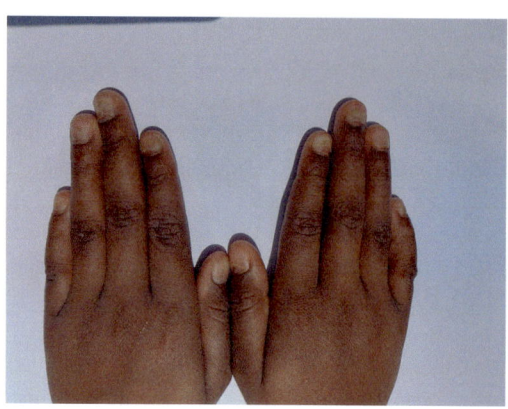

Fig. 6.14 Two hands

cal condition that is described. The author was involved in the management of this case, and most of the communication in this portion of the study is between the mother and patient and this author.

For the reader who may be short of time to read the detailed chronological presentation below, the summary is as follows:

Fever and a sore throat (12.11.2024) > infectious mononucleosis (18.11.2024) > nail shedding from late December (starting from 21.12.2024)

Further and detailed history and clinical presentation

On 12 November 2024, the patient and younger brother (still an infant) were taken to the hospital to consult the pediatrician because of fever that started about 3 days earlier; the patient's additional complaint was soreness of the throat while the brother had refused to feed. The pediatrician examined their throats, and both had hyperemia of the oropharynx while the patient had bilateral inflamed tonsils for which she was placed on a course of amoxicillin-clavulanate suspension (reconstituted from the powder). The hematological screen carried out the same day showed normal total white blood cell count with relative neutrophilia and lymphocytopenia, normal red blood cell count, normal hemoglobin concentration, reduced mean corpuscular volume, and reduced mean corpuscular hemoglobin, but a normal mean corpuscular hemoglobin concentration—these are shown in Fig. 6.15.

Microbiological examination with culture of a throat swab specimen revealed no bacterial growth within 24 h. The patient's mother was encouraged to continue the oral antibiotic therapy prescribed 2 days earlier despite the test results which excluded a bacterial infection.

On 15 November 2024, the patient developed rashes that are represented in the next three Figures—Figs. 6.16, 6.17, and 6.18.

Figure 6.16 shows multiple and discrete rashes on the dorsum of the left hand of the patient. From this image, the left fingernails that are visible are normal.

Figure 6.17 is a photograph of the lateral surface of the right wrist and hand of the patient.

Figure 6.18 is an enlargement of one of the small discrete rashes.

Based on the recent history of fever and sore throat, and the development of the rashes within 1 week, a diagnosis of infectious mononucleosis was made. This was despite the throat not showing the characteristic features of this viral disease when the child's throat was examined 3 days earlier.

The mother of the child was perturbed about the rashes, but she was informed that they would resolve soon but she should apply calamine lotion on the child at night and wash off in the morning.

On 21 December 2024, the mother of the patient complained that she noticed abnormal changes in the daughter's fingers; she stated that they were "worrisome." She enquired what they were as the parents of the child were disturbed about this unprecedented nail problem. The author advised them to take the child to the hospital where they normally attended and request for a pediatric dermatologist. At the hospital, the pediatrician examined and, from the findings, made a clinical diagnosis of onychomycosis. The author told them that the specific request for a pediatric dermatologist was because although he believed that the nail condition was a primary dermatological condition, it could be a systemic health challenge with a dermatological manifestation. The hospital did not have a pediatric dermatologist and so a pediatrician on duty during

Laboratory Test Result

NAME: ███████████████   EMR ID: ██████████   SEX: Female
AGE: 6years

LAB ID: ██████████████   SPECIMEN: Blood   TEST REQUESTED: ROUTINE
DATE REQUESTED: 12-Nov-2024 SPECIMEN RECEIVED: 12-Nov-2024 DATE UPLOADED: 12-Nov-2024

Haematology

FBC + COMPLETE DIFFERENTIAL (CHILD)

REFERENCE	RESULT	NORMAL RANGE
WBC	8.8	4.0-12.0 (10^9/L)
NEU	78	50.0-70.0 %
LYM	12	20.0-60.0 %
MON	10	3.0-12.0 %
EOS	0	0.5-5.0 %
BASO	0	0.0-1.0 %
RBC	4.8	3.5-5.2
HCT	36	35-50 %
HGB	122	120-160 g/L
MCV	76	80.0-100.0 fL
MCH	26	27.0-34.0 pg
MCHC	336	310-370 g/L
PLT	315	100-300 (10^9/L)
RDW-CV	13	11.0-16.0 %
RDW-SD	38	35.0-56.0 fl
MPV	7	6.5-12.0 fL
PDW	15	9.0-17.0 (10GSD)
PCT	2.3	1.08-2.82 mL/L

Fig. 6.15 Full blood count and white cell differential count

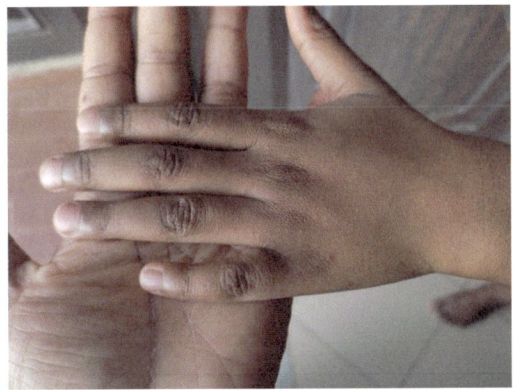

Fig. 6.16 The left hand of the patient is placed on that of the mother for this photograph

the Christmas season attended to the child. The child was given multiple bottles of Terbinafine.

The author advised that the parents should withhold reconstituting the oral antifungal or starting the treatment as he was not convinced that it was a fungal infection. He requested the following investigations on the same day based on a presumptive diagnosis of onychomadesis, with differential diagnoses as onychomycosis and onycholysis. The worried parents were advised to wait as the number of bottles of antifungal medication was evidence that the treatment would be a long one and so they should not be in a hurry to commence treatment although the

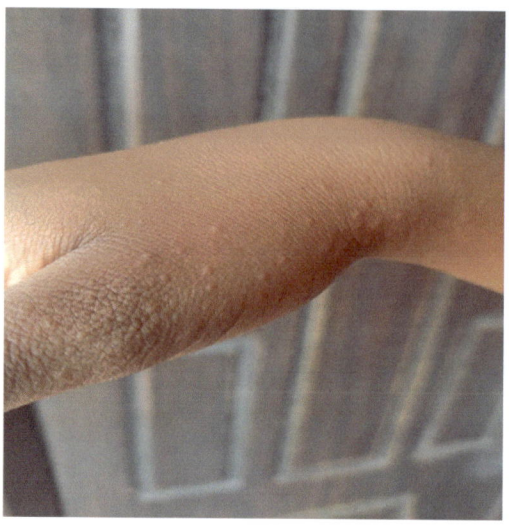

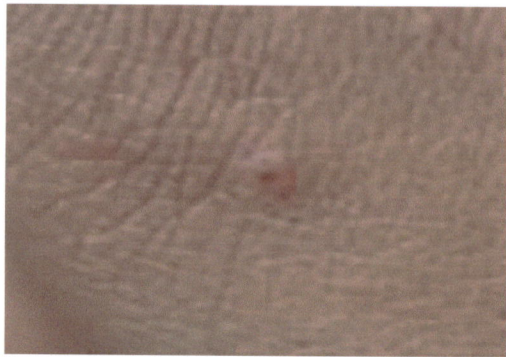

Fig. 6.18 An enlargement of one of the small discrete rashes

Fig. 6.17 The lateral surface of the right wrist and hand of the patient

drug had been dispensed—it would take a few days for the results to be ready. They acceded to the advice. The following are the investigations and their results:

On 21 December 2024, the patent's mother noticed the nail anomalies and that was when she complained the first time. The documentation in the earlier part of this presentation commenced on this date.

On 31 December 2024, additional laboratory test requests were as follows: nail plate specimen for mycological examination for fungal elements from KOH preparations, serum calcium, total protein, serum albumin, and a repeat complete blood count. These were based on a provisional diagnosis of onychomadesis with differential diagnoses as onychomycosis and onycholysis.

The test results were performed on 04 January 2025 and the test results were as shown in Fig. 6.19.

The author was not satisfied with the test result regarding serum calcium and requested the test in an ISO certified laboratory.

The test result was obtained on the same day, 06 January 2025. Whereas the serum calcium result in the first laboratory showed an elevated value, the test performed in the second laboratory showed a normal result although it was towards the lower end of the normal range.

The microbiological investigation on nail specimen was also conducted in the ISO certified laboratory as the first laboratory did not have the capacity to carry out the requested mycological investigation. The results of the test conducted on 06 January 2025 and reported on 07 January 2025 are as in Fig. 6.21.

By 17 January 2024, some nails of the right and left toes had become affected by this toe anomaly.

On 17 January 2024, she made the following observations about the fingernails of the left hand: The thumbnail was unaffected. The second to the fifth left fingernails were affected; out of the four affected fingers, two had their nail plates out. The little (fifth) fingernail plate fell off while she was in the school and that was the only extruded fingernail that caused her slight pain when it fell off, perhaps on contact with a part of her body or a classmate when they were playing.

These results showed the absence of fungal elements. Yeast-like organisms were scanty. There were no parasites.

Laboratory Test Result

NAME: ▮▮▮▮▮▮▮▮▮▮   EMR ID: ▮▮▮▮▮▮   SEX: Female
AGE: 6years

LAB ID: ▮▮▮▮▮▮▮▮▮   SPECIMEN: Blood, Blood   TEST REQUESTED: ROUTINE
DATE REQUESTED: 04-Jan-2025   SPECIMEN RECEIVED: 04-Jan-2025   DATE UPLOADED: 04-Jan-2025

Clinical Chemistry

LFT_LIVER FUNCTION TEST

REFERENCE	RESULT	NORMAL RANGE
ALBUMIN	4.7	3.5-5.2 g/dl
TOTAL PROTEIN	7.4	6.2-8.0 g/dl
AST (SGOT)	23	0.00-50.00 U/L
ALT (SGPT)	15	0.00-50.00 U/L
ALP	121	<935 U/L
DIRECT BILIRUBIN	0.1	UPTO 0.25mg/dl
TOTAL BILIRUBIN	0.4	0.0-1.4 mg/dl

Clinical Chemistry

SERUM CALCIUM (CA)

REFERENCE	RESULT	NORMAL RANGE
CALCIUM	12	8.5-10.5 mg/dl

Fig. 6.19 Liver function tests and Serum calcium

Report Details

Requisition Number	▮▮▮▮▮▮	Specimen Type	Ser
Order Reference		Comments	
Collection Date	12:03 06 Jan 2025	Diagnosis	
Request Date	12:07 06 Jan 2025	na	
Report Date	13:55 06 Jan 2025		
Report Updated Date	14:03 06 Jan 2025	Tests Resulted	
Report Type	FINAL REPORT	Albumin Serum; Calcium Serum; Full / Complete Blood Count	
Priority	ROUTINE		

Chemistry Results

Name	Result	Range	Units	Flag
Albumin Serum	45.1	35-50	g/L	
Calcium Serum:				
Calcium Serum	2.44	2.20-2.70	mmol/L	
Calcium Corrected	2.34	2.10-2.55	mmol/L	

Fig. 6.20 Chemistry results—Serum calcium and serum albumin

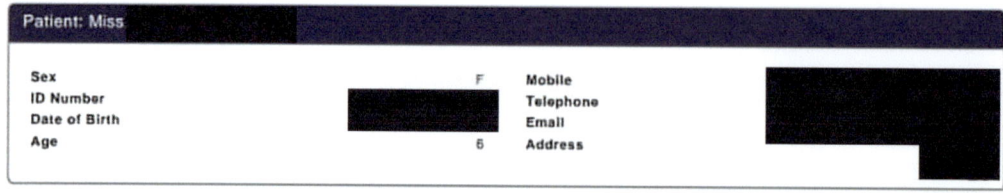

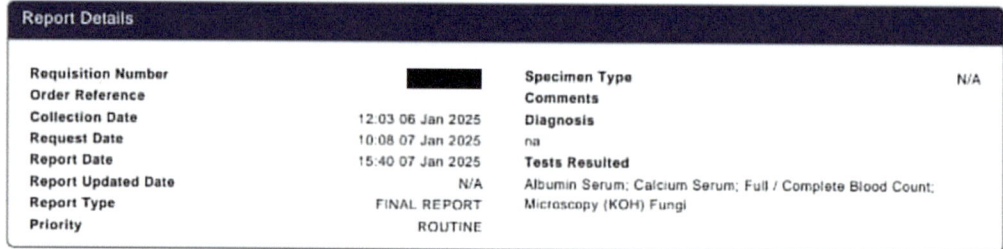

Microbiology Results

Test	Result	Reference Range / (Units)
Microscopy (KOH) Fungi		
Yeast-like Organisms	Scanty	
Fungal Elements	Absent	
Parasites	Absent	

End of Report

Fig. 6.21 Results of microbiology (mycological) test (KOH) on fingernail samples

Diagnosis

Onychomadesis

The author made the diagnosis of onychomadesis on 07 January 2024 on the basis of the absence of fungal elements in clipped samples of nails from the right fingers and the left fingers and the patient's clinic presentation (symptoms, history, and examination findings). He decided to discountenance the finding of scanty yeast-like organisms and opted to observe the patient.

On 17 January 2024, the mother reported that the right and left feet were affected. The right second toe seemed to have part of the nail plate out, and some of the toenails were discolored. The left fourth and fifth toenails were also affected.

Between 17 January 2024 and 21 January 2024, the patient's mother reported that three fingers of the right hand had their nail plates detached; the affected fingernails were of the index, middle, and little fingers. On 18 January 2024, she reported that the fourth fingernail of the right hand had also fallen off.

By the second week of February 2025, all the nails (fingernails and toenails) had been replaced with normal nails or were undergoing the healing process. The mother was glad that the new nails that replaced the detached ones appeared normal although they were still growing.

When this documentation was made, almost 8 weeks after the first report of the nail abnormalities, all the affected fingernails and toenails had detached and had been replaced with normally growing nails.

Treatment

Although the process involved in arriving at the diagnosis was long, the treatment was watching the nail grow.

The antifungal medications were not opened.

Prognosis

The prognosis of onychomadesis is good. This is evidenced in the index patient.

Follow-Up Care

The management of the condition in this child was challenging initially as the parents, particularly the mother, were worried and asked many questions. The questions were answered to the best of the author's ability to make the disease process and healing process clear. It was an opportunity to build confidence in the physician. It was gratifying to the patient, her parents, and this author to watch the growth of new, normal nails on both the fingers and toes.

Discussion

Onychomadesis is the separation of the proximal portion of the nail plate from its bed due to an arrest of the nail matrix temporarily [9]. This separation may result in the falling off of the nail plate with a concomitant formation of new nail.

Causes of onychomadesis include infections, mechanical trauma, severe medical illnesses, and autoimmune diseases. Onychomadesis is a sequel of hand-foot-mouth disease (HFMD) [10]. Medications like retinoids, azithromycin, and antineoplastic agents are well-known causes of onychomadesis. Idiopathic causes play a relatively minor role in onychomadesis.

Multiple-Choice Questions

1. Which of the following statements about alopecia is correct?
   A. Hair loss is always complete.
   B. In alopecia areata the lesions are usually irregular in shape.
   C. Surrounding hairs have the so-called "exclamation mark" appearance.
   D. It is treated with psoralens.

2. Paronychia: Which of the statements below is incorrect?
   A. It is a nail plate infection.
   B. It affects the nail fold.
   C. It is a fungal infection.
   D. It is a bacterial infection.

3. Which of the following statements is correct for hidradenitis suppurativa?
   A. Predilection is for skin the bears eccrine sweat glands
   B. It occurs commonly on the face and upper back
   C. Finasteride may not be used for treatment of initial stages
   D. Surgical excision is recommended soon after fistula formation

4. Which of the following statements about onychomycosis is correct?
   A. Non-dermatophyte molds are not implicated in etiology
   B. Pathology is limited to the nail plate
   C. Abnormality in pigmentation and shape of nail is a feature
   D. One-week course of itraconazole provides satisfactory treatment

5. A 25-year-old artisan presents with a painful 3-day bulbous swelling of the lateral and medial nail folds and a small area of fluctuance of the surface of the skin of the medial nail fold. Which of the following is the most appropriate investigation?
   A. Tzanck smear test
   B. Gram staining of an aspirate and microscopic examination
   C. Glycated hemoglobin estimation
   D. Scaping of the medial end of the nail plate for fungal studies

References

1. Estill MC, Ford A, Omeira R, Rodman M. Finasteride and dutasteride for the treatment of male androgenetic alopecia: a review of efficacy and reproductive adverse effects. Georgetown Med Rev. 2023;7(1). Available from: https://gmr.scholasticahq.com/article/88531-finasteride-and-dutasteride-for-the-treatment-of-male-androgenetic-alopecia-a-review-of-efficacy-and-reproductive-adverse-effects.

2. Zito PM, Raggio BS. Hair transplantation. In: StatPearls [Internet]; 2024. Available from: https://www.ncbi.nlm.nih.gov/books/NBK547740/#:~:text=.

3. Han SH, Byun JW, Lee WS, et al. Quality of life assessment in male patients with androgenetic alopecia: result of a prospective, multicenter study. Ann Dermatol. 2012;24(3):311–8. https://doi.org/10.5021/ad.2012.24.3.311. Google ScholarPubMed CentralPubMed.

4. Tobin DJ, Fenton DA, Kendall MD. Ultrastructural study of exclamation-mark hair shafts in alopecia areata. J Cutan Pathol. 1990;17(6):348–54. https://doi.org/10.1111/j.1600-0560.1990.tb00111.x. PMID: 2074281. Available from: https://pubmed.ncbi.nlm.nih.gov/2074281/#:~:text=.

5. Ballard K, Shuman VL. Hidradenitis suppurativa. In: StatPearls [Internet]; 2024. Available from: https://www.ncbi.nlm.nih.gov/books/NBK534867/.

6. Ovadja ZN, Jacobs W, Zugaj M, van der Horst CM, Lapid O. Recurrence rates following excision of hidradenitis suppurativa: a systematic review and meta-analysis. Dermatol Surg. 2020;46:e1–7. https://doi.org/10.1097/DSS.0000000000002403. [PubMed] [Google Scholar].

7. Smith SDB, Okoye GA, Sokumbi O. Histopathology of hidradenitis suppurativa: a systematic review. Dermatopathology. 2022;9(3). https://doi.org/10.3390/dermatopathology9030029. Available from: https://www.mdpi.com/2296-3529/9/3/29.

8. Miller IM, Ellervik C, Vinding GR, et al. Association of metabolic syndrome and hidradenitis suppurativa. JAMA Dermatol. 2014;150(12):1273–80.

9. Derek H, Rubin AI. Onychomadesis. Pediatr Clin N Am. 2014. Available from: https://www.sciencedirect.com/topics/medicine-and-dentistry/onychomadesis.

10. Chiu H, Liu M, Chung W. The mechanism of onychomadesis (nail shedding) and Beau's lines following hand-foot-mouth disease. Viruses. 2019;11(6):522. https://doi.org/10.3390/v11060522. Available from: https://pmc.ncbi.nlm.nih.gov/articles/PMC6630444/.

Miliaria

Symptoms

A 60-year-old woman complained of tiny rashes on the upper back and shoulders for about 1 week. There was no evidence of an increase in size but an increase in numbers. They were not pruritic. There was no pain in association with their appearance. There was no similar rash in any other part of the body. The rashes appeared during hot weather. She felt inconvenienced by them. She did not take any form of treatment.

Signs

On examination, the rashes were papules, multiple, and discrete. There was no scratch mark. There was no change compared with the surrounding skin pigmentation.

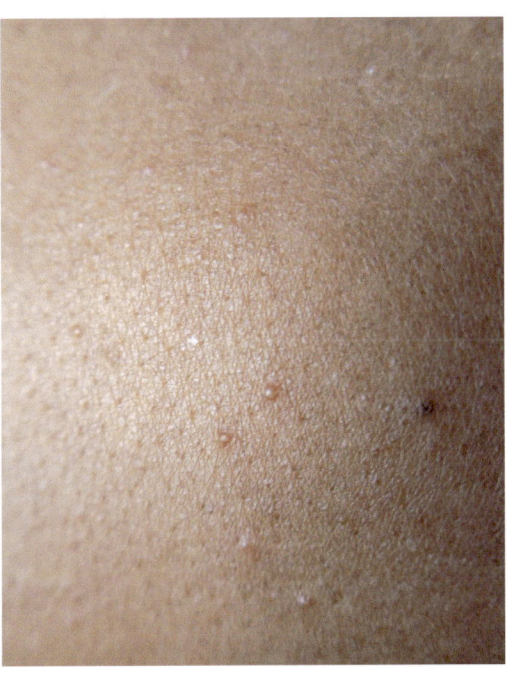

Fig. 7.1 The upper back of the patient

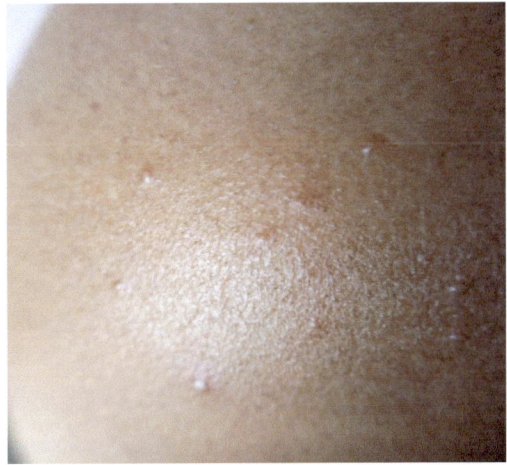

Fig. 7.2 The upper back of the same patient

I. Ukot, *Understanding Diseases in Skin of Color*, https://doi.org/10.1007/978-3-031-97503-5_7

Diagnosis

Miliaria (prickly heat, heat rashes)

Treatment

Treatment of miliaria crystallina may simply consist in exposing the affected part, avoiding occlusive dressing, having cool baths, using air-conditioning, or exposing to a cool environment. Calamine lotion helps some patients.

In cases of miliaria profunda, anhydrous lanolin cream suffices. In patients with miliaria rubra, mild-to-moderate topical corticosteroid creams may be applied to the affected part. When it is miliaria pustulosa, topical antibiotics should be applied.

Etiology

In miliaria, there is obstruction of the ducts of eccrine sweat glands; the result is leakage of sweat into the epidermis or dermis.

Discussion

Usual clinical features As indicated above, ductal obstruction explains the clinical presentation of miliaria. In patients with miliaria, there is usually excessive sweating, and this is aggravated by hot weather. There are different types of miliaria. Miliaria crystallina appears in the form of tiny, pinhead, vesicles that are fragile. The patient with miliaria crystallina is frequently asymptomatic, and the site of blockage of sweat is superficial, just below the stratum corneum and with minimal inflammation. Miliaria pustulosa is another but more severe form of miliaria [1]. When this form of miliaria is extensive, it may lead to heat

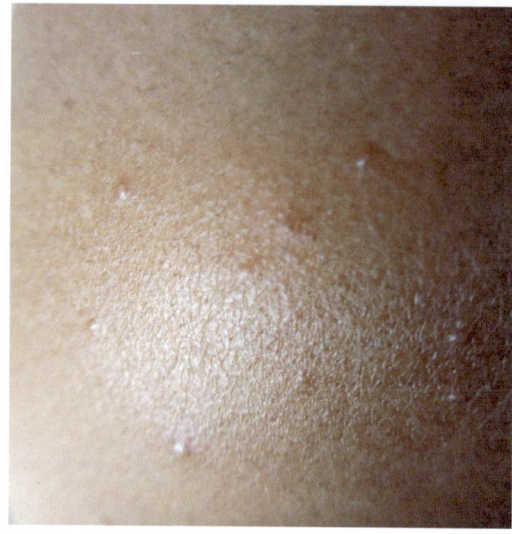

Fig. 7.3 The upper back of the same patient with rashes slightly enlarged

exhaustion; it requires early identification, diagnosis, and treatment. Other forms of miliaria are miliaria profunda with papular eruptions on the skin and miliaria rubra with erythematous rashes.

Investigations Investigations are usually not necessary in miliaria as the diagnosis is usually made on clinical grounds.

Prognosis

The prognosis of miliaria is good, especially miliaria crystallina which is usually asymptomatic and runs a self-limiting course.

Follow-Up Care

This patient and patients who, like her, have the mild form of miliaria may not require follow-up care.

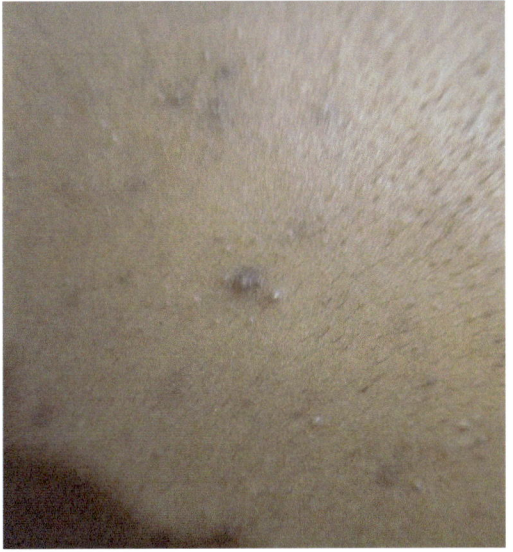

Fig. 7.4 The back of a 25-year-old female

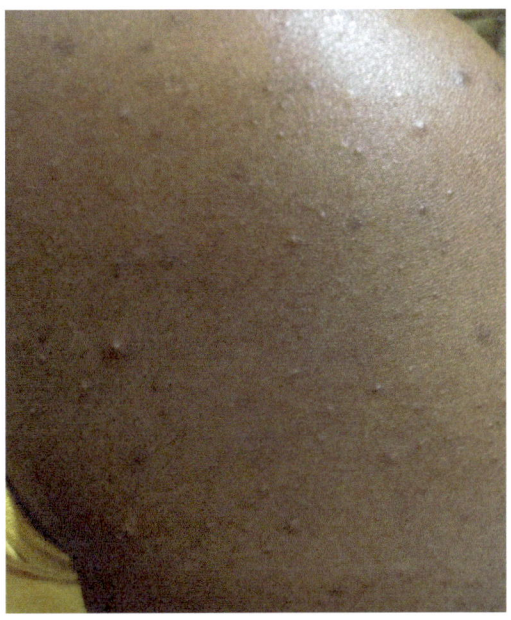

Fig. 7.5 The back of the 25-year-old female

Acne Vulgaris

Symptoms

A 25-year-old female consulted the physician with her main complaints being rashes on both shoulders. The rashes have been on for at least 1 year. The rashes also affected the upper and mid back. Only a few of the rashes were said to be recent. The rashes were only mildly pruritic, especially the ones on the back. The rashes on the back are the ones that she tends to scratch. There are no longer rashes on the face. The facial rashes started in the early part of puberty which was in high school; these were on-and-off only clearing in the last year. The rashes on the back seemed to have become aggravated coincidentally with amelioration of the ones on the face.

Signs

On examination, there were multiple discrete papules on the superior and posterior aspects of the shoulders. One of the rashes was a pustule. On the upper and mid back, there were similar pustules with the difference being that there were multiple hyperpigmented scars.

Diagnosis

Acne vulgaris

Treatment

Treatment is usually easy when the patient consults with a doctor early. In such patients, it is important that the doctor should explain the pathology to the patient or patient's parents. Simple things like using warm water to clean the affected areas, using simple bath soaps, avoiding using abrasive sponge on the rashes, and avoiding cutting, scratching, or pressing them are effective in allowing them to heal. When it becomes necessary, topical agents may suffice, e.g., benzoyl peroxide and retinoids. Some patients require oral antibiotics, e.g., doxycycline, minocycline, erythromycin, or clindamycin.

Etiology

Acne vulgaris is a papular rash that is caused by *Cutibacterium acnes*, formerly called *Propionibacterium acnes*. It is a Gram-positive anaerobe that has a commensal relationship with the human skin. It is a rod-shaped, slow-growing, nonspore-forming, and ubiquitous bacterium.

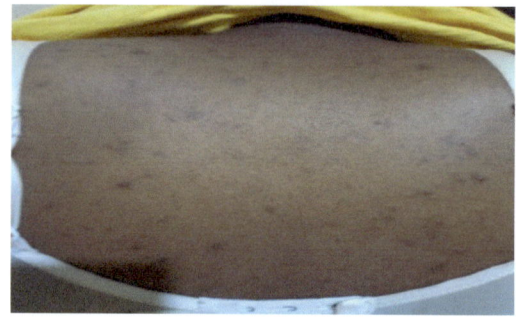

Fig. 7.7 Demonstrates the numerous scars on the upper back of the patient

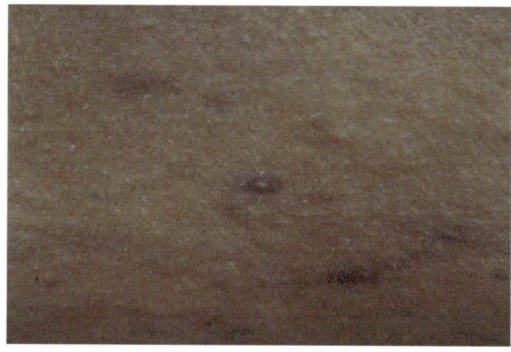

Fig. 7.8 Scar formation on the back (an enlarged image)

Discussion

Usual clinical features Usually, acne vulgaris appears around the pubertal period. It usually affects the face, upper chest, and upper back. Mild acne presents as comedones and a few papulopustules. As the patient gets into early adulthood, the rashes become fewer or they disappear; in some patients, they persist into this period of life and even beyond. The rashes are usually multiple and heal without scar formation. Scratching, pressing, or cutting the papules tends to lead to scar formation.

Investigations Acne vulgaris is essentially a clinical diagnosis and investigations are usually not necessary. A good history taking and physical examination suffice for making the diagnosis.

Fig. 7.6 The single pustule on the back of this patient is enlarged in this image

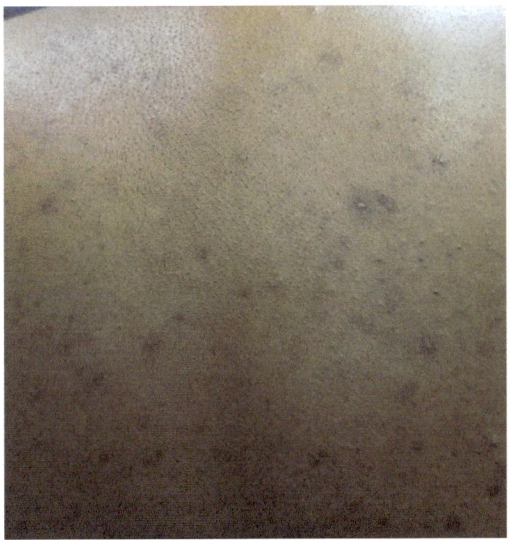

Fig. 7.9 Many patients have acne on more than one part of the body; this patient had just on the upper back and did not bother much about them

Prognosis

The prognosis of acne vulgaris is good in the majority of patients. However, in a few patients, the condition extends into an older age bracket—like in this patient. In such patients, the prognosis is worse if the lesions concentrated on the face, in which case the patient, especially, if a female may be more concerned than many male patients under similar circumstances. This patient had scars that were limited to the upper back, and she almost always covered that part except when she was at home. In some patients, there may be nodulocystic acne in which the nodules exceed 5 mm in diameter with associated comedones and inflammatory lesions; scarring is also a feature [2]. In comedonal acne, there is the absence of inflammatory papules and nodules. In moderate acne, there are inflammatory papules; other features are comedones and pustules.

Follow-Up Care

In acne vulgaris, follow-up care depends on the severity of the condition. A patient whose lesions respond satisfactorily to short-term or medium-term therapy and other home measures that prevent an aggravation of the lesions needs only a little follow-up care—unlike patients with severe cases who may need care by a dermatologist.

Nodular Acne

Symptoms

Figure 7.10 shows the face of a 30-year-old lady. The patient complained of facial rashes and roughness of her face since her teenage years. The rashes were like multiple "bumps" on her face, upper back, and upper chest. They had never given her a respite since onset within 1 year of her attaining puberty. They had a tendency of "coming and going" with little or no time interval prior to a repeat. If she did not have them on the back, she would have on the upper chest, the ones on the face were the most worrisome and the ones that made her come to this hospital—just as she had been attending other hospitals and clinics. She felt some comfort during her secondary school (high school) days because she had many classmates and schoolmates who had similar "pimples." Virtually, all the people who had these rashes at about the same time with her now have "smooth faces" making her situation stand out like a sore thumb. She felt embarrassed when they would ask her "Are you still having pimples?" She had applied numerous drugs in the form of creams, tablets, and capsules individually or in combination over the years and received only temporary relief. Even her younger siblings have "outgrown" pimples.

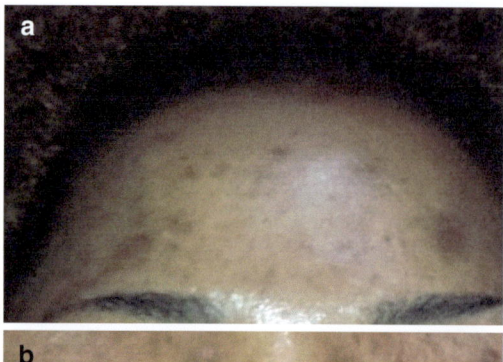

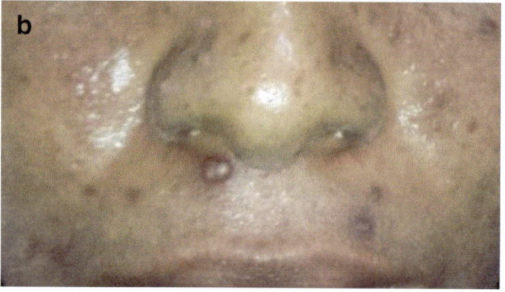

Fig. 7.10 (**a**, **b**) The face of a 30-year-old lady

Signs

This lady's face is masked, obliterating her eyes, and making her facial expression not obvious, but she looked unhappy.

Although she had applied powder on her face prior to leaving home for the hospital, her face was manifestly oily. There were multiple, discrete, hyperpigmented scars of various sizes. There was a single, prominent nodule on the nasolabial fold just inferior to the right nostril.

She was unwilling to expose her upper chest and upper back where, during providing the history of the presenting complaints, she had indicated that she had similar but fewer rashes of less concern as her clothes covered them.

Diagnosis

Nodular   acne   with   post-inflammatory hyperpigmentation.

Treatment

Testosterone plays a hormonal role in the etiology of acne vulgaris. With early and correct information on etiology, clinical course, and self-management of acne vulgaris coupled with diligent application of the information, most boys and girls should go through the period of its occurrence without eventually developing complications.

Treatment of scarring complications of acne vulgaris may not restore the face to a state of normalcy though there may be significant improvement. Focal acne scar treatment using CO_2 laser, injection of platelet-rich fibrin matrix which is platelet-rich plasma, and micro-needling are some means of treating atrophic scars. Punch techniques are surgical procedures used for treating patients with acne scarring.

Discussion

Here, attention is paid to severe and complicated acne vulgaris. Acne vulgaris typically starts in puberty and affects many boys and girls. The natural history is that it should no longer be a medical issue in early-to-mid-20s.

Sebaceous glands are appendages to hair follicles. A sebaceous gland produces sebum to lubricate its hair follicle and the skin. This means that the numerous sebaceous glands of the hairs on the body under normal conditions produce enough lubrication for hair and the skin, preventing dryness of the skin. The lubrication, when optimal, does not show as an excessively oily face contrary to the case with many patients with acne. Acne vulgaris is principally a result of excessive production of sebum. Not only is sebum production excessive, but there is also partial or total blockage of some of the sebaceous ducts. There is accumulation of sebum, dead skin epithelial cells, and a suitable environment is created for skin bacteria to act on the sebum and dead cells. This process leads to acne. A combination of this process and unhealthy habits, viz., picking and squeezing of the acne, cutting them, using abrasive sponge and "medicated soaps" that are available over the counter in many cities, etc., makes acne vulgaris prone to becoming complicated. Uncomplicated acne vulgaris presents as papules with blackheads or whiteheads. Healing is without scar formation.

Nodules and pustules are complications of acne vulgaris. They should not occur in people who practice correct care on acne vulgaris. Other presentations of complicated acne vulgaris are cysts and scarring. Scarring associated with acne vulgaris is not as common as the mild forms of acne, and they are not likely to occur in the early stages of acne. Repeated poor handling of acne vulgaris lesions means that the affected part is recurrently traumatized, undergoes inflammation, and does not heal properly before further damage is inflicted. Scarring therefore eventually results, and there are three types of atrophic scars—all of which are depressed— below skin level, viz., rolling scars, ice pick scars, and boxcar scars [3]. Rolling scar is a shallow and slope-edged scar, the result of scarring presenting as unevenness when the skin surface is palpated; ice pick scar is akin to applying a sharp ice pick to ice and removing it with the consequence of a deep, though small, hole/perforation within the scarred skin; boxcar scar is a wider depression in the skin and may have various shapes. While ice pick scars are generally maximum 2 mm wide, boxcar scars are wider but limited to 4 mm. These atrophic scars are mainly facial scars.

Patients who have complicated acne vulgaris are more prone to have issues with self-esteem partially because they become aware that their age-mates no longer have acne. Some of them listen to various opinions about treatment, including the ones with negative consequences. Patients, with or without acne complications, tend to seek medical attention after trying other forms of care or treatment. Complications of acne sometimes require plastic surgery intervention.

There may be evidence of social withdrawal in some patients with severe or complicated acne vulgaris making them feel uncomfortable at public functions including church services,

lecture halls, parties, etc. Some patients suffer from various degrees of depression. Acne should, therefore, be treated early and appropriately to avoid direct and indirect complications.

Prognosis

When compared with acne vulgaris, the prognosis is not good.

Follow-Up Care

This is essential and the patient should be advised to adhere to scheduled appointments.

Acne Keloidalis Nuchae

Symptoms

This male in the early 30s presented in the clinic with complaints of a "growth" at the back of his upper neck. The first time he noticed the small growth – the size of a rather firm pimple – was over one year earlier. It was painless and slightly itchy. There was a tendency for his fingers to go there, and occasionally when he had long nails, he would accidentally scratch it. In the past approximately 9 months, the growth had not only increased in number (now three) but also increased in size significantly. The growths had become more itchy and were causing him embarrassment although their location was at the back of his head and neck. Colleagues, friends, and family members were asking him questions about it, and some who had encountered a similar condition even proffered various solutions some of which he had tried without obtaining satisfactory relief. The purpose of his attendance at the clinic was to find a solution to the condition as he was getting worried that it could progress into a complication.

Signs

Examination of the occipital scalp and nuchal area of this male patient showed an irregularly inverted V-shaped three-in-one growth on the scalp just within the posterior hairline and the junction between the hairline and the nuchal area. They appeared to be three growths that had become linked to form the shape described. The "growth complex" was firm on palpation. It was not movable and appeared to be attached to the deeper structures especially during flexion of the neck.

Two hypopigmented areas were obvious. The hypopigmented areas were at the skin level, and palpating them gave a feel of thinness compared with the immediate surrounding unaffected skin—this was more obvious with the inferior one.

Diagnosis

Acne keloidalis nuchae

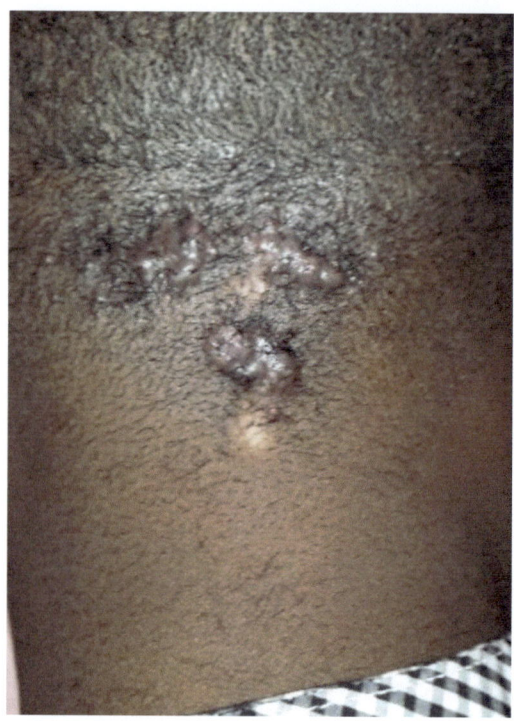

Fig. 7.11 The nape in a patient with acne keloidalis nuchae

Treatment

The management of acne keloidalis nuchae consists of the following:

- Microbiological studies with culture to ensure adequate antibiotic treatment only when there is pus or drainage.
- Advice to the patient on avoidance of pulling hair and scratching the lesion.
- Advice to the patient to avoid short haircuts and close shaving.
- Application of mild keratolytic agents; these may contain topical retinoids or α-hydroxy acids.
- Application of topical potent steroids; application of a combination of topical potent steroids with topical retinoids is very effective.
- Cryotherapy and targeted ultraviolet-B (290–320 nm) phototherapy have been used.
- In cases with late presentation, intralesional injection of methylprednisolone may be useful. The patient whose photograph is shown was given triamcinolone acetonide as an intralesional injection, and he developed the hypopigmented macular patches demonstrated in Fig. 7.11.
- Surgical intervention by laser ablation or surgical excision is also done. Wound healing by secondary intention results in fewer recurrences.

Etiology

Acne keloidalis nuchae is similar to, but not associated with, pseudo folliculitis barbae. It may result in people who frequently shave their scalp hair very close to the skin. It initially results from perifollicular inflammation, It features both acute and chronic granulomatous inflammation. It eventually presents as scarring and irreversible alopecia.

Prognosis

The prognosis of acne keloidalis nuchae depends on the extent of lesion and, to some extent, the timing of treatment. The latter usually depends on when the patient chooses to go to the hospital to consult with doctors. When it is small and is treated in the initial stages, the prognosis is good. The patient would do well to resist the urge to scratch, traumatize the lesion, and develop a bacterial infection.

Follow-Up Care

Follow-up care is usually warranted in patients who have undergone procedures or surgical interventions for acne keloidalis nuchae. In patients whose conditions and their treatment ought to be straightforward, the doctor may still want the patient to return to the clinic for review of treatment at least once.

Discussion

Acne keloidalis nuchae usually occurs at the nape and occipital scalp. In the initial stages of this condition, the patient with the lesions present have pruritus as the main symptom; an abundance of mast cells may be responsible for this symptom. The patient does not have pain; when there is pain, it is insignificant pain. Acne keloidalis nuchae does not affect non-hairy skin. Pustules are a common sign; these are follicular-based pustules. There are also papules which tend to coalesce, eventually forming plaques. Acne keloidalis nuchae is not synonymous with acne conglobata, but with scalp perifolliculitis and acne conglobata, it forms the follicular occlusion triad.

In acne keloidalis nuchae, tufts of hair within the lesion are a common finding. There is a predilection for the black race (and in males), rare in Caucasians, and occasionally found among Hispanics and Asians.

It is correct that acne keloidalis nuchae is keloid-like as the condition progresses; it forms plaques that look like keloids. Acne keloidalis

nuchae does not occur as a sequel to acne vulgaris, and it does not share histological features with acne vulgaris nor do the chronic cases present with hypertrophic scars.

Acne keloidalis nuchae may grow to the point of becoming disfiguring, and in advanced cases, discharging sinus tracts may develop just as the growth may result in abscesses.

Differential diagnoses Differential diagnoses of acne keloidalis nuchae include the following [4]:

- Acneiform eruption
- Acne vulgaris
- Acne conglobata
- Hidradenitis suppurativa
- Folliculitis decalvans

The differential diagnosis made may depend on the appearance of the skin lesion when the patient consults the doctor; if early, it may simulate acneiform eruption or acne vulgaris, but if much later, it may look like acne conglobata, hidradenitis suppurativa, or folliculitis decalvans.

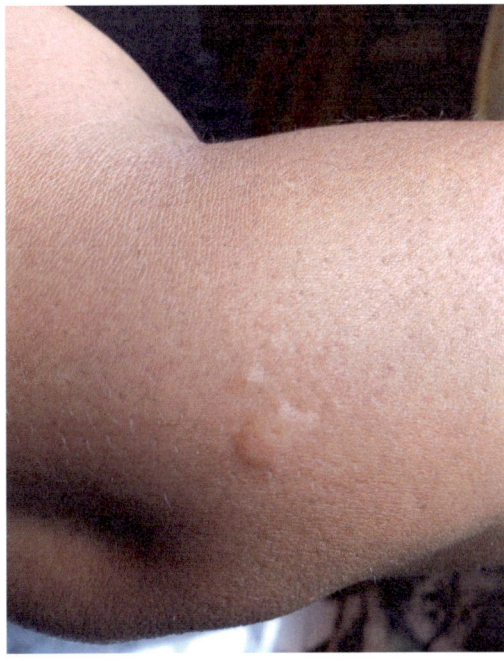

Fig. 7.12 The right forearm of a 60-year-old woman

Urticaria

Symptoms

She said that the single rash appeared after she felt an insect bite. She perceived the bite in the afternoon while in her bedroom which had an open door. She was surprised when she hit the affected part and found that she had just killed a mosquito; there was blood on the affected spot. She noticed at the bite site an itchy rash within 10 min of the bite. The rash was initially small, but within a few minutes, it increased in size to about 2 cm. The rash disappeared within 1 h after she applied hydrocortisone 1% cream to the rash. She keeps the cream because this was not the first time as she has had a similar rash, and the medication was prescribed by her doctor in the past. This patient observed that even when she gets bitten by mosquitoes in the night, her husband does not notice or complain of having been bitten by mosquitoes despite her killing mosquitoes that have perched on him while he slept; the husband has not had a similar rash. She does not have allergic conjunctivitis, allergic dermatitis, or

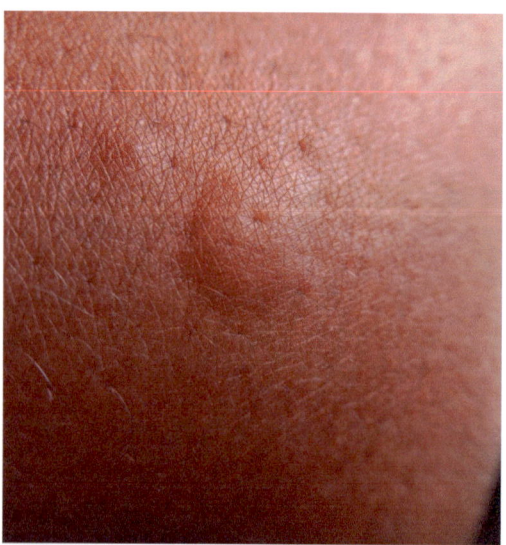

Fig. 7.13 An enlargement of the right forearm raised rash

bronchial asthma. There is a positive family history of allergy as her immediate elder brother is an asthmatic patient.

Signs

On examination, there was a 2 cm × 1 cm ovoid wheal on the lateral surface of the right forearm; there was a second but smaller wheal just beside the first one. There was no change in pigmentation of the skin over the rashes. There was no surrounding hyperemia. There was no similar rash on any other part of the body.

Diagnosis

Urticaria

Treatment

Based on the pathophysiology which includes degranulation of mast cells and release of histamine in urticaria, the treatment primarily entails use of non-sedating H1-receptor blocker antihistamines; examples include fexofenadine, cetirizine, levocetirizine, and loratadine. This is the treatment for mild cases as in the patient described above. The patient may, like the patient described, not need systemic therapy but topical therapy with antihistamine creams or mild corticosteroid creams, e.g., hydrocortisone 1% cream. Patients who do not mind drowsiness or a little more sleep may be prescribed chlorpheniramine or hydroxyzine. A patient with a more severe case or who is at risk of developing angioedema, hypotension, or anaphylaxis would need appropriate treatment for the severe presentation, apart from vital signs monitoring with or without ECG/EKG. In patients who develop the condition from avoidable exposure, e.g., environmental conditions, exposure to latex, pets, plants, food, or medications, urticaria can and should be prevented.

Etiology

Urticaria is an allergic reaction of the skin to environmental factors, foods, drugs, plants and animals, cosmetics, etc. Contact with skin may be obvious but it may not be. In this patient, it was from an insect bite. The allergic reaction basically consists of activation of H1 histamine receptors and H2 histamine receptors by released histamine. The result of H1 histamine receptor activation in smooth muscle cells and endothelial cells is an increase in capillary permeability; activation of H2 histamine receptors in these cells results in vasodilation in venules and arterioles.

Discussion

Usual clinical features Patients with urticaria may have wheals (also called welts) which in white skin looks red—in Black skin only the patients with light skin tone may have wheals that fit this description as many do not demonstrate it. These characteristically pruritic lesions that are elevated above surrounding unaffected skin may be small or large; single or multiple; circular, ovoid, or of irregular shape; and coalescent and affect one part of the body or many parts of the body. Large urticarial rashes are usually a coalescence of numerous small ones that appear almost simultaneously at the same site [5]. Acute urticarial rashes disappear with or without treatment within 6 weeks. In chronic urticaria, the rashes last longer than 6 weeks. When they are pressed, they demonstrate blanching. Urticaria tends to recur when the patient is exposed to the same allergen(s). A patient with urticaria does not have to develop the condition when there is exposure to all established causes of urticaria. The itchy rash heals without leaving a scar except in urticarial vasculitis in which there may be associated ecchymoses and hyperpigmentation at the site after healing.

Investigations From detailed history and a physical examination, the diagnosis of straightforward urticaria is usually made, especially in acute urticaria. Patients with chronic urticaria may require a full (complete) blood count, erythrocyte sedimentation rate (ESR), and antinuclear antibody test to rule out systemic diseases that may present with urticaria as a skin manifestation. Skin sensitivity testing may be required in some patients.

Prognosis

There is a good prognosis for urticaria. Rarely, a patient may develop angioedema, hypotension, or anaphylaxis. Urticaria may also run a chronic course.

Follow-Up Care

Follow-up care may be required when the patient's illness is severe or recurrent. When a patient is well-guided, they tend to identify and avoid the trigger agent(s)—in such cases, the recurrence rate is low; these patients may not require going for follow-up care as the frequency of episodes is minimized, and they can prevent their occurrence or mitigate them promptly.

Symptoms

In this patient, the symptoms were severe itching of sudden onset that woke her up from sleep in the afternoon. Prior to taking a nap that afternoon there was no complaint, and she could not figure out what caused the itching and accompanying extensive rash on her left forearm. She did not have any difficulty in breathing or pruritus in any other part of the body. She was careful not to scratch the lesion, but she rubbed it gently with the fingers of her right hand. It was not long since she made her hair and she and the author, who was nearby, surmised that it had to do with this most recent activity. The bedding was the same as the one she slept on the previous night. By the following morning, the rash were no longer visible. The patient has had a similar complaint, but it was a long time since it happened. She had a family history of allergy.

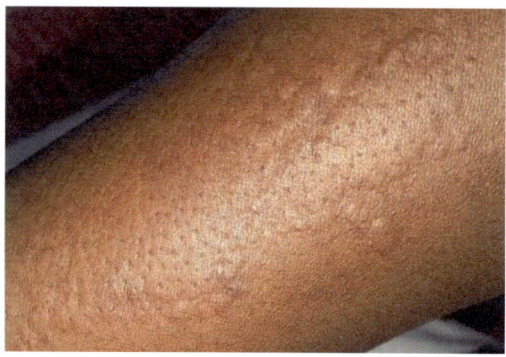

Fig. 7.14 The left forearm of a young woman under 25 years of age

Signs

On examination, the polymorphic wheal was long and measured about 15 cm × 4 cm. The raised rashes were clearly demarcated from the surrounding unaffected skin. The margins of the rashes were irregular. Figure 7.14 shows the outline of the extensive rash and "dimples" on it—these are absent from the normal skin. There was no erythematous area or any other difference between the affected part of the forearm skin and the rest of the forearm skin. The rash did not affect any other part of the body.

Diagnosis

Acute urticaria

Treatment

Levocetirizine 5 mg daily for 5 days

Etiology

With respect to etiology and pathophysiology of physical urticaria, the following have been implicated: vibration, water, cold, exercise, and dermographism. In dermographism, stroking the skin in some people results in an exaggerated response due to transudation of fluid from small blood vessels and edema in the skin over the area.

Histamine, leukotrienes, bradykinin, heparin, kallikrein, and substance-P are involved. Dermographism may be symptomatic (with pruritus) or asymptomatic. When symptomatic, triggers may be drugs, insect bites, etc., but dermographism is usually asymptomatic.

Vasoactive substances implicated in the pathophysiology of urticaria cause vasodilatation; the substances include prostaglandin D2, bradykinin, leukotriene C4, and histamine. In the pathophysiology of urticaria, mast cells play a significant role; mast cells are degranulated, leading to release of histamine. Basophils are involved. There is extravasation of plasma into the dermis. The presence of histamine is responsible for one of the most significant symptoms of urticaria, pruritus. Angioedema is progression of the events that occur in urticaria as there is extension of extravasation of plasma into the subcutaneous tissue or submucosal tissue.

In some patients with urticaria after visiting a hospital, latex in latex gloves worn by a doctor to examine the patient may be the cause. In other patients, antibiotic(s) prescribed for treating an infection may be the cause of urticaria related to serum sickness. Patients who receive blood transfusion may develop urticaria from a complement-mediated reaction.

Prognosis

The prognosis of acute urticaria is good.

Follow-Up Care

The patient may not need to return to the clinic for follow-up care when the response to treatment is within hours (even with oral medication).

Discussion

Urticaria occurs in all ages and both sexes; size is not a defining factor, and the widest diameter may be many centimeters just as it may under 5 cm; urticaria may present as just one rash, but when wheals are numerous, there may be conflu-ence. In patients with extensive urticaria, the wheals tend to be irregular in shape.

Acute urticaria can occur in young adults and children, but children are more prone; it occurs more commonly in patients with atopy. In acute urticaria, the lesions individually resolve within 24 h, and resolution may be within just a few hours. It is characterized by episodes that do not last up to 6 weeks. Angioedema or anaphylactic reaction may follow urticaria, but this is not usual. Acute urticaria may be spontaneous.

Clinical features of urticaria: The rashes are characterized by advancing edge and receding edge [6]. The patient experiences intense pruri-tus, application of pressure on the lesion(s) results in complete blanching, and there is no epi-dermal change.

Other features of urticaria include the fact that the lesions resolve leaving no scar; when urticaria is chronic, there are recurrent episodes that last more than 6 weeks.

When presented with a patient with rashes that are reminiscent of urticaria, the general practitio-ner should remember that management involves a detailed and organized history taking that should include food—in taking the history, questions should be asked to include ingestion of, and likely association with, tomatoes, shellfish, tree nuts, eggs, peanuts, etc. History taking should extend to occupation for those who are working and cir-cumstances in the school for students in hostels as exposure to the cause may be at work or at school, just as it may be at home. In the index patient, it is probable that the acute urticaria is related to a constituent of a hair product; she may have slept with her hair on top of her forearm.

Physical examination of the patient, with par-ticular attention to the rash(es), can lead to differ-entiation of urticaria from other skin conditions.

The diagnosis of urticaria is mainly clinical; laboratory and other investigations may assist in making a diagnosis, but they are not essential for arriving at the diagnosis if history taking and physical examination are thorough.

Symptoms

The patient was a 41-year-old woman. She com-plained of rashes that have been coming in crops within the past 6 months. The rashes affected the exposed parts of her body—the upper limbs and lower limbs; Figs. 7.15 and 7.16 are photographs of her right forearm and right arm. The rashes were said to be itchy and lasted for a few weeks each instance but not up to 6 weeks. She had taken drugs over the period and came to the clinic out of frustration with the recurrence of fresh rashes after healing of old ones, leaving dark-to-black flat scars. She could not predict when they would recur and could not associate them with anything; they would appear spontaneously. There was no positive family or occupational his-tory. She did not reside where she would be exposed to insect bites. She was not on any regular medication for a chronic medical condi-tion. There was no relevant history associated with food allergy. She did not come with any conspicuous jewelry and she worked where use

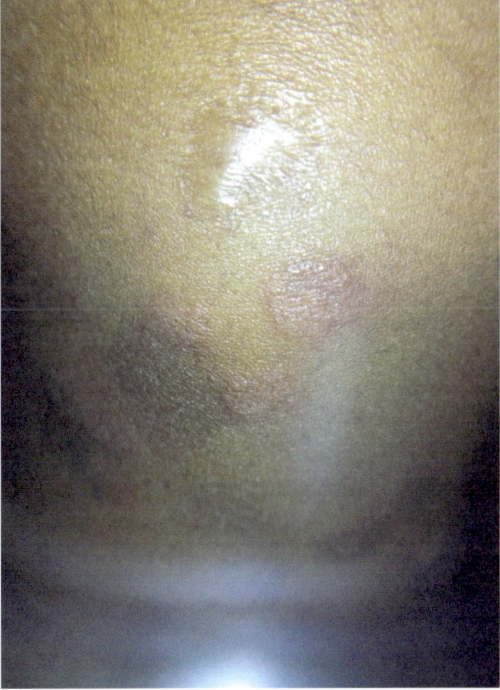

Fig. 7.15 The right forearm of a 42-year-old patient with recurrent rashes

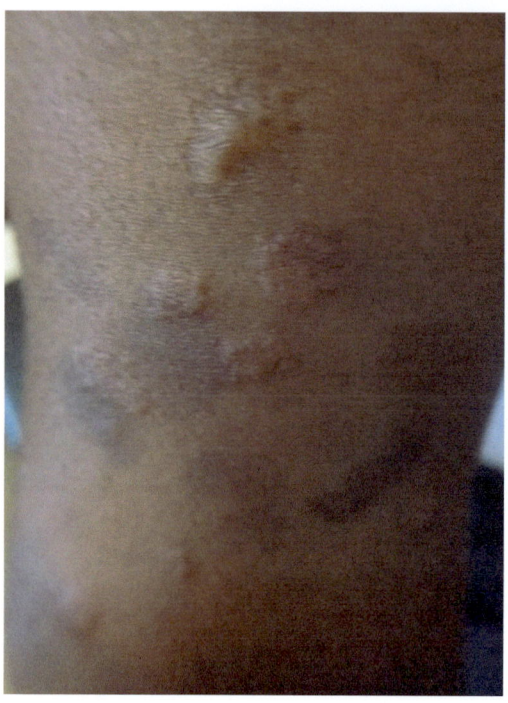

Fig. 7.16 The right forearm of the same 42-year-old patient with recurrent rashes

eter; they were irregularly-shaped violaceous plaques that were generally flat-topped except some with borders that had vesicles/papules. The older rashes were macules, were also multiple, but had greater irregularity in shape; these had healed, forming hyperpigmented scars. Some of the newer rashes were somewhat superimposed on the hyperpigmented scars. The most proximal of the skin lesions was a scar from a wound sustained in her childhood, unrelated to the pathological condition under consideration.

Diagnosis

Recurring urticaria

Treatment

This patient was placed on second-generation H1-antihistamines—the first line of pharmacological therapy.

Etiology

As documented for the earlier patient in this chapter, urticaria is an allergic reaction of the skin to external factors that may be environmental, foods, drugs, plants and animals, cosmetics, etc. Although urticaria frequently manifests with a wide range of areas of skin involvement (from one to multiple in a part of the body to single or multiple in various parts of the body) and is not specific in size or shape even in the same patient, it has a systemic pathogenesis.

Prognosis

The prognosis of urticaria seems to depend on factors some of which include the degree of severity of the patient's presentation, whether the trigger factor(s) are identifiable and identified or not, the efforts made by the patient to avoid trigger factors, the patient's emotional reaction of the skin condition, and adherence to prescribed drugs. Since chronic urticaria is commoner in women than

of such jewelry is discouraged. Her source of water was pipe-borne and she lived in government official quarters. History of exposure to mites or bed bugs was not sought. There was no history of antecedent or recurrent fever. The patient requested drug treatment but was told that a definitive diagnosis had to be made prior to commencement of therapy; she was booked for skin biopsy to be performed by the dermatologist. The patient came into the consulting room well covered and had to remove the additional clothing to show the affected part.

*By the time she returned in 1 week for skin biopsy, the lesions had resolved leaving only the previous scars. The procedure was not carried out, and the patient was to take the drugs she had been taking and to look out for trigger factor(s).

Signs

On examination, there were two sets of lesions. The dimensions of the recent rashes were multiple, each between 1 and 2 cm at the widest diam-

men, the patient whose condition is discussed here could be prone to developing chronic urticaria.

Follow-Up Care

In this patient, follow-up care happened to be a part of the presentation. It was when she returned for a scheduled skin biopsy that she reported that the rashes had subsided. If she chose not to return, the dermatologist and this author would have concluded wrongly that she defaulted and was "lost to follow-up." We appreciated her returning to inform us that the lesions had ceased.

Discussion

Usual clinical features Edema at the affected part(s) of the skin, pruritus, and erythema are the features of urticaria. In dark skinned persons, erythema may not be obvious. Pruritus may be moderate or intense, and the patient's assessment of the intensity may be subjective. Thankfully, urticarial lesions are usually transitory; this short-lived characteristic of acute urticaria makes it somewhat bearable, especially in patients in whom pruritus is also fleeting. Patients in whom the lesions and associated symptoms are recurrent (either in the acute form or chronic form) may feel distressed, and their quality of life may be impacted negatively. Many patients are unable to associate urticaria with a particular thing; it is usually after consulting a doctor that suggestions by the doctor may enable the patient to pin down the implicating agent(s).

Apart from acute urticaria with symptoms and lesions lasting between minutes and 6 weeks, there is chronic urticaria with features that exceed 6 weeks; for stable chronic urticaria, the features last as long as between 3 and 6 months. Two types of chronic urticaria are currently recognized, i.e., chronic spontaneous urticaria and chronic inducible urticaria. The features of chronic urticaria are the same as those of acute urticaria, but in the former, healing could leave hyperpigmented scars.

With both acute urticaria and chronic urticaria, there is stimulation of mast cells with release of vasoactive substances; vasodilatation, increased capillary permeability, extravasation of plasma, and inflammatory cells recruitment and eventual stimulation of sensory nerve cells result in wheals and pruritus that characterize these conditions. Autoimmune mechanism has been proposed for chronic urticaria.

In some patients, the symptoms resolve spontaneously.

Investigations Being a clinical diagnosis, investigations are usually superfluous. Only a few non-specific laboratory investigations may be considered unless the patient's history and findings during physical examination point towards other diseases that could be related, thus justifying more specific tests. If the case appears to be atypical, or there is doubt in refractory cases or certain chronic cases, skin biopsy may be justified.

Treatment As discussed in a preceding case report on urticaria, the first line of pharmacological therapy consists of the second-generation H1-antihistamines. Their standard doses can be increased fourfold to achieve symptom control in patients who do not receive a respite from standard doses. Novel drugs are expected to reduce the rate of symptom and lesion recurrence apart from shortening the time of their resolution.

Other drugs include first-generation H1-antihistamines, H2-antihistamines, high-potency antihistamines, leukotriene receptor antagonists, and short courses of corticosteroids.

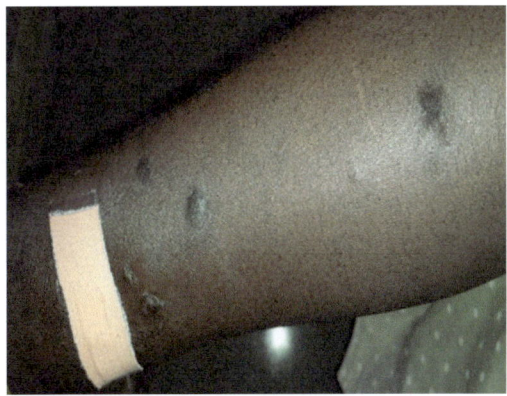

Fig. 7.17 The upper extremity of a 28-year-old female

For patients whose presentation fits chronic urticaria, cyclosporine and omalizumab are additional pharmacological agents.

Papular Urticaria

Symptoms

This 28-year-old female patient who lives in the rural area and engages in petty trading in her home in addition to farming both in her home and in a farm further from her home in the same village presented with a history of recurrent itchy rashes on the exposed parts of her body. These were the upper limbs and the distal portions of the lower limbs. She said that the symptoms have been there for about 8 years. The rashes were so pruritic that she occasionally cut them with her nails. The rashes were more than one at any time they occurred, and the rate of occurrence was frequent, mimicking the frequency of her going to farm in the distant farming site, especially when she was delayed in returning home. The rashes were usually on such evenings, and they would occasionally disturb her sleep because of the associated itching. Most times, the rashes would disappear, but she had some that persisted and many older rashes that healed and left scars. She was unhappy that as young as she was, she did not have a smooth skin, like her contemporaries who lived in the nearby city and returned home for weekends or for some communal festivities. Some people who engaged in work like hers had similar complaints.

When asked whether she was exposed to insect bites, she answered in the affirmative and stated that the bites were usually in the evenings. She could hardly see or ward off the insects prior to receiving insect bites. Some of the bites were associated with a tiny amount of blood at one or more sites.

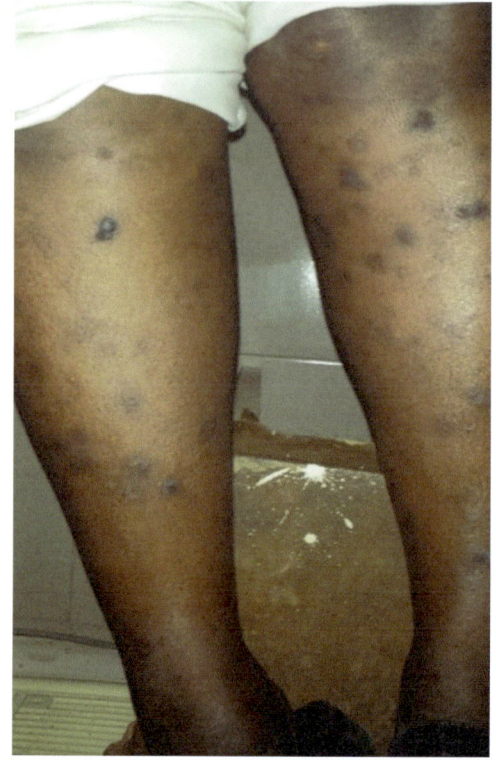

Fig. 7.18 The lower extremity of the patient

Signs

Examination of the affected parts of this patient's skin showed numerous scars that were discrete. The hyperpigmented scars were of diverse sizes and shapes. There was no obvious recent rash to which she had attributed a description of papules that followed initial small wheals. There were no scratch marks.

Diagnosis

Papular urticaria is the provisional diagnosis. This diagnosis is usually clinical following good, pointed, history taking, and physical examination.

Treatment

Treatment involves use of antihistamines (nond-rowsy during working or school hours and drowsy during the period of sleep). Details on antihistamines are available in the chapter on medications in dermatology.

Etiology

Papular urticaria is a skin hypersensitivity reaction to bites by arthropods. Arthropods belong to the phylum Arthropoda and the commonest culprits belong to the class Insecta. Flying insects, e.g., mosquitoes, commonly cause papular urticaria. Wingless insects like lice, e.g., *Pediculus humanus*, bed bugs (*Cimex lectularius*), and fleas, and arachnids of Acarina subclass, e.g., mites (*Sarcoptes scabiei*) and chiggers, are known to trigger papular urticaria. Winged insects by virtue of flying and their numbers—as well as repeated bites—tend to cause multiple lesions, while the slower arthropods may cause rashes that are limited to the areas they affect. However, areas affected are usually exposed parts of the body—exposed to the culprit.

Prognosis

The prognosis for recurrent acute urticaria is good if the patient can identify environmental, occupational, or other factors and control them.

Follow-Up Care

In a patient with papular urticaria, the follow-up care entails returning to the clinic for outpatient review and identification of the factors at home, workplace, and recreational habits/activities and religious services that could expose the patient to arthropods. Upon finding these factors or agents, the patient should make an aggressive effort to eliminate what deserves elimination and reduce exposure where a total separation from them is unavoidable.

Discussion

History History taking should concentrate on exposure as well as symptoms of the rashes. Exposure may not be at home but may be in places like school, dormitory, campgrounds, church, shopping area, open market, etc. depending on location of these places; the location of exposure to arthropods may also be elucidated from occupational history, e.g., working at housing or road construction sites; at other times, it is travel history that provides the location and nature of the exposure. Family history may or may not be useful—this is because members of the same family, equally exposed to an arthropod, may respond differently. When there is exposure to more than one causative arthropod, the picture may be different in terms of distribution, e.g., multiple from flying insects or limited to the trunk, or a part of it, from bed bugs.

Presentation While initially papular urticaria may appear like any other urticarial rash (i.e., small wheals 1 cm or less)—and some may regress over a short time—the rashes eventually become papules and last for weeks or months; they may then regress but could recur after a long time, especially with re-exposure to bites of the offending arthropod. The rashes are pruritic and, in some patients, may prevent sound sleep—like in this patient.

Investigation Scratching in response to pruritus may lead to hyperpigmentation and scarring—as shown. Occasionally, skin biopsy is required, e.g., this patient with plaster just had a biopsy done. Histopathological examination of skin biopsy enables the pathologist to provide a definitive diagnosis.

Control Environmental control of arthropods is both a preventive and control measure.

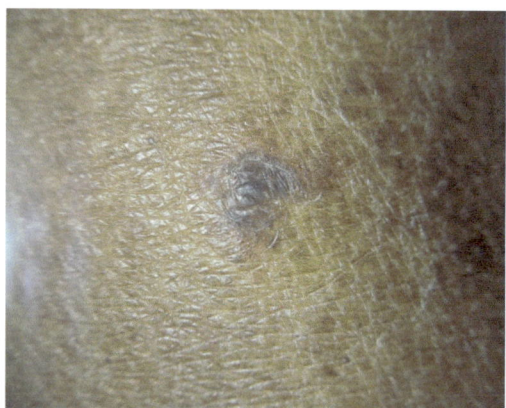

Fig. 7.19 Hyperpigmented rash on the proximal right thigh

Lichen Simplex Chronicus (Neurodermatitis)

Symptoms

The patient with this skin condition was in his mid-60s. He noticed the skin rash about 5 years earlier. The rash was moderately itchy, but the itching was usually transient, subsiding within 30 min even without treatment. He sometimes rubbed the skin to get some respite from the itching but had no cause to scratch with nails. The rash was the only one and appeared on the skin of the outer part of his upper thigh. The rash was said to be almost always there but only became itchy and darker during hot dry weather, especially during harmattan; at other times, it gave him no concern and he frequently forgot that the skin condition was there. It did not increase in size but seemed to decrease in size and become less dark when he applied hydrocortisone cream for a short period, usually less than 1 week. The rash did not spread and did not affect any other part of the body. There was no associated pain.

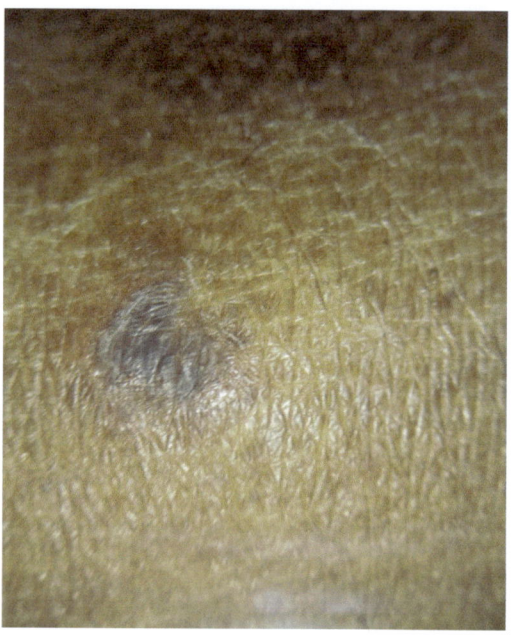

Fig. 7.20 An enlargement of the hyperpigmented rash on the proximal right thigh

Signs

On examination, the rash was a solitary hyperpigmented, "rough-surfaced" and scaly, macular eruption. It was 3 cm × 2.5 cm. The irregularly shaped macule was on the lateral aspect of the upper right thigh. It was clearly delineated from the surrounding skin. There was no fissuring and no signs of scratching of the affected or surrounding skin.

Diagnosis

Lichen simplex chronicus (neurodermatitis)

Treatment

Topical treatment with a low-potency corticosteroid (hydrocortisone 1% cream) and nondrowsy second-generation antihistamine (levocetirizine 5 mg orally daily).

Etiology

Lichen simplex chronicus, also known as neurodermatitis, is a chronic inflammatory skin condition with pruritic scaly patches of thickened skin from repetitive scratching or rubbing of the affected part.

Fig. 7.21 Further enlargement of the hyperpigmented rash

Prognosis

Prognosis in lichen simplex chronicus has a relationship between the patient's knowledge of, attitude to, and care for the condition. The patient should be made to know that the condition can recur and that the relapse or flare-up is usually linked to exposure to a trigger. In some patients, the chronicity of the lesions may lead to lifelong therapy.

Follow-Up Care

The patient should avoid triggers like skin irritants and stressful situations at home, workplace, and neighborhood. Injury to the lesions should be avoided and so the patient who obtains relief from scratching should be advised to obtain a similar relief from rubbing as the latter is unlikely to traumatize the affected parts of the skin. When a patient adheres to this line of follow-up care, the severity and recurrence of lichen simplex chronicus is less. The frequency of initiating the return to the clinic to consult the doctors is also minimized.

Discussion

Usual clinical features Lichen simplex chronicus presents as a pruritic, hyperpigmented, scaly, chronic skin condition which may present with lichenification (thickening of the skin), Koebner phenomenon (from scratching and wounding the affected skin), and fissuring. In early lesions, there is erythema, but this may not be obvious in dark-skinned people. The affected areas include exposed parts of the body like the neck and distal part of the legs and covered areas like the upper thigh in the case described. Other accessible sites are back of elbows, vulva, scrotum, and scalp; the sites of neurodermatitis are usually easy for the patient to reach and scratch. Sites of allergic contact dermatitis or irritant contact dermatitis may provide the background on which lichen simplex chronicus develops.

Investigations Though neurodermatitis can be diagnosed clinically by taking into consideration the history and findings on physical examination, it may be necessary to carry out investigations to rule out differential diagnoses.

- Patch skin testing is useful in excluding allergic contact dermatitis when the result is negative.
- Skin scraping and examination of specimen using KOH preparation is negative when it is not a fungal infection.
- Serum IgE level is expected to be normal in this inflammatory condition, unlike in atopic diathesis when the level is elevated.
- In elderly patients, like the index case, skin biopsy may be required to rule out psoriasis.
- Histological examination of skin biopsy specimen is positive in lichen simplex chronicus when it shows the characteristic finding of papillary dermal fibrosis in conjunction with vertical streaking of collagen bundles.

Management Depending on the site and size of the lesions, lichen simplex chronicus may require topical treatment or systemic treatment. Topical treatment is primarily with corticosteroids, and the potency of the chosen corticosteroid is determined by the location, e.g., mild for genital location and potent for a small, thick one on the extremities. When the lesion is thick and solitary, or just a few, and do(es) not respond to topical high potency corticosteroids, an intralesional high potency steroid like triamcinolone acetonide may be injected. Corticosteroids in the mid-potency range are useful in treating an acute inflammation of the lesion. When an enhancement of delivery of the drug, alongside preventing the patient from scratching, is required, occlusion dressing is used, and it also increases

the potency of the topical agent. Antipruritic creams may be required though corticosteroids play the twin role of reducing inflammation and reducing pruritus. Some patients who feel stressed may benefit from a short course of an anxiolytic, and those who need satisfactory sleep may benefit from a few tablets of a sedative.

Allergic Contact Dermatitis

Symptoms

The young lady whose hand is shown in Fig. 7.22 noticed itching over the raised lesions on the skin of her left hand on the precise area where black henna was applied. The rash that developed 2–3 days after application of black henna took an accurate shape of the design that she requested during the application of black henna dye at a beauty salon. She also showed a larger design on the right upper limb, proximal to the itchy rash. She did not complain of pain or itching at the time of presentation; she had slight irritation and itching on the day that she noticed the rashes. She came to complain about the rashes as they were still on her skin beyond the time they normally regress and disappear in people who do henna artwork on their skin. This was the first time she subjected herself to this beauty treatment as she was impressed by the design she had seen on one of her friends; the friend was the one who recommended the salon that the patient eventually patronized. She was unaware of having allergy to anything—food, jewelry, clothing, or medica-

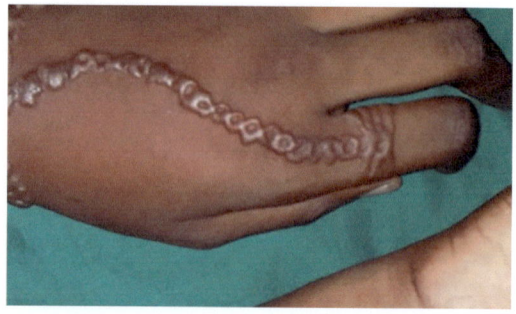

Fig. 7.22 The dorsum of the hand of a 19-year-old female

tions. She did not know if anyone in her family had an allergy, but her answer to asthma, frequent itchy or runny nose, or itching of the body was negative among any of her direct family members.

Signs

The dorsum of the left hand and index finger showed a chain-shaped design. At about the mid-portion of the left index finger, the design extended laterally and medially to create a wing shape that fanned out as four lines on each side. She had a much more intricate artistic design on the posterior surface of the distal left forearm and the left wrist. At the time she came to the clinic, every part of the linked rashes was raised, firm, and non-tender. The entire design had regular outlines and was continuous, and the larger ones that were proximal had additional shapes that the patient chose and the artist applied. The chain-shaped curvilinear design on the left hand and finger took the same pigmentation as the rest of the patient's skin. Parts of the intricate and more robust design on the left wrist and the distal end of the left forearm appeared slightly hyperpigmented. There were no scratch marks and there was no tenderness or erythema.

Diagnosis

Allergic contact dermatitis

Treatment

Treatment is application of corticosteroids topically for localized lesions or oral preparations for extensive rashes. The patient may require oral antihistamines or antibiotics depending on the presentation in terms of key features (e.g., pruritus or superimposed bacterial infection) and timing (early or late.)

Etiology

Allergy to henna due to addition of para-phenylenediamine (PPD) to natural henna with the resultant effect of darkening the color towards black, intensifying the stain, and extending the duration of the design on the skin, especially in tattoos. Some people develop an allergic reaction to PPD; it is a type IV delayed-type hypersensitivity reaction.

Prognosis

The prognosis is good, making explanation and reassurance sufficient for many patients.

Follow-Up Care

This manifestation of allergic reaction to application of henna is usually mild, and the patient may not require more than one follow-up visit to the physician for a review. The treatment is effective and the preventive measures that were discussed with the patient during the first consultation should be reemphasized, not just reiterated.

Discussion

The type of body art decorations that this young lady opted for is culturally accepted in some parts of Nigeria and other parts of the world and so the practice is widespread. Tourists sometimes find these designs which are supposed to last for a brief time attractive and subject themselves to receiving body painting or temporary tattoos. Henna is a plant that grows in hot climates. Its botanical name is *Lawsonia inermis*. The plant produces a brown, orange-brown, or reddish paste. The natural product infrequently causes problems to the skin, and people use it for skin painting and temporary tattoos. Natural henna extract stains the skin, and in approximately 3 weeks, it fades off without any intervention.

Pathophysiology The problem lies in adding para-phenylenediamine (PPD) to natural henna with the resultant effect of darkening the color towards black, intensifying the stain, and extending the duration of the design on the skin, especially in tattoos. Some people develop an allergic reaction to PPD; it is a type IV delayed-type hypersensitivity reaction. For patients who develop allergic reactions to henna dye, there may be an earlier initial sensitization to PPD or similar compounds, e.g., parabens, azo dyes, or para-amino benzoic acid. Slow acetylators tend to be more prone to developing skin sensitization to black henna. Previous sensitization may cause a rapid reaction in people when they use henna.

Usual clinical presentation In 1 or 2 weeks, the contact allergic reaction, a dermatitis, develops on the henna tattoo design as an eczematous eruption but may be urticarial, papular, and pustular or even take the form of blisters. Resolution occurs over time, but in some patients, a keloid may result.

Prevention This allergic contact dermatitis is preventable by avoiding exposure of skin to henna.

Chronic Chemical Irritant Contact Dermatitis

Symptoms

The patient with the condition described in this chapter is a mechanic who owns and runs his business. He handles a variety of vehicles that use petroleum products like gasoline (premium motor spirit or petrol), diesel, engine oil, automatic transmission fluid, manual gear-box gear oil, brake fluid, engine radiator coolant, grease, and "condemned oil." In Nigeria, "condemned oil" is the name given to engine oil that is discharged from a vehicle's engine sump during servicing; this usually blackened engine oil contacts the mechanic's hands for short or prolonged periods and is either discarded improperly or kept aside to be used for other purposes.

He had over the past 2–3 years noticed gradual changes in his skin. The changes consisted of itching, dryness, rashes, darkening, and thickening. The changes were limited to the upper limbs, from the fingers up to the elbows. He became more concerned because the itching became more frequent and more intense recently, neces-

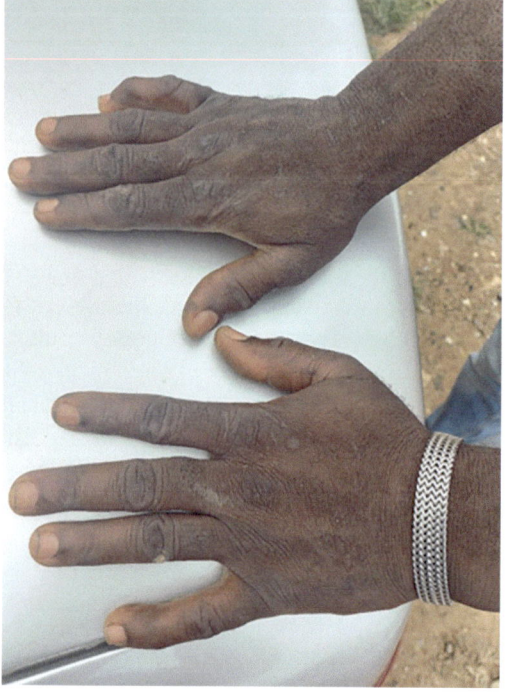

Fig. 7.23 The dorsi of a mechanic's hands

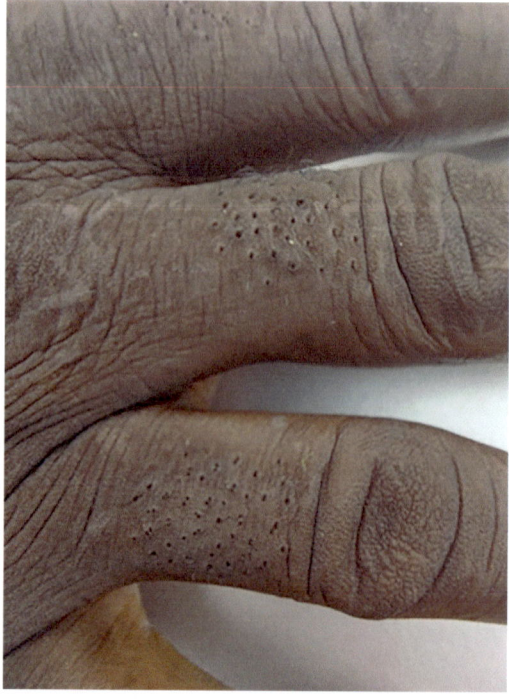

Fig. 7.24 An enlargement of a part of the dorsum of the right hand and fingers

sitating the consultation. He was used to the other skin changes as he had attributed them to his work as a mechanic.

The patient is a mechanic with many years of experience. Occupational history showed that as at the time of consultation he had been working as a mechanic for slightly over 20 years. He used a coverall that covered his body and the upper limbs up to the elbows. He did not practice the wearing of gloves or use of any form of personal protective equipment (PPE) for his hands or forearms. He did not use goggles. He did not use face masks even when he worked on or emptied petrol tanks of cars. He did not protect his body in any way when he drained car tanks to work on them and when he refilled fuel tanks with the fuel that he stored temporarily in a jerry can. He acknowledged that his hands and forearms were exposed to petroleum products especially when he worked on vehicle engines. He had inadequate supply of water for washing his upper limbs periodically while working, especially when petroleum products made direct contact with his skin. He made no provision for whole body washing before leaving the workplace for home, but he usually left his coveralls at the mechanic workshop. He removed and changed his clothes when he returned home from work. He washed his hands before eating at home, but inadequacy of water in the workplace did not allow him to do that during working hours; in that circumstance, he used cutlery to eat as much as was reasonably practicable. At home, he tried to separate his work clothes from clean clothes. He washed his entire body before going to bed.

Signs

Figure 7.25: Examination of the affected parts showed stained palms with "roughness" and thickening of the palms and dorsi of the hands. There were hyperpigmented scars of the hands, wrists, and forearms up to the proximal one-third of the forearms both anteriorly and posteriorly, especially posteriorly. There were healed scratch marks. There was no fissure. The palms were stained. On enquiry during the physical examina-

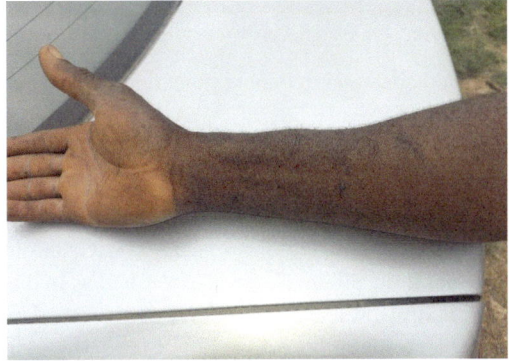

Fig. 7.25 The anterior surfaces of the patient's right forearm, wrist, and hand

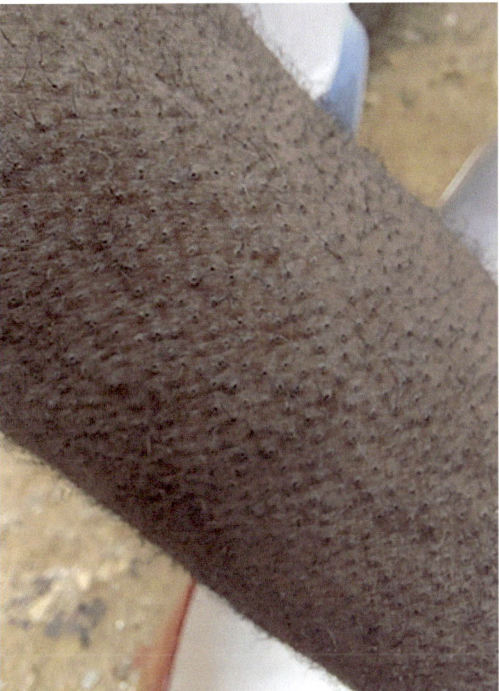

Fig. 7.26 An enlargement of a portion of the anterior surface of the right forearm

tion, the patient said that the hyperpigmented scars were from scratching of the skin and not from traumatic injury in the workplace.

Figure 7.26: The forearms were dry and dusky; the posterior parts had scanty and unusually short hairs. Both anterior and posterior forearms demonstrated prominent elevated areas surrounding the hairs.

Diagnosis

Chronic chemical irritant contact dermatitis

Treatment

Treatment consists of topical corticosteroid creams. If the affected area is extensive, as in this patient, it is preferred to use oral corticosteroids. Emollients and moisturizers should be applied to the affected areas. The prescription for this patient was hydrocortisone 1% cream. He was asked to apply a mild body lotion mixed equally or 2 to 1 with pure glycerin especially at night before going to sleep.

Etiology

Irritant contact dermatitis results from a direct cytotoxic trauma to the skin. In this patient, the insult was from repetitive exposure for a long time to chemicals that are present in petroleum products.

Prognosis

The prognosis of irritant contact dermatitis is good in patients whose exposure is once or a few times with long intervening periods that allow healing to occur and be complete. In the patient discussed, and similar patients whose exposure is regular due to their occupation, a change of occupation may be the solution in severe cases; in others, adjustment in the workplace and work procedures that minimize or eliminate direct contact of the irritant with the patient's skin can make the prognosis favorable.

Follow-Up Care

This patient did not return for follow-up care. The author's suspicion, based on this patient's expression and attitude during the consultation especially when the remedying approach and actions he was required to make is that he did not accept any disruption of his routine and occupational practices. When a general physician faces this situation, the best thing is to refer the patient to the dermatologist. Unfortunately, this patient did not even keep the first follow-up appointment for referral to be considered, offered, and made.

Discussion

Crude oil is the natural resource from which petroleum products are manufactured. Petroleum products are hydrocarbons; hydrocarbons are made up of the basic building blocks—hydrogen and carbon. The mixture of hydrogen atoms and carbon atoms in a variety of combinations and chemical linkages with other atoms produces the wide range of hydrocarbons currently in use.

Petroleum products may be in gaseous, liquid, or semisolid form, and so they may come as cooking gas and other types of gas, diesel, or gasoline (petrol), engine oil, grease, asphalt (bitumen), etc. These products may therefore be in forms that are inhaled in the air we breathe, e.g., cooking gas or gasoline if they are released to the environment where human beings are present; it is imperative for these to be contained in cylinders (for gases) or tanks and other containers (e.g., for petrol that is a liquid that evaporates).

Apart from safety considerations, petroleum products pose health concerns when they are not handled or used in the way they are supposed to be.

Usual clinical features Features of chronic irritant contact dermatitis include pruritus, ill-defined areas of involvement, lichenification, and fissuring. When the disruption of the stratum corneum caused by the irritant heals, the skin changes may be restored. When frequent re-exposure does not allow the natural healing process to occur or be complete, there may not only be lichenification but also scar formation.

Investigations A patient who does not know the provoking agent or is exposed to multiple agents that could cause contact dermatitis may require patch skin testing to determine the precise cause as a patient may have both allergic contact dermatitis and irritant contact dermatitis. In chronic irritant contact dermatitis, a skin biopsy followed by histopathological examination of the specimen aids in making the diagnosis. When contact dermatitis is acute, an observant patient can associate the acute onset of the skin condition with contact with the irritant.

Avoidance of exposure When it is possible, e.g., accidental, or occasional exposure to the irritant without the knowledge of it as the causative agent, as soon as possible after the doctor identifies the cause, the patient should stop the exposure. In occupational settings, appropriate personal protective equipment must be used.

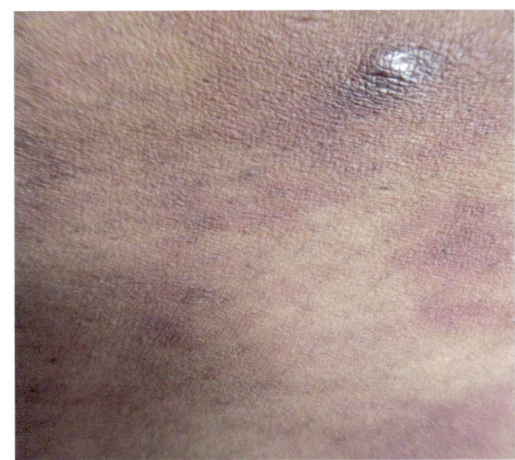

Fig. 7.27 The upper back of the patient

Skin Bleaching

Symptoms

This patient, in her early 50s, had been using a combination of body creams and lotions for many years; she did this either sequentially or at the same time. Over the years, she observed that the skin products she used to "maintain her complexion" had caused severe changes to the uniformity of her skin color and additionally affected her skin texture. Her skin had become much whiter in certain places than she desired, and in others the skin had become either unchanged in color or had become darker. Unfortunately, some parts of her body in proximity, e.g., her hands and fingers, showed this opposing color changes. This had become a cause of embarrassment to her in the presence of friends and family members.

Signs

Figure 7.27 is a photograph of the patient's upper back. On examination of her upper back, there was an island of marked lightening with extensive areas of surrounding hyperemia. The skin did not show evidence of shrinking, thinning, or sagging.

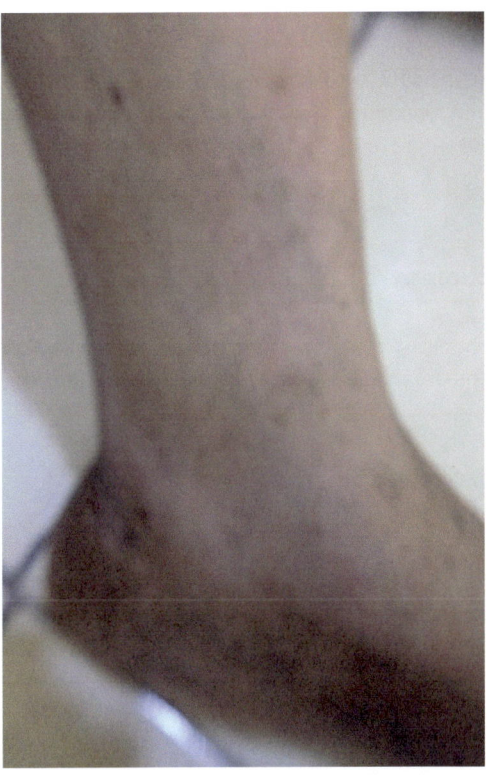

Fig. 7.28 The medial aspect of a patient's left leg and foot

Figure 7.28 is a photograph of the distal part of the left leg of this patient. Examination of this part of her body showed a clear difference in skin pigmentation; while the lower leg just above the ankle and the ankle were very light in skin pigmentation, the medial aspects of the foot and heel had multiple patches of hyperpigmentation. A close look at the lower leg shows bluish streaks demonstrating superficial veins that ordinarily should not be visible except the skin has become thin.

Diagnosis

Skin Bleaching

Treatment

Though this condition is irreversible, it may be managed by using products that can mask the most exposed part(s) of the body when the patient is in public.

Patients with high blood levels of mercury should undergo chelation treatment, but this does not improve the lightening effect of mercury on the skin.

Etiology

The basic etiology of skin bleaching is destruction or prevention of the production of melanin.

Prognosis

The prognosis of skin bleaching may be favorable in the very early stages if use of the implicating product is discontinued. It could also be fair if the active ingredient is single and affects only the skin and use of the product is promptly terminated.

Follow-Up Care

Follow-up care is essential when managing patients who have had significant damage to their skin like in skin bleaching. Each visit should be spaced appropriately to encourage the patient to keep the appointment(s) and enable the physician to obtain essential elements that point to improvement or otherwise regarding the treatment.

Discussion

Skin bleaching also goes by the more fanciful names "skin lightening" and "skin whitening." It involves the exposure of the skin, usually by application of creams or lotions, to chemical agents that have the propensity to not only reduce the numbers of melanin but also diminish the ability of melanocytes to synthesize melanin. It results from long-term use of these agents. Cosmetic products, e.g., creams, lotions, soaps, that contain bleaching agents have any or a combination of the following:

- Mercury (usually inorganic)—FDA allowable limit of mercury is 1 ppm, but many harmful products exceed this ceiling. Mercurous chloride and mercurous oxide are toxic and should not be used in cosmetic preparations.
- Hydroquinone—Topical use of hydroquinone (cream) is not associated with any significant toxicity. It is useful in the treatment of conditions with hyperpigmentation, e.g., post-inflammatory hyperpigmentation, freckles, melasma, solar lentigines, and chloasma [7]. However, indiscriminate and prolonged use of hydroquinone outside the recommended purposes may result in damage to skin. Hydroquinone has adverse effects that include skin inflammation, xeroderma, and erythema; it also tends to cause a false rise in glucose levels when capillary blood sample is used, e.g., glucometer as it interferes with a reagent.
- Clobetasol—This is a potent corticosteroid and, over time, may cause elevation of blood pressure and blood glucose or impede blood pressure and blood sugar control.
- Cortisone.
- Vitamin A.

Some bleaching agents come in the form of oral preparations.

Usual clinical features The skin of a person who achieves the desire of skin bleaching is a lighter-than-natural skin pigmentation of that patient. Occasionally, the patient discovers that the reduced pigmentation of the skin is not as originally envisaged. For other patients, the new pigmentation was never intended as the patient just wanted "toning" of the skin. For yet other patients, they were totally oblivious of the constituents of the skin products they have been using, especially at the beginning. Some of the patients knew that they would, over the months and years of using the cosmetic creams and lotions, achieve lightening of their skin but did not plan for or anticipate the extent and irreversibility of the depigmentation of their skin. Many patients do not know of any other effect of these products on the skin (or other parts of the body). The patients are usually women, but recently men are patients too.

The skin lightening may be uniform or variegated; in the latter, mottling in skin color is an esthetic embarrassment for some patients, especially when it occurs in exposed parts like the dorsi of hands where the knuckles tend to be more resistant to color change than other portions.

Another feature of skin bleaching is thinning of the skin; the thinning in some patients could be severe enough for a close look to reveal the outline of superficial veins. Such thinned skin is susceptible to bruising and other forms of injury.

Striae distensae (stretch marks) are associated features of skin bleaching in certain patients.

Some patients achieve skin lightening from laser therapy.

Investigations When required, investigations are not to make a diagnosis as this can be achieved from history of the condition and physical findings on examination.

Investigations may be carried out to find out the effects of some of the products, e.g., on kidney function. Blood and urine tests can demonstrate high levels of mercury. Serum electrolytes, urea, and creatinine and urinalysis may show alteration in renal function indicating damage to the kidneys. A complete blood count may show changes in blood cells. Liver function tests may determine if the liver has been affected or not. A suspicious area of the skin may require a skin biopsy and histopathological examination for skin cancer.

Segmental Vitiligo

Symptoms

This patient who was just over 20 years old came to the hospital with complaints of progressive, painless, non-itchy, multiple, white patches of the skin of his face for over 2 years. He felt distraught about the rashes that were essentially limited to one part of the body—his face; he would have preferred them to affect an inconspicuous part of the body. He knew that the rashes were not of sudden onset but could not satisfactorily describe the degree of progression of this condition with a gradual onset.

He did not complain about numbness or tingling over the affected part but rather believed that he had normal sensation of pain, touch, and vibration like on the unaffected part of the face and other parts of his body. He was the only person in the family who had this condition. He was not happy with the fact that his age mates shunned him and some felt that he had leprosy or some other infectious disease. He came for this consultation with the hope that he would receive effective treatment as everything he had tried in the form of orthodox and traditional medicine has proved inefficacious.

Signs

Figure 7.29: There is an extensive whitish but irregularly shaped macule on the right side of the face. The superior border of the macular lesion is just below the root of the nose which is a part of the nasal bridge. It covers the right side of the ridge of the nose, the right ala of the nose, the right nasolabial fold, the malar area, and the cheek (part of which has a peninsula of normal skin). Just beyond (medial to) the pen-

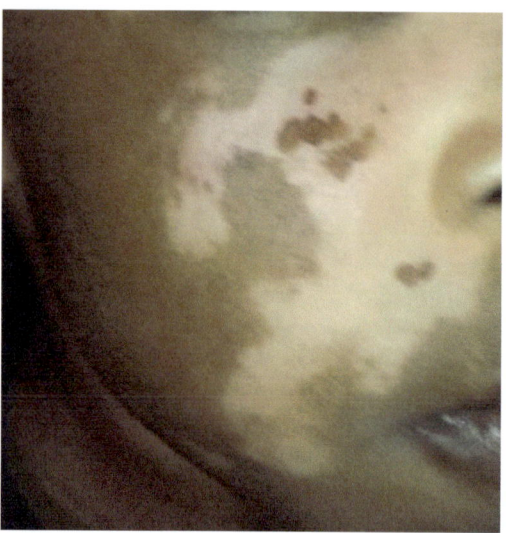

Fig. 7.29 Lesions on the face of an adult male

insula, the macule spares five islands of normally pigmented skin—three are large while the remaining two are tiny.

The lesion was non-tender and there was no anesthesia or dysesthesia.

Diagnosis

Segmental vitiligo

Treatment

This patient needed treatment by dermatologists as they are better equipped to choose the form of treatment and reevaluate the patient's response to therapy.

Treatment options include topical drugs, phototherapy, laser therapy, surgical therapy, etc. Drug treatment includes topical steroids and calcineurin inhibitors, e.g., tacrolimus and cyclosporine. Phototherapy with narrowband ultraviolet (UV)-B phototherapy may be administered.

However, since patients show variable results to treatment, it is wise for the patient to be informed of this variability among patients.

Prognosis

With extensive vitiligo, the prognosis is not good; the dermatologist requires patience and the ability to transmit their confidence and expertise to the patient for the patient to get encouragement. The patient needs resilience and hope to get a satisfactory response to treatment.

Follow-Up Care

Follow-up care for selected patients may require the input of behavioral physicians, and so such patients should be referred to these specialists timeously.

Discussion

The patient is a young person, but vitiligo can affect people at any age and no gender is spared.

Types In this patient with the rashes essentially limited to one side or part of the body, the lesion is called segmental vitiligo. When it affects a small part of the body or just one portion, it is referred to as focal vitiligo. When the rashes are widespread and affect a significant portion of the body, it is generalized and, when the distribution is on both sides of the body, it is symmetrical.

Unlike alopecia, vitiligo presents as an absence of skin pigmentation, while alopecia features normal skin pigmentation. Like alopecia, vitiligo has an autoimmune etiology. Damage to structure and/or function of melanocytes leads to loss/lack of melanin. Any part of the skin may be affected, and mucosa may be affected too, e.g., nasal and buccal mucosa; moreover, the skin that is frequently initially affected is of the extremities and the face. Hair on the affected parts of the skin can also be de-pigmented, e.g., scalp hair, eyebrows, and eyelashes. The retina may also be affected.

Usual symptoms and signs The symptom is gradual loss of pigmentation of the skin usually in

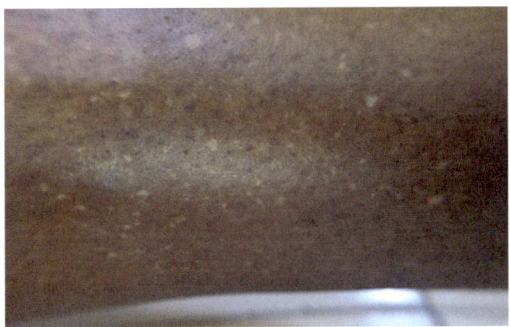

Fig. 7.30 The right leg of a 51-year-old female

a patchy manner; the progression is indeterminate and may thus be gradual in one person and relatively fast in another patient. The rashes are not pruritic or painful. There is no paresthesia or dysesthesias. In terms of signs, these macules are depigmented (whitish), irregular in shape, non-scaly, and initially patchy. Since the rashes, even when few and focal, tend to occur in visible parts of the body like the face and hands, patients must deal with the associated psychological impact. Family members, friends, classmates, schoolmates, and colleagues may not understand that the condition is benign and noncontagious and may subject the patients to covert or overt stigma.

Disseminated Lenticular Leukoderma (Idiopathic Guttate Hypomelanosis)

Symptoms

The first (female) patient complained of whitish spots on both legs. The rashes were initially few but had, over the 2-year duration since onset, gradually increased in number significantly. The "spots" did not seem to increase in size. There were no complaints of pruritus, pain, or other symptoms. Neither her face, upper limbs, nor other parts of her body were affected. She had not been using skin lightening cream. She felt embarrassed by their large number and attention-attracting color. This was a secondary condition as she came to the clinic with another skin condition that occasioned the consultation.

Signs

On examination, there were numerous small hypopigmented macules of various sizes and shapes but majorly under 5 mm. Each had a clear demarcation with normal skin. No other part of the body was involved.

This second patient is a man in his mid-60s. The two whitish rashes have been there for about 1 year, were asymptomatic, had neither increased in size nor number, and did not give the elderly man any concern; they were just skin color changes not found anywhere else on the body. Figure 7.33 is a close-up photograph of the upper rash shown in Fig. 7.32.

On examination of the hypopigmented rashes, there was loss of hair in these tiny rashes that were roughly circular and measured about 4 mm each.

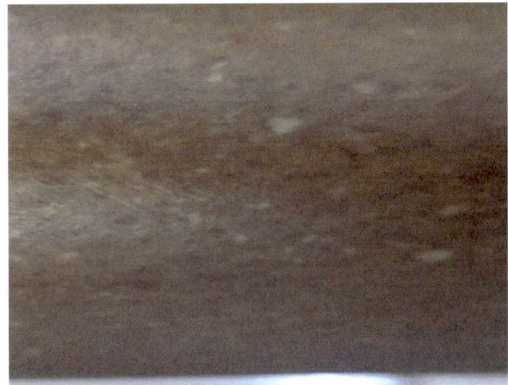

Fig. 7.31 The right leg of the same patient

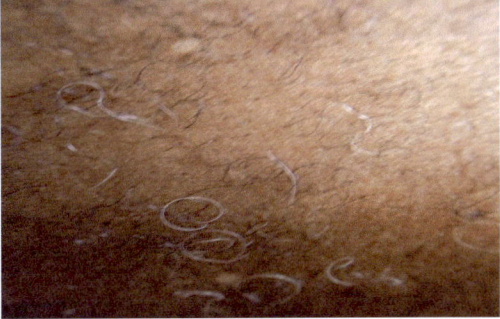

Fig. 7.32 Lateral aspect of the right mid-thigh of a man

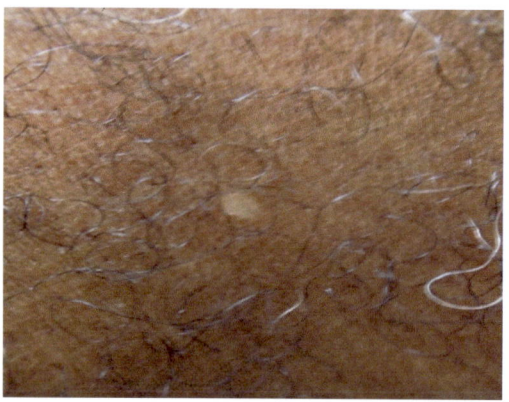

Fig. 7.33 Lateral aspect of the right mid-thigh of a man

Diagnosis

Disseminated lenticular leukoderma (idiopathic guttate hypomelanosis)

Treatment

Primary therapy consists of masking the lesions with skin coloring and significantly reducing the duration and intensity of exposure to sunlight. Drug therapy, when required, entails using topical agents like corticosteroids and retinoids, e.g., Retin-A®, tretinoin cream, or gel especially when the lesions are not extensive and the patient is concerned with the aesthetic blemish to exposed skin. Intralesional corticosteroids may be given. Some patients may require cryotherapy or dermabrasion. For many patients, treatment may not be required and the physician may simply explain the relationship between the condition and the environment. Apart from minimizing exposure to sunlight, prevention entails advice to young women to avoid tanning their legs; this may be more relevant for girls and young women who have a family history of this condition.

Etiology

As at the time of writing, the etiology of this skin condition is unknown. However, it is believed that it is related to prolonged exposure to the sun with consequent deleterious effects on melanocytes. It may be multifactorial in etiology with an admixture of environmental and genetic factors. It is, however, a benign leukoderma.

Prognosis

The prognosis of idiopathic guttate hypomelanosis is good in so far as it is an asymptomatic and benign condition that can be tolerated by the patient without treatment or treated with satisfactory result.

Follow-Up Care

Not many patients require more than one or a few appointments for follow-up care.

Discussion

Disseminated lenticular leukoderma is a well-known cause of acquired leukoderma.

Usual clinical features Hypopigmentation of patches of the skin occurs in both light-skinned and dark-skinned individuals as they grow older. The condition is commoner from middle age onwards, and the lesions tend to increase in number as the affected persons grow older. Men and women are affected, but it tends to be commoner in women. Exposed parts of the body also tend to be more affected though lesions are uncommon on the face and neck. It is not only benign but also asymptomatic. Patients usually present because of aesthetic concerns.

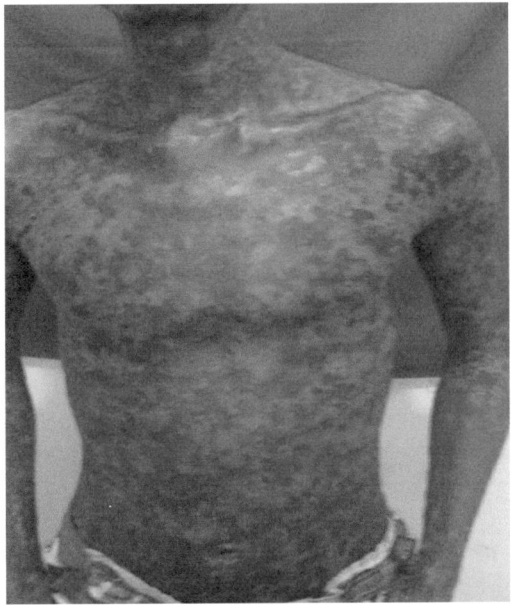

Fig. 7.34 A young man in his early 20s with extensive rashes

Investigations Idiopathic guttate hypomelanosis usually does not require investigations as it is largely a clinical diagnosis. In the early stages of the condition, dermoscopy shows nebuloid morphology with indistinct, smudged borders. Skin biopsy of the lesion is not usual; when done, histopathological examination of the affected lesions shows decrease in the total number of DOPA oxidase-positive melanocytes in the stratum basale of the epidermis. This is not the case in vitiligo in which there is complete absence of melanocytes.

Erythroderma (Generalized Exfoliative Dermatitis)

Symptoms

Generalized rashes affecting the body from the face to the feet and the neck to the heel. The patient said that he developed febrile illness for which he purchased some drugs in "a chemist shop." He did not know the names of the medications, but the person who operated the shop mixed some drugs for him to go home and take when he laid his complaints of fever and body pains to the man. When he got home, he took the drugs as he was directed, and he felt better by the next day. He took the rest of the drugs as dispensed and instructed and was well within 5 days. However, within 2 weeks of taking the medications, he developed these unprecedented rashes. His entire body was itchy, and the rashes developed rapidly to envelop most parts of his skin within a few days. His hitherto smooth skin became scaly. He loathed his current looks, and his friends were shocked to see the exposed parts of his body. He had never had any skin illness resembling his current illness in any form; he was unaware of anybody in his family or neighborhood with this type of disease. He was unaware of having allergy to any food or drugs. He did not take any herbal preparation prior to or during the current febrile illness. He decided to come to the hospital as soon as he could gather the funds as he concluded that this illness was something beyond the chemist shops in his community. He hoped that he would receive satisfactory treatment in the hospital and wished that he would not have a recurrence of this skin condition.

Signs

This patient's general condition belied the severity of his condition; this was because he walked into the consulting room when it was his turn to be attended to. It is unclear why he did not opt for treatment in the emergency room. On examination, virtually the entire body was involved, from face to the feet anteriorly and the entire trunk posteriorly. There was scaling of the lesions. At the time he came for consultation, there was no evidence of being in the acute phase as the findings were scaly lesions that had fallen off leaving a generalized area of hypopigmentation with interspersed normal skin.

Diagnosis

Erythroderma (generalized exfoliative dermatitis)

The doctors in a clinic of the general outpatient department promptly referred this patient to the dermatologist. The dermatologist made a diagnosis of erythroderma and took over the management of this patient.

Treatment

The treatment of a patient with the diagnosis of erythroderma may involve the following [8]:

- Admission into the wards for satisfactory monitoring—thus temperature monitoring will help prevent the patient from becoming hypothermic, and fluid input and output monitoring will assist in preventing the development of either dehydration or cardiac failure.
- Maintenance of skin moisture—application of wet gauze dressings with the use of topical steroids underneath the dressing, tepid bathing, and later application of emollients.
- Good nutrition, especially high protein to counter protein loss from skin desquamation.
- Treatment of the identified etiology, e.g., psoriasis—this encourages early resolution of erythroderma. The doctor should do this, ensuring avoidance of unnecessary drugs.
- Avoidance of scratching to prevent bacterial infection—clipping the patient's nails short and use of oral antihistamines are helpful.
- Prevention of complications or prompt and effective treatment of complications if the patient presented with them.

Etiology

There are many potential causes of exfoliative dermatitis. Attempts at elucidating the etiology of exfoliative dermatitis may yield positive results, but in many cases, they do not—about 30% of cases are idiopathic. The following are some of the causes: drug allergy, seborrheic dermatitis, psoriasis, lichen planus, lupus erythematosus, atopic dermatitis, contact dermatitis, dermatophytosis, etc. The etiology may be systemic diseases associated with some of the listed skin conditions; the systemic diseases include cancers, e.g., leukemia, lymphoma, cancer of the rectum, and non-cancers, e.g., HIV infection, mycosis fungoides, and reactive arthritis. There are numerous drugs that have been implicated in the etiology of exfoliative dermatitis, and so the doctor should enquire about current and recent drug exposure—in some instances, the patient may have forgotten about having taken the drug in one form or another.

Prognosis

The prognosis of generalized exfoliative dermatitis is not good if the trigger factor is a preexisting systemic disease like psoriasis or if there are complications like high-output cardiac failure and sepsis from severe secondary bacterial infection.

Follow-Up Care

The physician advises the patient to return to the clinic for review of their condition, explaining why. In this patient, it was necessary to be followed up by the dermatologist.

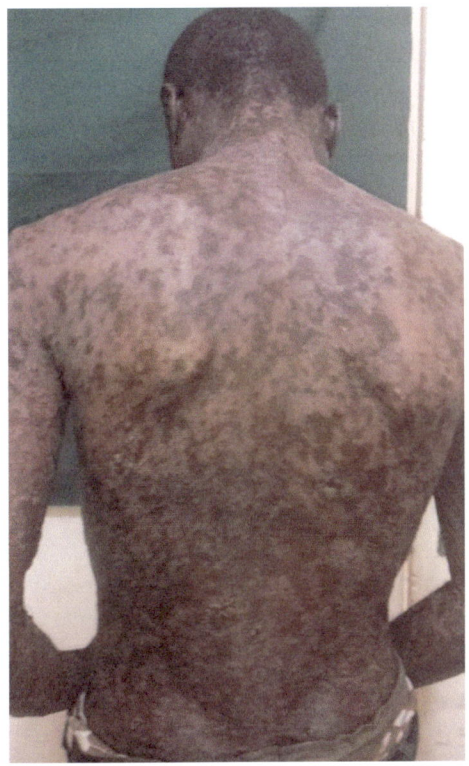

Fig. 7.35 The same young man with extensive rashes

Discussion

Erythroderma is generalized exfoliative dermatitis. Males are at least twice more likely to develop exfoliative dermatitis, and the age may reflect the underlying disease entity though most patients are at least in their fifth decade of life. There is usually a precipitating entity; however, this resultant clinical presentation may overshadow or overwhelm the precipitant.

History The physician should be patient and aim at taking a comprehensive history. Since the patient with erythroderma may have had a dermatological condition that now seems to pale into insignificance as the etiology, it is necessary for the patient to help the physician unearth such conditions, e.g., atopic dermatitis or contact dermatitis. Alternatively, since the patient may have used medications orally or in injection form, enquiry should be made directly for a list of drug names or indirectly for illnesses for which the patient was treated with drugs—those prescribed by physicians, "suggested" or "recommended" by nonmedical people, and purchased over the counter or herbal preparations made locally or sold in some pharmaceutical outlets.

Clinical presentation The presentation is a patient with generalized erythematous eruption; within 1 week, exfoliation which manifests as loss of skin with peeling and scaling follows. In the Black skin, the inflammatory process does not present as erythematous eruption except in the patient with light skin tone. Exfoliation usually starts from flexural surfaces; scratching, because of itching, leads to excoriation. Within a couple of weeks loss of hair and nail may result. As the condition progresses, there may be changes in pigmentation of the skin as seen in the patient above who had extensive areas of skin hypopigmentation. There may be lymphadenopathy. Careful and detailed physical examination of the patient may show features of the underlying skin disease, e.g., psoriasis, lichen planus, etc.

Investigations After detailed history taking and physical examination, the investigations for patients with suspected erythroderma may include the following:

- Full blood count for anemia
- Erythrocyte sedimentation rate for elevation
- Serum protein for hypoalbuminemia and hyperglobulinemia—e.g., IgE (in atopic dermatitis)
- Peripheral blood smear and bone marrow studies for cell morphology for leukemia
- HIV infection detection by polymerase chain reaction
- Skin scrapings for fungal studies or for the mite, *Sarcoptes scabiei* var hominis
- Appropriate cultures for herpes simplex virus or for overgrowth of bacteria

Other tests may be performed for cancer as the etiology, depending on the age and sex of the patient, e.g.:

- Papanicolaou smear test for cancer of the cervix
- Mammography for cancer of the breast
- Prostate-specific antigen and digital rectal examination for cancer of the prostate
- Stool examination for occult blood for upper gastrointestinal cancers
- Sigmoidoscopy for lower gastrointestinal cancers

Drug and nondrug contact allergens may be sought for by carrying out patch skin tests when the patient is in remission. Histology shows chronic or subacute dermatitis, but biopsy results may indicate the underlying skin disease. These and other tests may be repeated in some patients during the management of erythroderma.

Complications The complications of erythroderma include the following:

- Temperature dysregulation (e.g., hypothermia) from extensive loss of the skin—prevention of hypothermia may be achieved by the use of Bair hugger systems to warm patients
- High-output cardiac failure
- Dehydration
- Electrolyte imbalance
- Secondary bacterial infection

Other complications have a bearing on the etiology of erythroderma in the index patient.

Toxic Epidermal Necrolysis

Symptoms

The patient, in her early 40s, was rushed to the emergency room of the hospital. The husband, who brought her, indicated that she was ill about 2 weeks earlier and purchased medications over the counter from a small drug store in the community. The person who operates the outlet listened to her complaint of fever and severe body pains and gave her a combination of drugs that consisted of tablets and a capsule. It was as she completed the last of the medications that she noticed that her entire body was itchy, and, within 24 h, she developed rashes from various parts of the body. By the next day, blisters covered an extensive portion of her body, and she became darker than her normal complexion. There was associated pain as the rashes continued to increase in size. It was not possible for her to adopt any position that would give her rest. She felt more ill than she had ever felt. The husband could not attend to his business because of the wife's deterioration in health. He took her to the nearest health center, but the healthcare personnel said that they could not handle the extensive burns that his wife had developed. They simply gave her injection for paid and itching and asked him to take her to a "big hospital" where they would admit her for proper medical treatment. They said that they do not hospitalize patients and did not know how to handle her condition.

The history was obtained after the doctors-on-call quickly evaluated her; put her on oxygen delivered by mask, opioid analgesic, intravenous broad-spectrum antibiotic, and intravenous infusion of metronidazole; provided other urgent care; and referred her to both the dermatology unit of the department of medicine and burns unit of the department or surgery.

Signs

The patient was conscious, in pain, restless but could not turn her body from the pain, and tachypneic. It was difficult to check her temperature or her conjunctivae, but she had dry lips, tongue, and mouth. Her pulse rate was high, but her blood pressure was in the normal range. There was nowhere on the arms to connect the sphygmomanometer because of the involvement of both upper limbs; however, the doctor spotted an area in the lower limb which was suitable for tying the cuff. The doctors and nurses decided to leave the sphygmomanometer in situ, thus devoting the apparatus for her sole use.

She had more than 85% superficial burns that affected the head and neck, the trunk anteriorly and posteriorly, the upper limbs, and lower limbs. The lesions were hyperpigmented where there were bullae and vesicles but hyperemic where she had lost superficial skin from sloughing. On the trunk, there was evidence of recent break of some vesicles and bullae with fluid that looks serum while in other parts of the body there was dried, crusted, and discharged.

Since the presentation was the same everywhere in her body, the description of Fig. 7.36 represents the other Figures. Only the ones that demonstrate additional features are briefly described.

Figure 7.36 is the left side of the face and neck of a woman with plaited hair. There is hyperpigmentation of the skin. There is irregularity of the surface of the skin at the left forehead; the skin at that site is not only hyperpigmented but is black, just like her hair. On the lateral part of the left

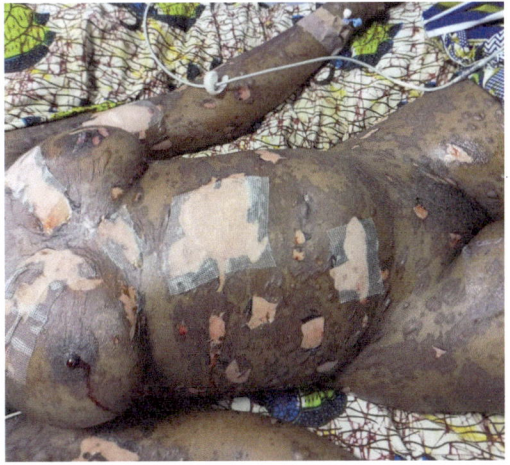

Fig. 7.37 Frontal view of most of the patient's body

side of the frontal scalp skin (mid-way between the left ear and the top left end of the image), there is a light-yellow crusted skin with flipping of the skin anteriorly.

Every part of the left ear is involved in the lesion with loss of skin and exposure of the ear cartilages at the helix, antihelix, crura of the antihelix, antitragus, and lobule. Detached skin covers the upper part of the lobule, concha (cavum and cymba), intertragal notch (incisura), and the tragus. Parts of the skin over the temporal area and the submandibular area are also detached, but not completely.

Of the seven selected photographs, Figs. 7.37 and 7.42 are significantly different as they show nipple hemorrhage.

The rest of the Figures are to illustrate the extent of skin coverage by this condition.

Diagnosis

Toxic epidermal necrolysis

Treatment

Despite the care that healthcare providers in the emergency unit gave the patient, neither the burns nor dermatology units could do much for her as she died within 72 h after arrival in the hospital.

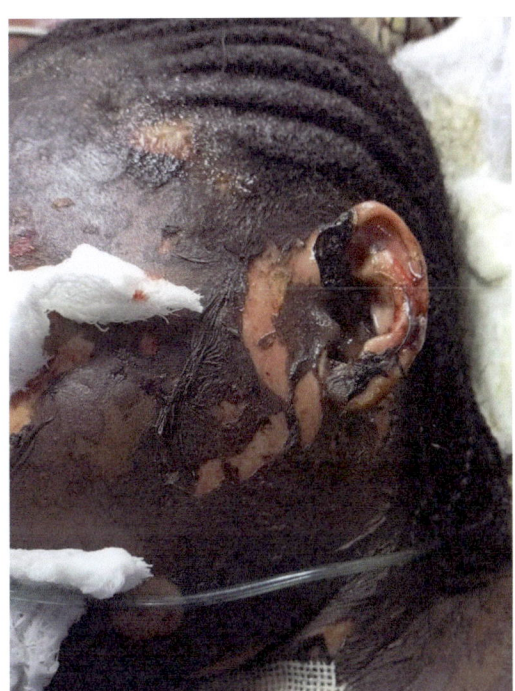

Fig. 7.36 Left side of the patient's head

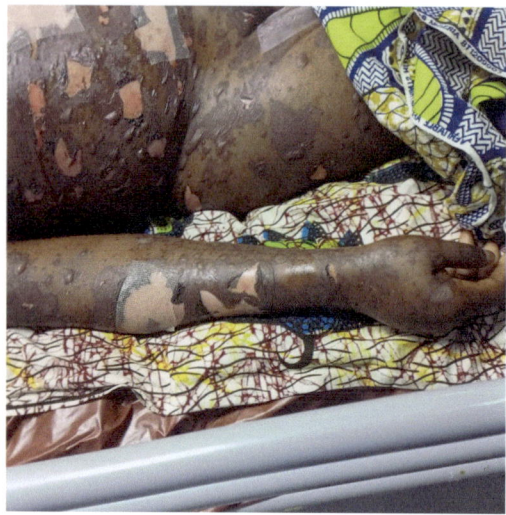

Fig. 7.38 Right half of the patient's body

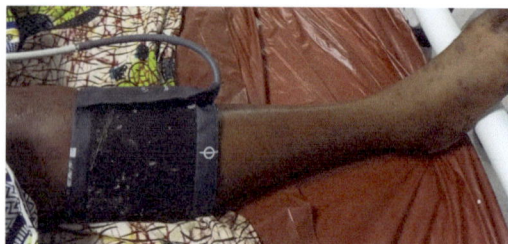

Fig. 7.39 Blood pressure monitoring using the patient's right leg

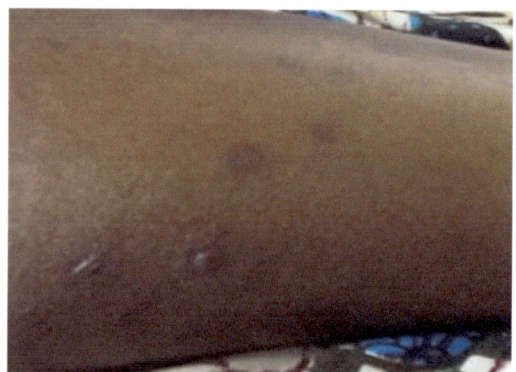

Fig. 7.40 Target lesions on the patient's leg

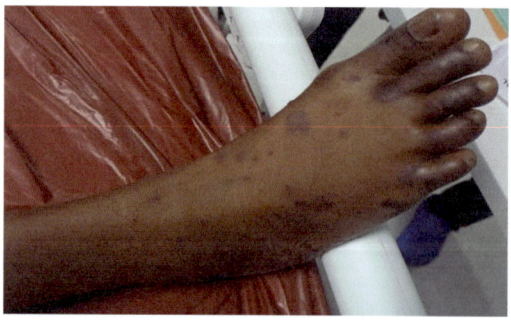

Fig. 7.41 Involvement of the ankles, foot, and toes

Etiology

The etiology of toxic epidermal necrolysis (TEN) is exaggerated apoptosis of keratinocytes. The condition is characterized by extensive detachment of the skin.

Prognosis

The prognosis of toxic epidermal necrolysis is not good; it was not, particularly for the patient whose condition the author describes in this case study. The starting point of her treatment was late, and her chances of survival were slim. Unfortunately, she died.

Follow-Up Care

For this patient, follow-up care was out of the question.

For patients who survive, multiple units or teams in the hospital would comanage their condition, and they are eventually discharged from the wards, with great caution. The follow-up care would involve specialists in the specialties that provided care during hospitalization.

There was no suitable place on the upper limb to do blood pressure monitoring.

Figure 7.40 shows an enlargement of the right leg to demonstrate healing target lesions on the skin.

Figure 7.41: The photographed portion of the right lower limb shows mild-to-moderate skin lesions compared to the ones on the trunk. The macular eruptions on the dorsi of the right toes are hyperpigmented.

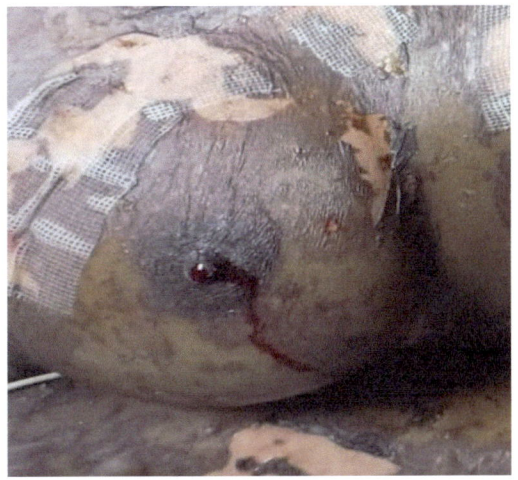

Fig. 7.42 Hemorrhage from the nipple of the right breast

Figure 7.42 shows hemorrhaging right nipple.

Discussion

Toxic epidermal necrolysis is an acute inflammatory disorder that focuses on the epidermis and mucous membranes. This uncommon but severe condition with a relatively high mortality rate presents as extensive bullae and vesicles; it is so severe and acute that in a short period the affected skin and mucous membrane is shed in large sheets; on the skin the extent of damage is visible, but mucosal membrane may be underestimated as these are present in parts of the body that are internal.

In toxic epidermal necrolysis (TEN), there is excessive apoptosis of keratinocytes. This severe dermatological condition is characterized by extensive detachment of the skin. It is a dermatological emergency with complications that may cause death; the mortality is about 30%. TEN is frequently linked with drugs, but it may be an idiosyncratic reaction.

Success in the management of toxic epidermal necrolysis (TEN) is predicated on making a timely diagnosis. In the practice setting where this condition is reported, this becomes a herculean task because due to poverty, preference of alternative healing methods, opting for "chemist shops" (these outlets for sale of drugs over the counter with no need for prescription, other than the recommendation of the seller are right there in the rural areas), a high reliance on hope for spiritual healing, and the distance required to be traversed to arrive at and access care in the appropriate hospitals, acutely and severely ill patients hardly arrive in the time required to receive expert medical services.

Treatment principles include the following [9]:

- Hospitalization, preferably in the intensive care unit (ICUF)
- Hospitalization to continue in other wards with emphasis on which body system is most greatly impacted
- Fluid and electrolyte management
- Pain management
- Nutritional support preferably with involvement of a nutritionist/dietician
- Surgical dressings to protect denuded skin
- Satisfactory antibiotic cover to prevent or treat infections, including anaerobic infection
- Care by teams of specialists

The investigations that should be carried out are similar to the ones listed for erythroderma (an earlier topic in this chapter).

Fixed Drug Eruption

Symptoms

Figure 7.43 shows a 4-year-old female. The mother complained of severe generalized itching, while the child was receiving treatment for a febrile illness with a presumptive diagnoses of sore throat and malaria. The itching involved the head soon followed by rashes that appeared on dark patches that she had about 1 year earlier; this time, however, the rashes were more as she developed rashes at other parts of the skin where there were none. The rashes affected much of the body and involved the head, trunk (anterior and posterior), and the extremities. History obtained from the patient's mother was that

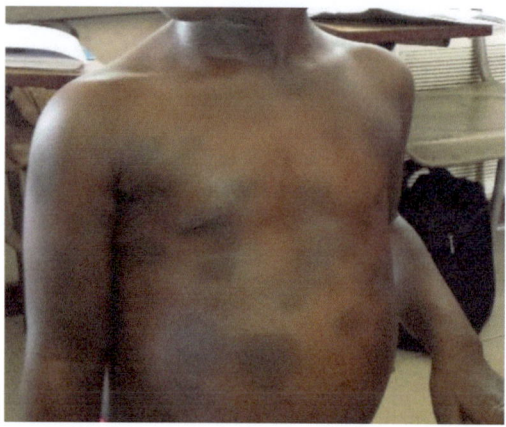

Fig. 7.43 The upper extremities and anterior trunk of a 4-year-old female

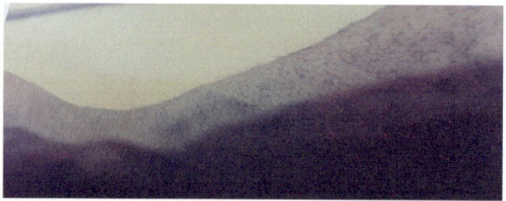

Fig. 7.44 The right forearm of a young adult male patient

she had recently received treatment with a sulfonamide. She did not have any other symptoms. There were no systemic features.

Figure 7.44 shows the forearm of a young adult male patient. He came to the clinic to make complaints that were not related to a dermatological condition. He was attended to regarding the current illness. However, during physical examination, the large black patch on his right forearm attracted the doctor. Enquiry about the skin lesion showed that the patient took medication from a local chemist shop for fever about 1 year earlier. Within 1 week of taking the single dose of the medication, he developed the patch on the same spot where he had a first patch at least 6 months earlier. This time, the patch was larger by the time it healed. In each instance, he had severe itching. He had made up his mind not to purchase medications from non-doctors; this was one of the reasons he came to the hospital with the current health challenge.

Signs

Figure 7.43: Multiple discrete, irregularly shaped, hyperpigmented macular eruptions on the face, neck, chest wall, abdominal wall, upper limbs, and lower limbs. A close examination of the child's photograph shows involvement of her lips. The macules have clearly defined margins and were black even in this child with Black skin with moderate tone. A few of the rashes have a regular outline and are oval or circular. There is a large patch on her neck and over the left mandible. The mandibular part of this large patch is about 5 cm × 2 cm at the widest diameters, while the one on the neck is about 8 cm × 2.5 cm in length and height.

Figure 7.44: A single longitudinal hyperpigmented macular patch of the skin on the lateral aspect of the distal right forearm and the wrist. The rash in this patient with Black skin of deep tone is black; it is much more hyperpigmented than the patient's normal skin. The rash measures 14 cm × 6 cm at the widest diameters.

Diagnosis

Fixed drug eruptions for the child and fixed drug eruption for the man.

Treatment

Loratadine syrup, although this is more expensive than the drugs in the first generation promethazine and chlorpheniramine that cause drowsiness in patients.

The adult patient did not require any medication as the black patch was not what brought him to the hospital for consultation.

Etiology

Regarding the etiology and pathophysiology of fixed drug eruptions,

- The offending drug has affinity for keratino-cytes in the stratum basale; the drug functions as a hapten.
- Memory T cells and CD8⁺ effector cells con-tribute significantly to reactivation of lesions of fixed drug eruptions when the incriminating drug is used, usually parenterally or orally.
- Locally there is upregulation of intercellular adhesion molecule-1 (ICAM-1) by keratinocytes.
- Keratinocytes liberate tumor necrosis factor-α. Tumor necrosis factor-α is one of the cyto-kines released by keratinocytes in fixed drug eruption.
- CD8 cells survive an episode, and this is from interleukin expression by keratinocytes; CD8 cells survival ensures storage of memory which is rapidly expressed when the drug is reused resulting in a more rapid manifestation of the lesions at the same site.

Prognosis

The prognosis of fixed drug eruption is good when the condition is not severe and does not leave permanent black patches on the skin.

Prognosis is also good when the patient or caregivers of the patient identify the trigger and ensure that the patient avoids them.

When the patient has many lesions, like the pediatric patient, the patient should be referred to a dermatologist to manage the condition. This child was ultimately under the care of a dermatologist.

Follow-Up Care

A general medical practitioner may provide the first follow-up care; if the lesions heal (or are healing) without any cosmetic repercussions, the general practitioner should reiterate the preven-tive measures and advise further follow-up care at the patient's discretion. If, however, the lesions are extensive and they are healing leaving hyper-pigmentation, the general medical practitioner should refer promptly to the dermatologist for follow-up care if the dermatologist was not involved in the initial care either by a prompt referral or by inviting the specialist to manage the condition in a private medical practitioner's facility.

Discussion

During history taking, the general medical practi-tioner should ask questions for the following are expected with regards to fixed drug eruptions:

- Parents who are unfamiliar with this skin con-dition, especially the trigger factors or precipi-tating agents, hardly pinpoint the offending drug except the child was taking just one med-ication at, or just before, the onset.
- A personal past medical history of drug reaction.
- History of ingestion of a combination of drugs with undisclosed names, purchased over the counter for fever and body pains.
- A positive family history of atopy.
- Occurrence after ingesting another drug but of the same class as a known culprit.

Fixed drug eruption may be sequel to the use of the following drugs by the patient:

- Sedatives
- Antibiotics
- Analgesics
- Anticonvulsants
- Muscle relaxants

Examples of antibiotics are those in the peni-cillin and quinolone classes; for analgesics, examples are nonsteroidal anti-inflammatory drugs (NSAIDs); examples of anticonvulsants are phenothiazines. Eruptions that are reminis-cent of fixed drug eruptions sometimes occur in patients for whom a thorough drug history excludes fixed drug eruptions; in such cases, a detailed food history should be obtained as nuts and food supplements may be sources of expo-sure. Food items that are implicated include pea-nuts, cashews, crabs, licorice, kiwi, strawberries, shellfish, lentils, and asparagus—in such cases the diagnosis is fixed food eruption (FFE) [10].

Symptoms associated with fixed drug eruptions include fever, malaise, anorexia, abdominal cramps, and itching. Pruritus is almost a constant symptom at the beginning of the disorder; the other symptoms are known to occur in patients with fixed drug eruption, but infrequently.

Initial exposure to the offending drug is expected to cause onset of eruption(s) later than 6 h but within approximately 2 weeks. The eruption may heal without affecting the patient's skin pigmentation. Re-exposure to the cause results in a more rapid development of the eruption; appearance of skin eruption following re-exposure may be within 1 h in some cases but may extend to 18 h.

Regarding fixed drug eruptions, the lesions may initially be erythematous in light-skinned patients with Black skin. When the lesion is single or they are few, the eruptions are usually circular or oval. The lips and the genitalia are common sites of fixed drug eruptions; other common sites are the upper extremity and hip sacral area and the lower back. Residual skin hyperpigmentation is a common finding; in patients in whom resolution occurs, many months may elapse before hyperpigmentation disappears.

Fixed drug eruptions are not limited to the exact previous site(s) as additional rashes occur when a patient is re-exposed. A fixed drug eruption is usually less than 10 cm. They may be as few as 1 and as many as 20 in 1 patient

Differential diagnoses Differential diagnoses of fixed drug eruptions include the following:

- Erythema multiforme
- Acute urticaria
- Pityriasis rosea
- Post-inflammatory hyperpigmentation

Principles of management Regarding the management of fixed drug eruptions, the physician should bear the following in mind and go on to ascertain their implementation:

- Oral antihistamines should be prescribed to patients who need them—patients who have pruritic lesions need oral antihistamines, preferably the second-generation antihistamines. These are more expensive but do not cause drowsiness that is a common side effect of the first-generation antihistamines.
- In extensive cases like in the above pediatric patient, topical application of corticosteroids on the eruptions is strongly discouraged—prescription and application of topical corticosteroids should be avoided; rather, parenteral route of administration of a defined safe dose of corticosteroid as a short course is preferred to avoid overdose via skin absorption. The parents of the child may be overenthusiastic and apply the entire tube of hydrocortisone 1% cream just once or twice. In some practice settings, the parents may go to a shop staffed by a nonprofessional who may recommend "something stronger," and not realizing who the patient is or how extensive the lesions are, the "recommended" cream may contain a fluorinated steroid which, when used on an extensive area in children, may lead to the pediatric patient developing toxic effects. There are also instances that parents keep the empty tube of the cream to enable them to purchase more, rather than returning to the hospital as the experience is traumatic for them and their children in terms of time to, at, and from the hospital coupled with absence from work for the parent and school for the child (if of school age).
- Some patients with superimposed bacterial infection may require antibiotic therapy.
- In severe cases, the patient may require hospitalization.
- Avoidance of an established causative agent is a preventive measure—the general medical practitioner should recommend this; when the risk factors have not been identified, the physician should suggest them to the patient and ask the adult to be on the lookout for them, or the parents of a minor to try and link a drug or a food to the eruption if it recurs.

Multiple-Choice Questions

1. Acne vulgaris: Which of the statements below is correct?
   A. It takes the form of papules, pustules, and nodules.
   B. It usually has its onset in middle age.
   C. It is hardly complicated by scar formation.
   D. It commonly affects the abdomen.

2. Which of the following relationships pertaining to miliaria is correct?
   A. Miliaria profunda—Superficial tiny lesions
   B. Miliaria rubra—Uncommon in infants
   C. Miliaria pustulosa—Synonymous with impetigo contagiosa
   D. Miliaria crystallina—Tiny, clear vesicles

3. Which of the following statements about miliaria is correct?
   A. Typically ductal blockage prevents sweat production
   B. Sweat duct blockage explains presentation
   C. Miliaria pustulosa does not cause heat exhaustion
   D. Inflammatory reaction is remarkable in miliaria crystallina

4. Which of the following relationships pertaining to acne vulgaris is correct?
   A. Mild acne—Comedones and many papulopustules
   B. Comedonal acne—Presence of inflammatory papules and macules
   C. Nodulocystic acne—Scarring associated with nodules >5 mm diameter
   D. Moderate acne—Absence of inflammatory papules

5. Which of the following associations regarding urticaria is correct?
   A. Bradykinin—Contributory vasoactive substance
   B. Sedentary lifestyle—Predisposing factor
   C. Wheals that do not blanch—Characteristic
   D. Avoidance of allergen—Last line of management

References

1. Guerra KC, Toncar A, Krishnamurthy K. Miliaria. In: StatPearls [Internet]; 2024. Available from: https://www.ncbi.nlm.nih.gov/books/NBK537176/#:~:text=.
2. Jaggi RJ. Acne vulgaris. Dermatology. Medscape. 2020. Available from: https://emedicine.medscape.com/article/1069804-overview#:~:text=.
3. Sun C, Lim D. Trichloroacetic acid paint for boxcar and polymorphic acne scars. Dermatologic Surg. 2022;48(2):214–8. https://doi.org/10.1097/DSS.0000000000003339. PMID: 34923523. Available from: https://pubmed.ncbi.nlm.nih.gov/34923523/#:~:text=.
4. Satter EK. Acne keloidalis nuchae (AKN) differential diagnoses. Dermatology. 2024. Available from: https://emedicine.medscape.com/article/1072149-differential.
5. Schaefer P. Urticaria: evaluation and treatment. Am Fam Physician. 2011;83(9):1078–84. Available from: https://www.aafp.org/pubs/afp/issues/2011/0501/p1078.html.
6. Wong HK. Acute urticaria. Allergy Immunol. Medscape. 2023. Available from: https://emedicine.medscape.com/article/137362-overview.
7. Schwartz C, Jan A, Zito PM. Hydroquinone. In: StatPearls [Internet]; 2023. Available from: https://www.ncbi.nlm.nih.gov/books/NBK539693/.
8. Umar SH. Erythroderma (generalized exfoliative dermatitis) treatment & management. Dermatology. Medscape. 2024. Available from: https://emedicine.medscape.com/article/1106906-treatment.
9. Jellinek-Cohen SP. Toxic epidermal necrolysis (TEN) treatment & management. Infect Dis. 2024. Available from: https://emedicine.medscape.com/article/229698-treatment#:~:text=.
10. Anderson HJ, Jason B, Lee JB. A review of fixed drug eruption with a special focus on generalized bullous fixed drug eruption. Medicina (Kaunas). 2021;57(9):925. https://doi.org/10.3390/medicina57090925. PMCID: PMC8468217. PMID: 34577848. Available from: https://pmc.ncbi.nlm.nih.gov/articles/PMC8468217/#:~:text=.

Papulosquamous disorders that are discussed in this chapter are three; they are seborrheic dermatitis, psoriasis, and lichen planus. These are conditions that general medical practitioners, the target audience of this book, need to recognize. Seborrheic dermatitis is prevalent in childhood, and in this chapter, the condition is described in the neonatal period and infancy. Psoriasis is a condition that dermatologists attend to; it runs a chronic course but still needs to get to the specialists as soon as possible after the patient reports the initial features. Getting a typical dermatologist's attention is usually by a referral by the primary care physician. How will the patient take themselves to these few and busy specialists if the patient does not go to the hospital soon after observing the signs of psoriasis; or if they observe the signs and consult the general practitioner, but the general practitioner does not make a provisional diagnosis, or do a prompt referral? The general practitioner is, therefore, an essential bridge between the patient and the dermatologist. It is also important to recognize psoriasis as a condition with involvement of multiple organs in some patients; therefore, when a general medial practitioner identifies the skin manifestations of psoriasis and refers the patient to the dermatologist, the patient with psoriasis is promptly on their journey of investigations to know the organs that might be affected by this condition. What is written on psoriasis can be extrapolated to lichen planus.

Infantile (Neonatal) Seborrheic Dermatitis

Symptoms

Figures 8.1 and 8.2 pertain to the first of the two children with the condition that is also called infantile seborrheic dermatitis (ISD). According to the mother, the 3-month-old boy developed the rashes at age 3 weeks. The rashes started at the back and soon developed on the chest, abdomen, and buttocks. Other parts of the body that were affected were the face, upper limbs, and lower limbs. The baby was not irritable even ab initio

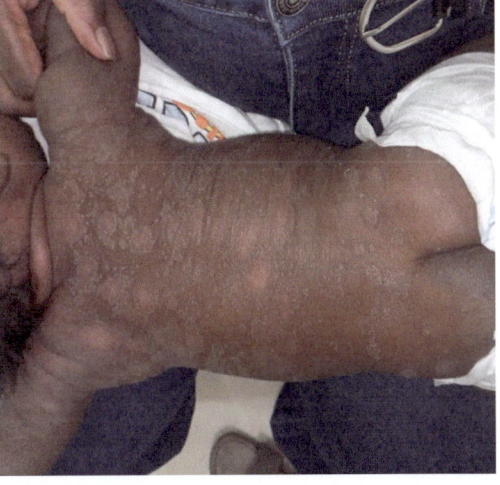

Fig. 8.1 The back, neck, arms, and buttocks of a 3-month-old boy

© The Author(s), under exclusive license to Springer Nature Switzerland AG 2025   141
I. Ukot, *Understanding Diseases in Skin of Color*, https://doi.org/10.1007/978-3-031-97503-5_8

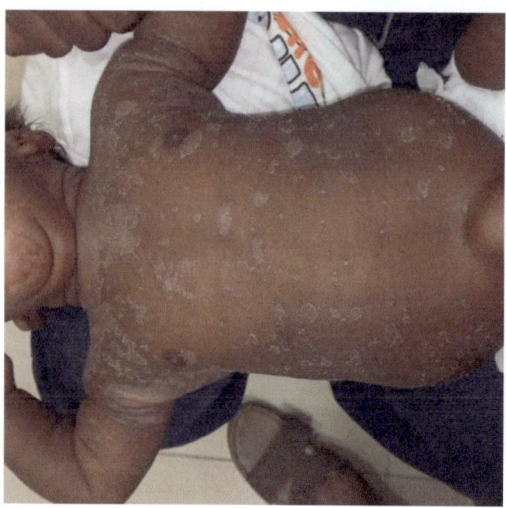

Fig. 8.2 The neck, upper limbs, chest, and abdomen of the 3-month-old boy

and there was no evidence of pain. The baby breastfed well and slept well despite the increasing number of the rashes. Since the mother did not bring the child to the hospital soon after the onset of the lesions, an enquiry was made as to the reason and what she had done; her response was that she went to a chemist shop and the attendant prescribed and sold a cream by name "triple action" for her to use on the baby. She applied the cream on the child but up to that time she had been applying a local agent called *ndom* which is a chalky substance mixed with water to form a light emulsion paste. She brought the son when there was no satisfactory response to the two modalities of treatment.

Signs

On examination, the baby had numerous irregularly shaped, slightly scaly, and grayish macules. The slight change in pigmentation was more of hypopigmentation when compared with the infant's moderate tone of the Black skin. There was extensive skin involvement of the posterior

trunk as demonstrated in Fig. 8.1; apart from the upper and lower back, the posterior and superior surfaces of the proximal arms were involved, with the buttocks least affected. The anterior trunk (chest and abdomen) had fewer rashes though they were still plentiful. The rashes as shown in Fig. 8.2 were of similar configuration as the ones on the back and affected the chest, abdomen, neck, axillae (right more than left), and the lower part of the face. Though not captured by any of the photographs, the rashes also affected the upper thighs bilaterally. The baby was not irritable during history taking until the clothes were removed and the baby was examined and later positioned for the photographs.

Figure 8.3 is a close-up photograph of the neck, chest, and upper abdomen of the same child in Figs. 8.1 and 8.2. It shows confluence of the macules on the upper chest with very irregular margins. This photograph shows slight hypopigmentation of the large rash when compared with surrounding skin.

Figures 8.3, 8.4 and 8.5 demonstrate the same skin condition in the second patient. This child had a similar presentation as the first child but the lesions were fewer and covered less skin area. The back shows more rashes than the front of the torso.

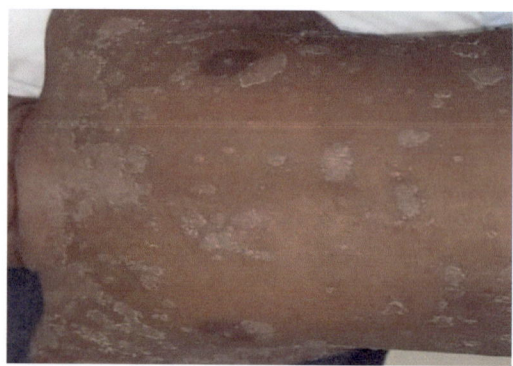

Fig. 8.3 The anterior neck, proximal arms, chest and abdominal wall of a baby showing extensive areas of irregularly-shaped, coalescent, hypopigmented, macular eruptions with associated flaking

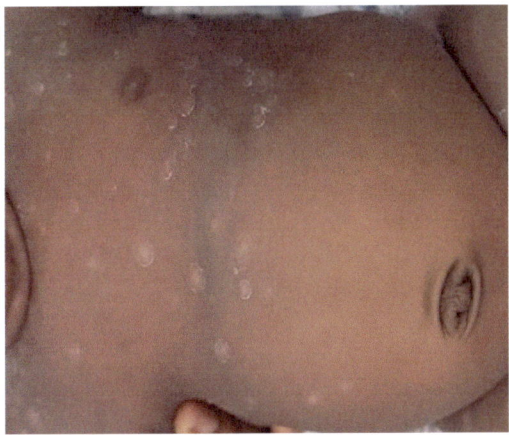

Fig. 8.4 The chest and abdomen of another infant

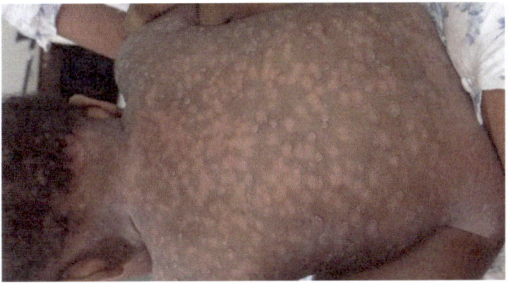

Fig. 8.5 The back and left thigh of the second infant

Diagnosis

Infantile (neonatal) seborrheic dermatitis

Treatment

An infant with a few lesions may not require any treatment. Treatment may not alter the course of the condition in this age group, and the risk-benefit considerations regarding some medications may not justify instituting and continuing treatment. Drugs include emollients, topical antifungal agents, and topical corticosteroids; if corticosteroids are considered for prescription, the fluorinated ones should be avoided. For babies with cradle cap, shampooing of the hair followed with gentle, non-abrasive combing is an effective means of removing the scaly lesions mechanically.

*The cream that the first child's mother was asked by the chemist attendant to apply on her son contains three drugs—an antibiotic, an antifungal, and a fluorinated corticosteroid. For a child at this age, application of the cream on such a wide skin area is inimical to the health of the patient as it has a potent steroid. Unrestricted availability and sale of drugs is one of the challenges in medical practice in this practice setting. In this case, the cost of the drug prevented the mother from using the cream for a long time—unlike the local remedy (*ndom*) which is cost-friendly. The mother applied the local preparation for a long time without a reprieve and only recently commenced using the cream purchased over the counter.

Etiology

The etiological agent is assumed to be the normal skin flora *Malassezia furfur* (*Pityrosporum ovale*), but overgrowth of this yeast may just be an association with other factors like abundance of sebum containing oils produced naturally by sebaceous glands in the infant coupled with susceptibility of the individual [1]. Even the amount of sebum that the skin produces (and, consequently, the amount of unsaturated fatty acids on the skin surface) and the concentration of the implicated yeast do not appear to be critical factors in the etiology of seborrheic dermatitis [2]. Maternal hormones that are still in circulation in the neonate or young infant may also be contributing factors to the development of infantile seborrheic dermatitis.

Prognosis

With infantile seborrheic dermatitis, being a self-limiting disease, a favorable prognosis is the norm and parents of the patients should be so advised. Doing so encourages the parents to achieve lessened anxiety while they apply the prescribed medications on the patients and await the disease to run its natural course.

Follow-Up Care

It is necessary to let the anxious parents know that seborrheic dermatitis in infancy is a self-limiting condition and that, even when it does not resolve as early as the parents would want, it usually subsides by the time the child celebrates the first birthday. Since parents tend to be worried, when the doctor gives them an appointment for follow-up care for their babies, it is well received. The doctor's appointment sends the positive message that the clinician is interested in the progress of treatment and desires a quick recovery for their child.

Discussion

The peak of infantile seborrheic dermatitis (ISD) is between 2 weeks and 12 months of age [2]. There does not seem to be sex predilection, and the condition is found in all climatic zones and all races and ethnic groups.

Usual clinical features The scalp is frequently involved in infantile seborrheic dermatitis, and scalp disease in this age group is known as cradle cap—neither of the babies' condition described included cradle cap. In cradle cap, the lesions may go slightly beyond the scalp and involve postauricular skin, nape, and forehead.

ISD can, however, affect other parts of the body, like in one of the infants in the case described in this chapter in whom most of the body was involved. ISD affects the diaper area (commonly called nappy area), posterior surface of the ears, and the eyebrows.

The multiple, irregularly shaped, scaly macules are neither painful nor pruritic, and the baby is usually not irritable.

It is a principally scaly inflammatory skin condition that occurs soon after birth and usually within the first 3 months of life; it could occur later but frequently resolves on its own prior the child's first birthday and uncommonly beyond age 2 years. In children that there is no sign of resolution, rather the condition becoming more extensive, treatment may be required.

Parents are usually worried when the lesions are extensive or resolve gradually.

It is worth noting that in older patients in the age group when seborrheic dermatitis peaks (adolescence and the age range 30–60 years), seborrheic dermatitis may be as mild as in mild cases of dandruff and as severe as exfoliative erythroderma—it has a wide spectrum of presentation [3].

Investigations The diagnosis is usually clinical and investigations are not required. The scaliness of the lesions, except in intertriginous areas like the axillae and skin folds in the baby's neck where they may be moist, and their distribution on the body provide reasonable lead to making a right diagnosis.

Differential diagnosis An important differential diagnosis of infantile seborrheic dermatitis is atopic eczema in this age group. In atopic eczema, the lesions also appear in the flexural areas, but the baby is irritable from the pruritic nature of atopic eczema; the intense itching provokes scratching which may be evidenced by marks on the patient's skin.

Psoriasis

Symptoms

The patient from whom the photograph in Fig. 8.6 was taken was an adult female in her mid-50s. She complained of having severely itchy, multiple black growths on her body within a time frame of at least 2 years—the itching was severe enough to make her scratch frequently, sometimes without realizing that she was doing so. She was careful not to traumatize the lesions—she maintained short nails to ensure this even when she scratched without realizing it [4]. Scaling of the lesions occurred but it was minimal [4]. There was no pain, but she occasionally felt discomfort over the lesions when she bent the elbows. The lesions developed gradually and affected various parts of her skin, viz., the thighs, both legs, and the back of both elbows [5]. Apart from Fig. 8.6 that shows the

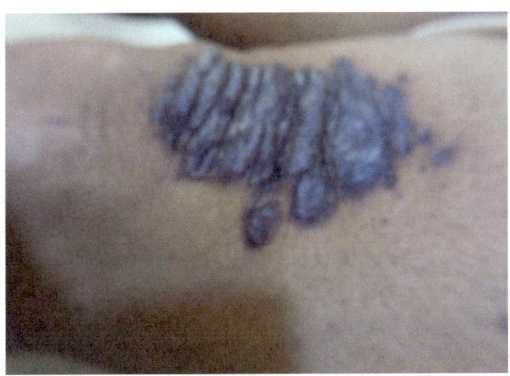

Fig. 8.6 Distal part of the anterior surface of the right thigh just falling short of the knee

largest of the lesions, which was on her thigh, she had them in different sizes. She did not have the same or similar growths in the past and was the only person in her family with the condition. She did not take any unprescribed drugs before the onset of the growths. She took various medications prescribed for this condition and augmented them with herbal preparations as the former did not provide the expected level of relief. Her work did not entail physical contact with chemicals.

One of the greatest concerns she had was the unsightly appearance of the growths, and she made efforts to wear clothes that would not expose the affected parts in public, but it was difficult to consistently cover her elbows. The second greatest bother was severe, almost unrelenting itching that necessitated the consultation—it was particularly itching of the growths on the back of the elbows. She had had several hospital visits since the gradual onset and progression of the skin disease and had received a variety of medications to no avail. She did not know the reason for the skin condition, did not know what would eventually happen to her, and had a deep-seated wish to obtain a permanent solution to the problem. Her adult daughter who accompanied her for the consultation was unhappy about the recalcitrant nature of the skin problem that was almost disfiguring her mother. She almost countered her mother's ready acceptance to give consent for

the photographs to be taken but eventually agreed with the mother and consent was written and signed.

Signs

Examination of the thigh, which was one of the parts that the patient was willing to expose for the photographs, showed an 8 cm × 3.5 cm black, firm, growth with irregular outline and irregular surface demonstrating whorls. The growth was an aggregation of a series of ridges and crevices; there was no complete fissuring as normal skin was not visible between them. There was no bleeding. Scratch marks were not evident. The above is a description of the lesion on the distal part of the anterior surface of the right thigh just falling short of the knee, Fig. 8.6. Palpation showed that the growth was firm and immovable. In this patient with light-to-moderate tone Black skin, there was no complaint of erythematous scaly lesions at any time, and she did not present with any during this consultation and physical examination.

The lesions were much smaller, many were confluent, some were solitary, but they all had almost different sizes with the largest measuring 3 cm. Each of them had a consistency like the thigh lesion. There was no tenderness.

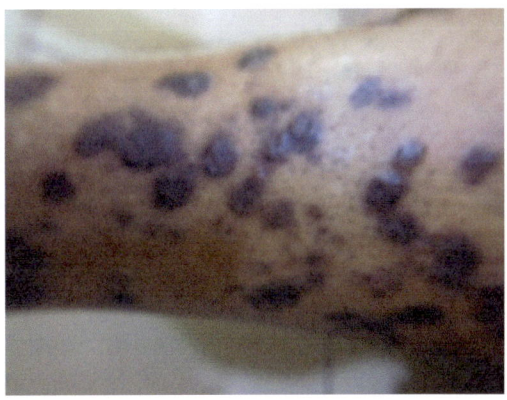

Fig. 8.7 Black lesions on the patient's left leg

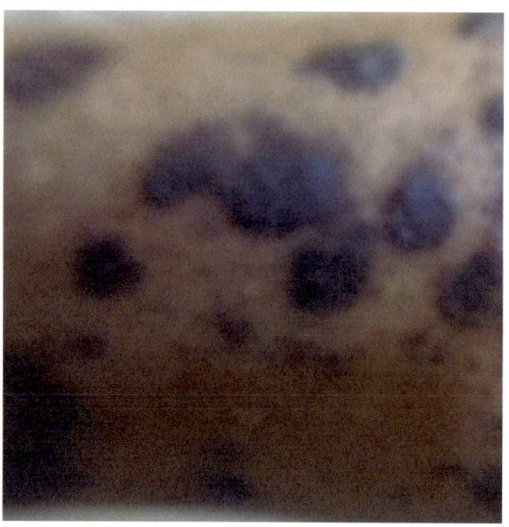

Fig. 8.8 A close-up image of a portion of Fig. 8.7

Diagnosis

Psoriasis

Treatment

Generally, patients with psoriasis should be encouraged to reduce emotional and physical stress and do some form of mild-to-moderate physical exercises. Since psoriasis may affect other parts of the body further, examination should be carried out for evidence of non-dermatologic presentation. The general physician who may not be adequately equipped in skill or equipment should refer the patient to specialists for specialist review.

Patients with mild or moderate skin disease may obtain satisfactory respite from application of topical agents; these are preparations to reduce inflammation by using steroidal anti-inflammatory agents and pruritus by using anti-pruritic lotions and creams. Topical corticosteroid preparations are the mainstay and first line of treatment of psoriasis of the skin; they suppress the migration of polymorphonuclear leukocytes (neutrophils) and reverse the increased permeability of capillaries which are features of inflam-

mation. Reduction of epithelial turnover rate is achieved with retinoids. Other useful drugs are moisturizers. Keratolytic drugs like anthralin and salicylic acid play a role in treatment as they remove scales from the lesions and make other topical agents accessible to the lesion [6]. Vitamin D analogs like calcitriol and calcipotriene prevent thinning of the skin and are beneficial for patients with psoriasis; the foams and solutions are beneficial in scalp psoriasis. Coal tar is an antipruritic as well as an inhibitor of deregulated proliferation of the epidermis and infiltration of the dermis; the shampoos are useful in scalp psoriasis [6].

When a patient has a severe case, injectables like corticosteroids are used. Immunomodulators like tacrolimus and antimetabolites like methotrexate and cyclosporine are needed. Interleukin inhibitors like brodalumab and similar drugs and phosphodiesterase-4 inhibitors exemplified by apremilast are useful [6].

For patients with dry eyes in ophthalmic presentation of psoriasis, the use of "artificial tears" that contain hydroxymethylcellulose, hydroxypropyl cellulose, hydroxypropyl methylcellulose, carboxymethylcellulose, sodium carmellose, sodium hyaluronate, etc. may be applicable. Cicatricial ectropion and trichiasis require surgical treatment by ophthalmologists.

Depending on the presentation of the patient, orthopedic surgeons, rheumatologists, psychologists, etc. may be needed to provide satisfactory management of the patients with psoriasis.

In summary, moderate-to-severe cases of psoriasis should be treated by dermatologists who may guide their general medical practice colleagues in caring for the patients in between follow-up appointments for specialist review [6]. For the milder cases with evidence of limitation to the skin, it is possible to treat with topicals (creams and systemic drugs as mentioned in this sub-heading), stress reduction, phototherapy, and even climatotherapy [6]. Adjunctive treatment may entail the use of moisturizers and keratolytics like salicylic acid and urea. Sunshine is a recommended source of therapy [6]. There is abundance of sunshine in the tropics where people with Black skin are indigenous to and reside; when they emigrate to cold parts of the world, they may make the best of the available sunshine by ensuring adequate exposure to it.

Etiology

Psoriasis is a chronic inflammatory dermatological disease. The fundamental pathology is epidermal keratinocyte hyperproliferation. Excessive turnover rate of epidermal cells with accumulation of the cells and lichenification at the involved sites is the result. The disease is multifactorial, and immunology, genetics, and the environment are contributory.

Prognosis

The patient should be made aware of the fact that psoriasis is a chronic disease. The prognosis in this condition depends on factors such as the time of presentation for the diagnosis to be made and commencement of satisfactory treatment, whether the disease is mild, moderate, or severe, and the patient's commitment to playing their part in the management of the condition.

Follow-Up Care

Follow-up care is essential and the dermatologist provided it. The specialist discussed with the patient and arrived at a mutually convenient date for the next appointment. In between specialist appointments, care may be carried out by the nonspecialist under a specialist's prescription's guidance.

Discussion

Although psoriasis can occur in any part of the skin, there are high-impact sites for psoriasis; the number and size of the lesions at these sites are immaterial for the mere presence of the papulo-squamous lesions there is enough to create a negative impact on the patient's quality of life. The sites are as follows [5]:

- Face
- Genitalia
- Scalp
- Hands, feet, and nails
- Skin folds

Usual clinical presentation Psoriasis with primarily skin presentation may affect various parts of the skin, e.g., scalp, lumbosacral region, parts of the skin prone to friction, and pressure like the extensor surfaces exemplified by the posterior surface of the elbows and anterior surface of the knees. It also affects the joints, intergluteal clefts, and glabrous skin (i.e., non-hair-bearing parts of the body) like the glans penis, soles, palms, and nails—the latter being one of the skin appendages. There is a wide range in presentation of this disease as in one patient it may be mild, while in others it may be moderate or severe—this is in terms of symptomatology, area(s) of skin covered, and non-skin parts of the body like joints, eyes, etc. There may be pain, fever, and pruritus. Pruritus may be severe enough to provoke scratching that may lead to scratch marks and bleeding. In some patients, there may be scaling, lichenification, and fissuring of the skin [4]. Patients with eye involvement may present with conjunctivitis or blepharitis. Joint pain is a feature of psoriatic arthritis. The psyche of patients with severe disease may be impacted upon negatively.

The diagnosis of psoriasis is usually made on clinical grounds especially when the presentation is dermatological; it is imperative to take a good history and carry out a detailed examination of the lesions.

Investigations If the general medical practitioner who makes the diagnosis based on clinical features has access to equipment to carry out investigations on patients with psoriasis, it is still important to refer to a dermatologist to care for the patient or commence treatment.

Investigations that the nonspecialist requests need not be complicated or extensive as there is no specific test for diagnosing psoriasis [7]. The blood test, erythrocyte sedimentation rate (ESR), which is a nonspecific test of an inflammatory process in the body, may prove useful; the test is simple, available in laboratories in every practice setting, and affordable to most patients. ESR is usually normal in patients other than those with pustular psoriasis and erythrodermic psoriasis in whom their blood specimens show high levels; in these conditions, white blood cell count is concomitantly elevated [7]. Blood tests help to rule out differential diagnoses like gout and rheumatoid arthritis in patients with joint disease [7]. In patients who have features of fungal disease like onychomycosis, fungal studies are appropriate [7]. Radiographs of joints may help in patients who have arthritis. Other tests like joint scans can identify early joint involvement, and histopathological examination of skin biopsy may be diagnostic—these and other advanced investigation modalities should be left for relevant specialists to determine their necessity [7].

Lichen Planus

Symptoms

This patient, in her late 20s, developed generalized itchy rashes that commenced from the flexures at the knees and elbows; the rashes became generalized within 3 months. The rashes covered almost every part of the body as shown in the Figures on this topic. There was no antecedent systemic disease with fever, malaise, and muscular or joint pain. There was no anorexia, weakness, nausea, or vomiting. She did not believe that she had lost weight. The patient considered the rashes unsightly and embarrassing. She had not seen or heard of this type of rashes on anybody in her family and neither did she know of anyone throughout her time at school or any neighborhood where she had lived so far. She wondered how she acquired the disorder and hoped that it was not a sinister disease that would prevent her from marrying or giving birth to children. The disorder did not prevent her from carrying out work

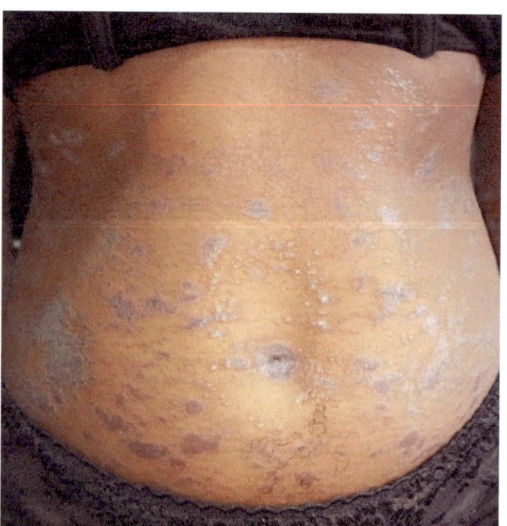

Fig. 8.9 Involvement of the patient's abdominal wall skin

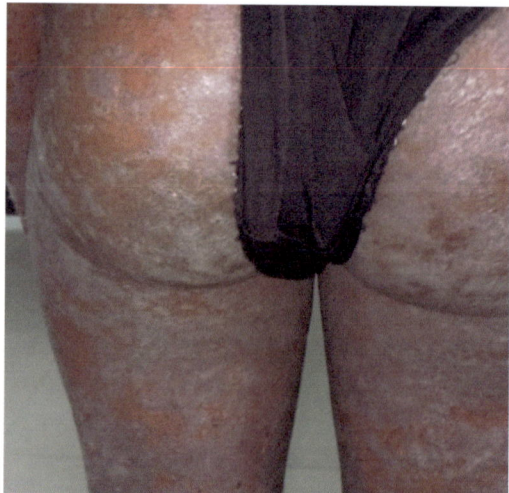

Fig. 8.10 Buttocks and posterior aspect of the patient's thighs

in the house but she had become restricted to the home and found it difficult to cover all the rashes with clothes to enable her to go to church or to seek employment.

Signs

Examination showed a generalized eruption of grayish-white plaques with shapes that could be described as polymorphic and variable sizes. Some of the lesions were so large and irregular in shape that they must have been the result of coalescence of initially not-so-large plaques. Only a few of them measured less than 3 cm. The rashes were not tender and there was no area of hyperemia in the few uninvolved portions of her skin.

This patient was neither febrile nor pale. She walked into the consulting room unassisted and traveled to the teaching hospital unaccompanied.

Diagnosis

Lichen planus

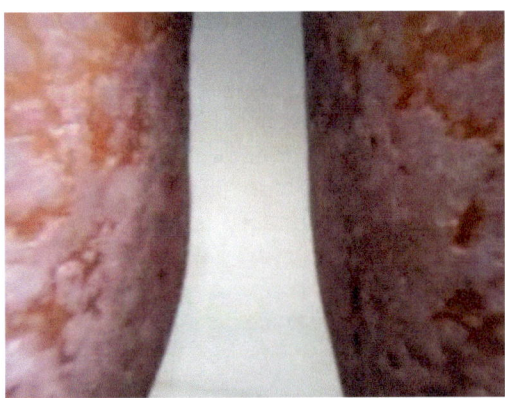

Fig. 8.12 Close-up image of the patient's thighs (anterior)

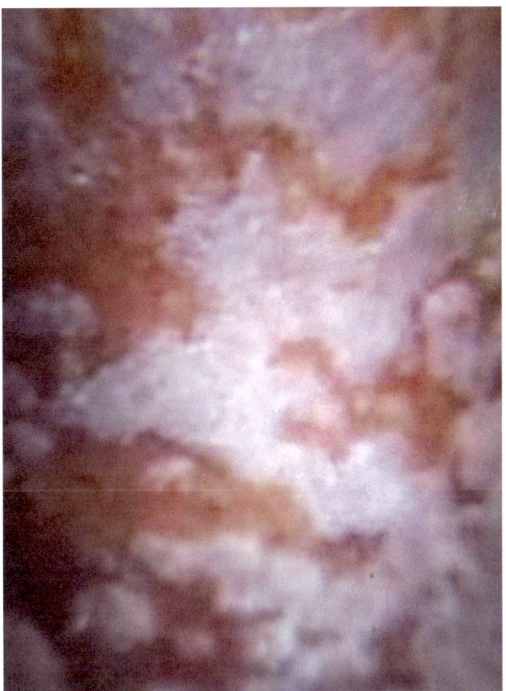

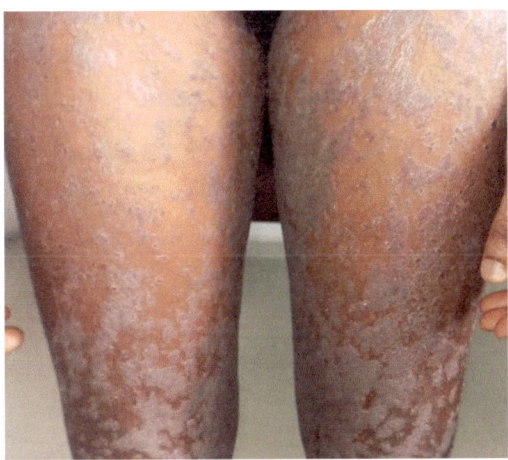

Fig. 8.11 The lesions on the anterior aspect of the patient's thighs

Fig. 8.13 Close-up image of the rashes on the patient's right thigh, close to the knee

Treatment

Spontaneous resolution is the norm in patients who have cutaneous lichen planus; it occurs within 2 years [8]. The principles that determine treatment is amelioration of pruritus for patients who have distressing pruritus; this is done while awaiting resolution of the lesions [8].

This patient had diffuse lichen planus and the treatment for her was the tablet form of Prednisolone 30 mg daily initially but tapered until she was on 10 mg daily to complete 6 weeks.

Patients whose lesions are not extensive need the superpotent steroid Clobetasol 0.05% administered topically twice daily for 2 to 4 weeks. When the response is not satisfactory, intralesional steroid injections like triamcinolone acetonide are administered into the most problematic lesions.

Etiology

Although its origin is unknown, lichen planus is an immunological disorder. The pathway ends with activation of cytotoxic T cells with keratinocyte apoptosis in the epidermis [8]. Individuals who are seropositive to hepatitis C virus (HCV) and people who are seropositive to the human immunodeficiency virus (HIV) are more prone to developing lichen planus [8].

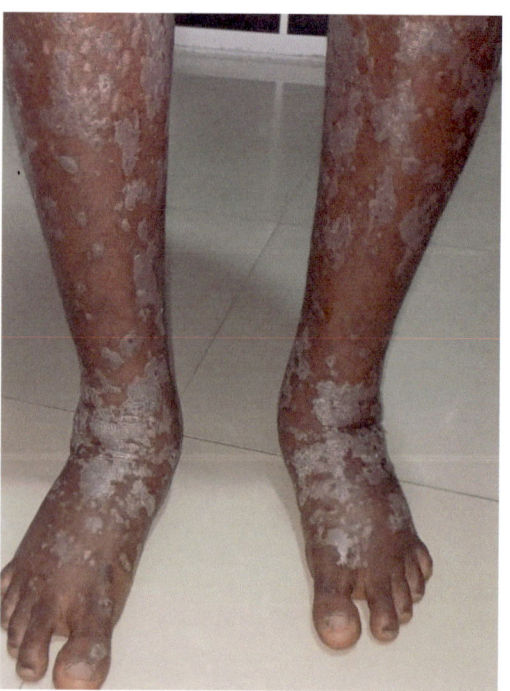

Fig. 8.14 The same patient—lesions on the legs (anterior) and feet (dorsi)

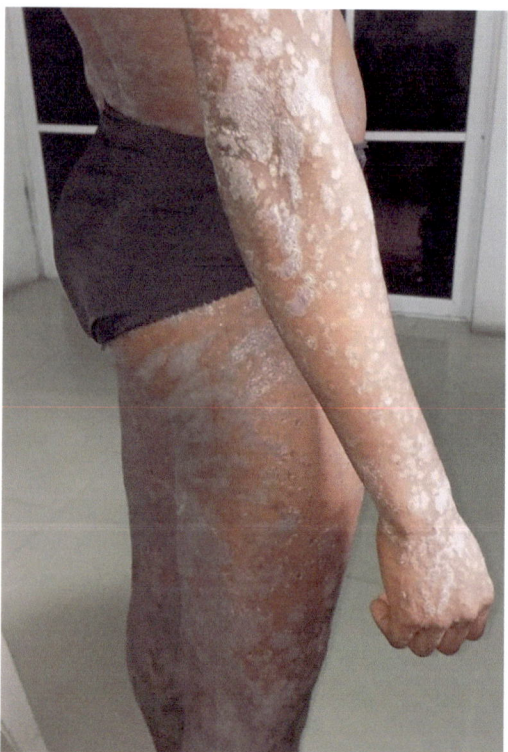

Fig. 8.15 Lesions on the lateral aspects of both right limbs and parts of the trunk

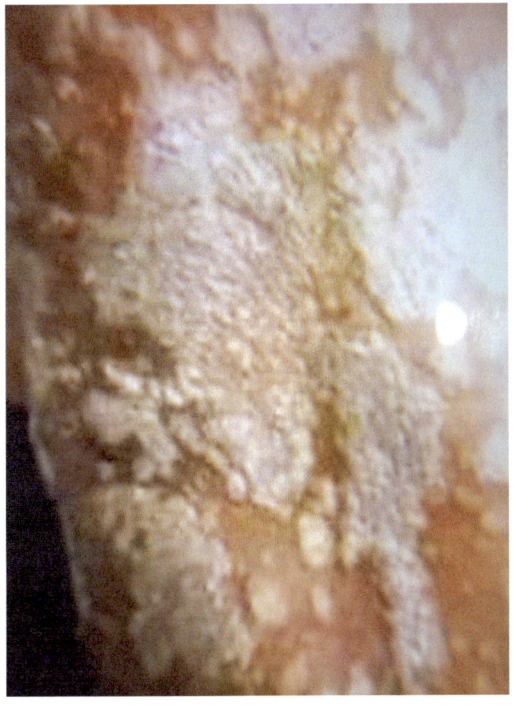

Fig. 8.16 Close-up image of the lateral aspect of the right upper limb lesions

Prognosis

The prognosis of lichen planus is considered good because of the potential of resolution within 2 years, but this period is long for a patient who is emotionally traumatized by this disorder. The prognosis is not favorable in patients who have mucous membrane involvement or patients who have pain and moderate or severe pruritus [8].

Follow-Up Care

Follow-up care was a necessity in this patient. As earlier documented, she felt very distraught with the condition of her skin. She kept the appointments for follow-up care with the dermatologist. There was improvement to treatment by the time of this report.

Discussion

Lichen planus is a self-limiting disease, but it may run a course of months to years [9]. It may be found in patients who have diseases with altered immunity like myasthenia gravis, alopecia areata, or vitiligo [9]. Lichen planus usually first appears on flexural surfaces and the rashes continue to erupt, covering the body in about 18 weeks [9]. Lichen planus also presents as a systemic disorder, but the lesions of the dermatological form usually resolve by 18 months, about 85% of them [9].

In this patient with light-to-moderate tone of Black skin, the lesions were polygonal, planar, pruritic, and plaques and did not have the other two *P*s that are descriptive of lichen planus [10]. In the patient, rather than purple, the lesions were grayish-white and there was no papule.

Multiple-Choice Questions

1. Which of the following statements about seborrheic dermatitis is correct?
   A. It is common on the lower extremities
   B. Dandruff is seborrheic dermatitis of the scalp
   C. There is an association with a *Corynebacterium*
   D. Treatment is with long-term fluorinated steroids
2. Which of the following statements about psoriasis is correct?
   A. There is hyperproliferation of melanocytes
   B. Exposure to sun aggravates the condition
   C. It is uncommon in childhood and teenage group
   D. Moisturizers produce symptomatic relief
3. Which of the following is a correct association in psoriasis?
   A. Plaque psoriasis—Rare form
   B. Distribution—Asymmetric
   C. Nail psoriasis—Pitting
   D. Facial involvement—More in adults

4. Which of the following statements about lichen planus is correct?
   A. Skin lesions are usually polygonal
   B. Most patients are asymptomatic
   C. Wickham's striae are purple plaques
   D. Intralesional corticosteroids are best used in extensive, multiple lesions
5. A 25-year-old man with a deep tone of Black skin presents with lichen planus. Which of the following statements is incorrect?
   A. The lesions are pruritic
   B. The rashes cover a significant portion of his skin
   C. He feels distraught with the lesions and request treatment for prompt recovery
   D. The lesions are purple

References

1. Tucker D, Masood S. Seborrheic dermatitis. In: StatPearls [Internet]; 2024. Available from: https://www.ncbi.nlm.nih.gov/books/NBK551707/#article-28811.r5.
2. Wikramanayake TC, Borda LJ, Miteva M, Paus R. Seborrheic dermatitis—looking beyond *Malassezia*. Exp Dermatol. 2019. https://doi.org/10.1111/exd.14006. Available from: https://onlinelibrary.wiley.com/doi/10.1111/exd.14006.
3. Handler MZ. Seborrheic dermatitis. Dermatology. Medscape. 2023. Available from: https://emedicine.medscape.com/article/1108312-overview.
4. American Academy of Dermatology Association. Psoriasis: signs and symptoms. Available from: https://www.aad.org/public/diseases/psoriasis/what/symptoms.
5. National Psoriasis Foundation. Locations and types. Available from: https://www.psoriasis.org/locations-and-types/.
6. NIH. National Institute of Arthritis and Musculoskeletal and Skin Diseases. Psoriasis: diagnosis, treatment, and steps to take. 2023. Available from: https://www.niams.nih.gov/health-topics/psoriasis/diagnosis-treatment-and-steps-to-take#:~:text=.
7. Habashy J. Psoriasis. Dermatology. Medscape. 2024. Available from: https://emedicine.medscape.com/article/1943419-treatment.
8. Arnold DL, Krishnamurthy K. Lichen planus. In: StatPearls [Internet]. Available from: https://www.ncbi.nlm.nih.gov/books/NBK526126/.
9. Hoffpauir LA. Lichen planus. Dermatology. Medscape. 2025. Available from: https://emedicine.medscape.com/article/1123213-overview.
10. Usatine RP, Tinitigan M. Diagnosis and treatment of lichen planus. Am Fam Physician. 2011;84(1):53–60. Available from: https://www.aafp.org/pubs/afp/issues/2011/0701/p53.html#:~:text=.

Cutaneous Neoplasms: Benign and Malignant

This chapter covers a selection of benign neoplasms and just one malignant neoplasm of the skin. The selection contains congenital and acquired neoplasia. Some new growths on the body cause great concern to parents of their baby, e.g., melanocytic nevi and, especially, giant congenital melanocytic nevi. Some of the growths hardly qualify as growths for they tend to stay the same for long periods; an example of this is capillary hemangioma. A benign growth, like keloids, may have a defined etiology while others have what may be considered associations and they have varieties—of which neurofibromatosis is an example. Alteration to normal chemistry in the body may cause or be associated with some growths, and this is exemplified by penile calcinosis cutis. The only condition that is malignant is malignant melanoma; malignant melanoma is one of the conditions that deserve to be in this book that dwells on disease in skin of color, specifically the Black skin.

The topics in this book, in the order that they appear, are Campbell de Morgan spots (capillary hemangioma), pyogenic granuloma, melanocytic nevi, giant congenital melanocytic naevus, keloids, penile calcinosis cutis, neurofibromatosis Type 1 (von Recklinghausen's disease), and malignant melanoma.

Campbell de Morgan Spots (Capillary hemangioma)

Symptoms

The elderly patient in his mid-60s presented with the complaint of a single bright red rash on the inner aspect of his upper right thigh. The rash was small, pinhead sized, painless, and not itchy. He said that he noticed the solitary rash when he was about to apply body lotion on the affected part after having a shower. He could not say when the rash appeared but was certain that he did not see it in the 3 days prior, although he carried out the same routine on those days and other days. This was the first time that he had such a rash. He did not have it in any other part of his skin. He could not figure out what caused this sudden-onset rash and made the complaint out of curiosity. He wanted to know the reason and desired to have a solution to it. There was no history of eating unfamiliar cooked food, fresh fruits or vegetables, nuts, or taking a drink recently. He did not take any drug outside the prescribed ones for his multiple medical conditions. He was not bitten by any insect in or outside his house, and he did not have any social or religious activity outdoors

I. Ukot, *Understanding Diseases in Skin of Color*, https://doi.org/10.1007/978-3-031-97503-5_9

in the past 1 week. His work was principally indoors. No member of his household had a similar rash. He was HIV-negative.

Signs

Figure 9.1: When examined, there was a solitary, bright red, round-to-ovoid soft papule on the medial aspect of the patient's upper thigh. The rash was very distinct and did not gradually fade in color to take the normal pigmentation of the surrounding skin. It was 1.5 mm in diameter. There was neither tenderness nor blanching.

Figure 9.2: When reviewed 2 days later, the color had changed to oxblood, the size was unchanged, and the lesion was still single. The photographs were taken at this review. As there

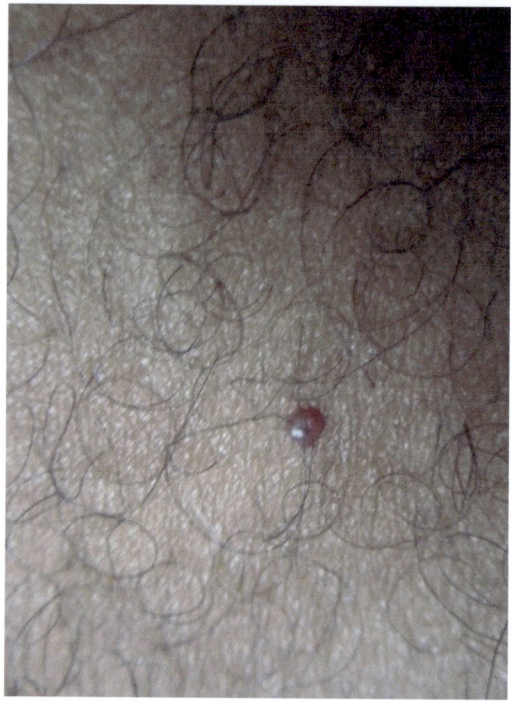

Fig. 9.2 The solitary papule on the thigh

was still no associated symptom, the patient was encouraged to observe further. He reported that by 5 days after he first noticed the rash, it had resolved spontaneously after turning brown.

Diagnosis

Campbell de Morgan spots (capillary hemangioma)

More on Symptoms: About 3 months after the patient said that he was certain that growth had "disappeared," he noticed it again at the same spot with the same characteristics as the first one. The patient observed this recurrence of the growth.

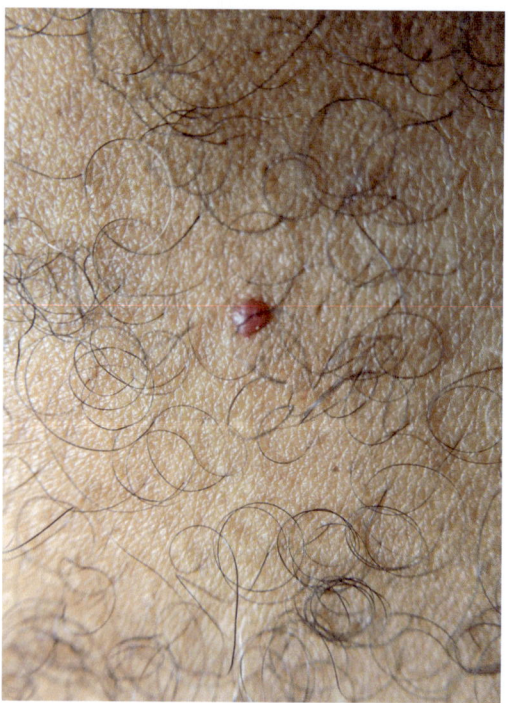

Fig. 9.1 The little growth on Day 1—the day the patient first noticed it

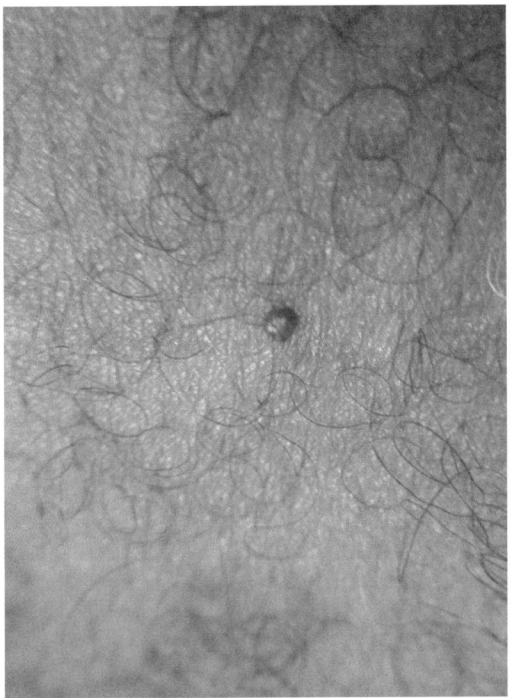

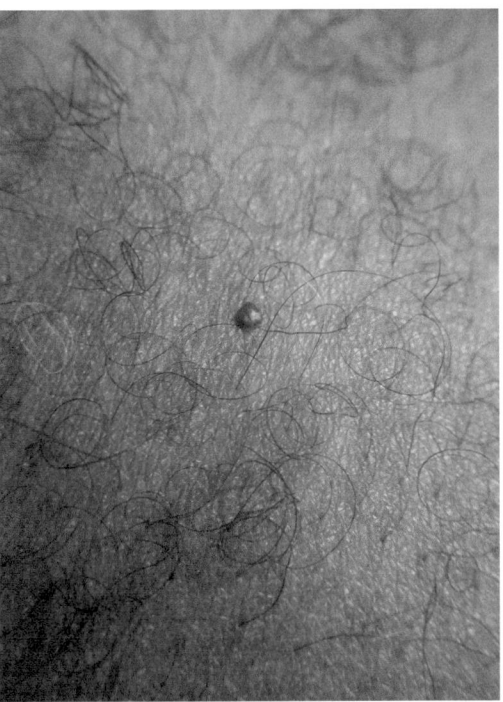

Fig. 9.3 Rash on the same spot 3 months after it purportedly "disappeared"

Fig. 9.4 The same growth in Fig. 9.3 after 4–5 months after recurrence

Treatment

Realizing that this condition is not a threat in any way, the patient was not prepared to have any of the treatment options.

Etiology

The etiology of Campbell de Morgan spots (also known as cherry angiomas, adult hemangiomas, senile angiomas, and ruby spots) is unclear, and it is believed to be part of the aging process. There also appears to be association with pregnancy, diabetes mellitus, human papillomavirus 8, and immunosuppressive states; it is also associated with drugs such as alkylating agents (class of antineoplastic drugs), e.g., the nitrogen mustards like ifosfamide, cyclophosphamide, and chlorambucil. Other drugs associated with their etiology are cyclosporine and tamsulosin.

The growth was essentially of the original size with the only difference being that its shape was now diamond-shaped unlike the original lesion in Fig. 9.1 or the one that recurred in Fig. 9.3.

Prognosis

The prognosis of senile angiomas is good. Treatment may leave scars, especially of the relatively large lesions.

Follow-Up Care

The patient did not see the need to have follow-up care after the first that is mentioned in the history, but due to the disappearance and reappearance he was willing to have reviews. Review findings are documented in the figures up to Fig. 9.6 at 14 months later. The findings were that the color of the lesion remained red and the

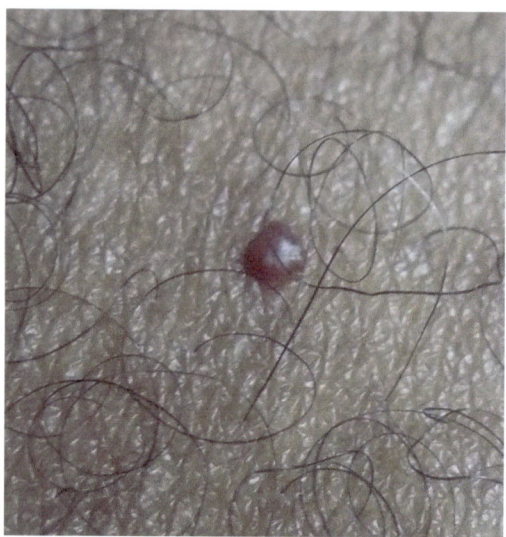

Fig. 9.5 Growth at 9–10 months after it was first noticed—an enlarged image

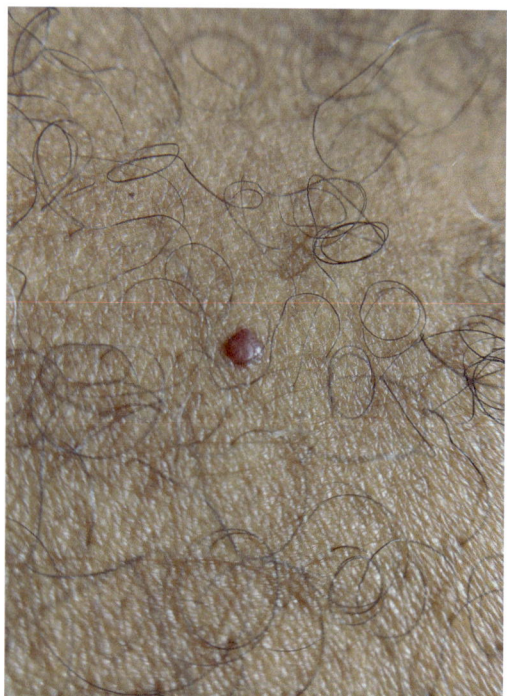

Fig. 9.6 The solitary growth maintaining diamond shape 14 months later

lesion had not increased in size; curiously, however, it appeared that the lesion had a mild alteration in shape from round to diamond shaped. The patient was reviewed 14 months after he first noticed the lesion. The lesion is as shown in Fig. 9.6.

Discussion

Usual clinical presentation The patient with Campbell de Morgan spots is usually an adult but may be a teenager or young adult. They complain of multiple painless and non-itchy spots or papules that are bright red. The spots usually start as small macules; they become small red papules that are about 1 mm but could grow to 5 mm. The papules may be dome shaped. There may be a pale halo. They are usually multiple and tend to increase in size as the patient ages or in older patients. The lesions affect the trunk (anterior more than posterior) and the proximal part of the upper or lower extremities. They hardly affect the face, palms, or soles. Blanching may occur on palpation.

In this patient who reported not seeing the lesion 5 days after he first noticed it, it was curious as although these lesions are known to resolve spontaneously, it should not be within 1 week. The author is still of the opinion that the tiny growth may have been on the site for months without the patient realizing it.

Investigations Adult hemangiomas are usually diagnosed on clinical grounds from the history and their appearance. Optical coherence tomography assesses how deep the lesions are. When it is carried out, histopathological examination shows newly formed capillaries (neovascularization) that demonstrate narrowing of capillary lumina initially but eventually their dilatation; there is also endothelial cell proliferation and concomitant atrophy (thinning) of the epidermis. It is a form of capillary telangiectasia. Findings on dermoscopy are multiple well-defined red lacunae, white fibrous stroma that separates the lacunae. There are Individual vessels that are not identifiable or small vessels that are located peripherally [1].

Treatment The reason for treatment may be cosmetic, and it could be to prevent bleeding from accidental trauma to the lesions. Small angiomas are treated with electrocauterization. The bases of the larger ones are also treated with electrocautery after shave excision of their surfaces. Curettage, carbon dioxide laser therapy, and cryotherapy are treatment modalities. Treatment with intense pulse light or pulsed dye laser also provides good results. Treatment is usually not required unless there is infection, a cosmetic embarrassment when the lesion is present in a conspicuous site, or the growth erodes into the epidermis or it undergoes maceration [2]. This patient was not willing to undergo treatment, especially as the lesion was in an inconspicuous part of the body.

Pyogenic Granuloma

Symptoms

The patient, a 45-year-old artisan working at a building construction site, injured his right hand with the little finger being the most severely injured part. There was bleeding at the affected little finger and he had excruciating pain at the finger; the pain was disproportionately more than the size of the injury. The pain was throbbing, especially when he lay down to sleep, and disturbed his sleep on the first couple of days following the injury at the workplace—a private building under construction. About 2 weeks after he decided to treat himself, because he did not have enough money at the time to go to a hospital, he noticed that the wound developed a growth rather than healing the way he expected. He had had injuries in the past, right from childhood, and did not have a similar experience as the current one. When he noticed that the bleeding that had stopped recurred and he was still bleeding slightly by the next day, he opted to absent himself from work and attend to the current health concern. He was a daily-paid worker and so he could not continue going to work and ignoring his health just because of the little income he knew he would lose for the day; he made the sacrifice and that was why he consulted a doctor for the first time regarding the injury and subsequent growth.

Signs

Figure 9.7 shows the right little finger of a middle-aged man who had trauma to the affected finger less than 2 weeks earlier. The skin over the dorsum of the proximal nail fold of the right little finger is swollen, bulbous, and hyperpigmented. There is an irregularly shaped whitish growth from the elevated proximal nail fold and extending distally towards the beginning of the nail plate. There is an irregularly shaped meaty growth that extends from the distal end of the whitish growth to cover the proximal part of the nail plate. This reddish-brown growth terminates on the nail plate forming a rough V or L. The distal margins of the growth cover more of the medial portion (upper in the image) of the proximal nail plate than the lateral portion (lower in the image). Perhaps due to the angulation of the involved finger for the purpose of taking this photograph, there is blood collection in the superficial "gutter" formed between the medial end of the nail plate and the medial nail fold. There is no similar blood pooling on the remaining margins of the nail (the lateral nail fold or the free edge of

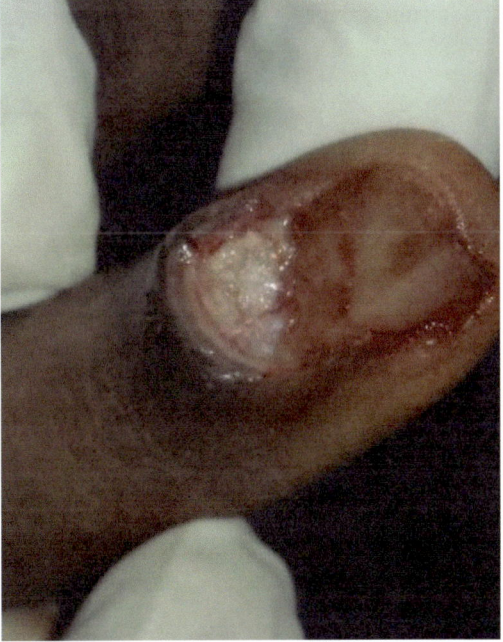

Fig. 9.7 The right little finger of a middle-aged man

the nail plate). The growth was tender but the tenderness was mild. The patient came to the hospital with the growth uncovered.

Diagnosis

Pyogenic granuloma.
The diagnosis is usually made on clinical grounds.

Treatment

The treatment for this patient was tetanus toxoid, oral antibiotics to cover staphylococcal organisms, metronidazole for likely anaerobic infection, analgesics orally, ascorbic acid, and wound dressing. Wound dressing was done. Due to skin and nail involvement, the patient was referred to the dermatology clinic which did not hold on the day the patient came for consultation; he was booked for the next dermatology clinic.

Prognosis

Posttreatment, scar formation, bleeding, or recurrence is possible.

Follow-Up Care

The follow-up care was to be provided by the dermatologist. If, however, the dermatologist after the consultation felt that another specialist was needed, they would do a further referral.

Discussion

Fingers are very important to every person, and traumatic injuries to the fingers have a variety of limitations that they impose on the injured person. The injured person may be a child, young adult, or older person; the person may, therefore, be an infant grappling with the challenges of attaining the pediatric milestones, be a pupil or student who needs to write and do other things in school, be an adult who needs complete fingers to function optimally occupationally, or be a retiree who needs to attend to, at the least, activities of daily living. The limitation imposed by injury to a finger depends on the affected finger as fingers have various degrees of importance in terms of their contribution to dexterity, e.g., the little finger when compared with the thumb. Limitation arising from injury could be for a few days or last for months or years. Trauma that is principally surgical or orthopedic and the one that is primarily dermatological have different weight ratings in terms of overall impact on function, time for recovery, cost of treatment, and a need for rehabilitation.

Pyogenic granuloma is a dermatological condition that arises from traumatic injury to the fingers.

Apart from the initial severe pain and associated bleeding which the patient treated with analgesics and arrest of the bleeding, the patient later observed a growth developing on the affected finger.

Pyogenic granuloma usually has trauma as a precursor. It affects the skin and frequently involves parts of the body with mucous membranes. The name seems to be a misnomer from the fact that it is not the result of a primarily infectious process just as it is not granulomatous, in the usual pathological description of granulomas. It is a capillary hemangioma.

Pyogenic granuloma is a fleshy, rapidly growing globular skin growth, which takes the semblance of a polyp. Pyogenic granuloma is discrete and solitary. It tends to bleed easily because of the hemangiomatous characteristics of the lesion. In Fig. 9.7, there is blood at the medial side of the affected little fingernail with a little pool of blood between the surface of the nail plate and the medial skin fold. Pyogenic granuloma that is regressing features extensive fibrosis [3].

Regarding pyogenic granuloma of the skin, the fingers and face are the usual sites, but other parts of the skin can be involved. Gums, lips, and the tongue are parts with mucous membranes that pyogenic granuloma frequently affects.

Investigations Investigations, including skin biopsy, may be required especially when there is recurrence. In some cases, the growth may show evidence of infection—like discharge—and in such cases, microbiological examination of a swab specimen accompanied by culture and antibiotic sensitivity tests is required. When indicated, the patient may benefit from appropriate antibiotics.

Differential diagnoses Differential diagnoses of pyogenic granuloma include capillary hemangioma, venous stasis, and nevi that have been traumatized, acrodermatitis, warts, glomus tumors, Kaposi sarcoma, bacillary angiomatosis, and reactive angioendotheliomatosis.

Histology Part of its histological features includes central branching capillaries that are surrounded by endothelial cells and lobular vascular proliferation that is reminiscent of granulation tissue because of inflammation and edema. The peripheral portions of the growth demonstrate hyperkeratosis and acanthosis.

Treatment Treatment may not be required if it is a tiny growth as it may heal without treatment. When treatment is required, this may include cryotherapy, laser therapy, electrocautery, or surgical excision.

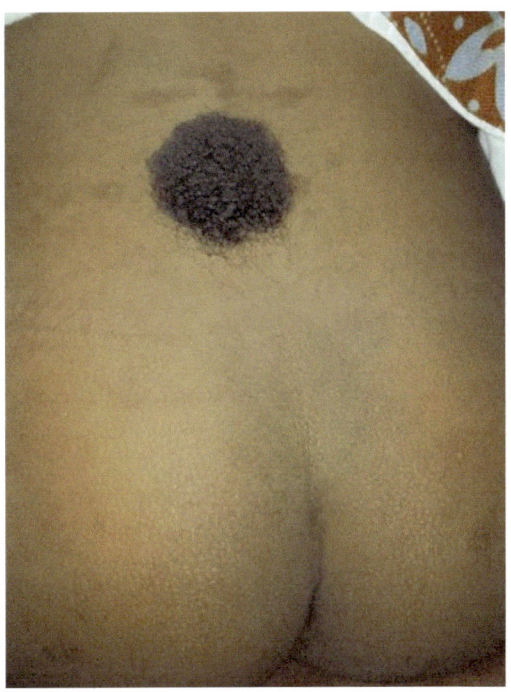

Fig. 9.8 A black skin patch on the lower back skin of a baby

Congenital Melanocytic Nevus

Symptoms

The mother of this 3-month-old baby brought the child to the hospital to complain of a black and hairy spot on the back of the baby. She said that the patch was there at birth. She came because she had not seen that kind of black area on any baby, and family members from her side and the husband's side were surprised. There was no family history of a similar skin condition. The patient's mother believed that the black spot did not inconvenience the baby as the baby did not scratch the area or cry when lying on the back. The mother could not say if the patch was increasing in size, but she felt that it was growing with the baby.

Signs

On examination of the baby, there was a single 3 cm × 3 cm hairy, jet black, circular patch on the lower back (approximately the upper lumbar spine). The black patch of the skin was clearly delineated from normal skin. There was no other rash on the body. There was no obvious skin defect. There was no loss of sensation of touch or pressure. The baby's palms and soles, in between the toes, and scalp were not involved.

Diagnosis

Congenital melanocytic nevus

Treatment

For this baby, the treatment was observation and documentation of the findings during follow-up consultations visits. The findings showed no indication for investigation, e.g., skin biopsy.

Etiology

Neural crest cells give rise to nevomelanocytic nevus cells which are found in pigmented nevi [4]. These new cells can synthesize melanin just like melanocytes that are normal features of skin.

Embryologically, Mongolian spots are considered anomalous development, and these malformations are believed to be hamartomas as they are like hamartomas. In congenital melanocytic nevi, melanocytes predominate. Concurrently, they have an increase in other types of cells nor-

mally found in the skin. The result is an exaggeration in the number and size of hair follicles, or an increase in other appendages of the skin.

Prognosis

The prognosis of congenital melanocytic nevi is good, especially when they are single as in this patient.

Follow-Up Care

Follow-up care is essential. This is done by both the parents of the patient and the doctor. It is advisable to refer the patient to a dermatologist to do the follow-up care. When the parents are informed that the growth is benign but should be watched for increase in size, they get relieved. They also adhere to the dermatologist's request for keeping follow-up appointments when they are made to know that the doctor will be examining not only the lesion(s) but also other parts of the body when necessary. The dermatologist makes a comparison between the sizes documented between the previous initial and previous follow-up visit(s) and the current one for increase in size. In addition, the body is inspected for an increase in number for patients who have multiple nevi.

Acquired Melanocytic Nevus With Leukotrichia

Figures 9.9, 9.10, 9.11, and 9.12 are photographs of a black spot on the left shoulder of an elderly male patient. He had a similar spot on the skin over the flexor muscles of the left arm. He also had a few others on other parts of the body. He had had them for many years and did not remember the first time he noticed them. They caused him no concern as they were asymptomatic, and they had neither increased in size nor in number. The one shown in the photograph was the only one through which hair grew and recently had gray hair just like hair in other parts of his body.

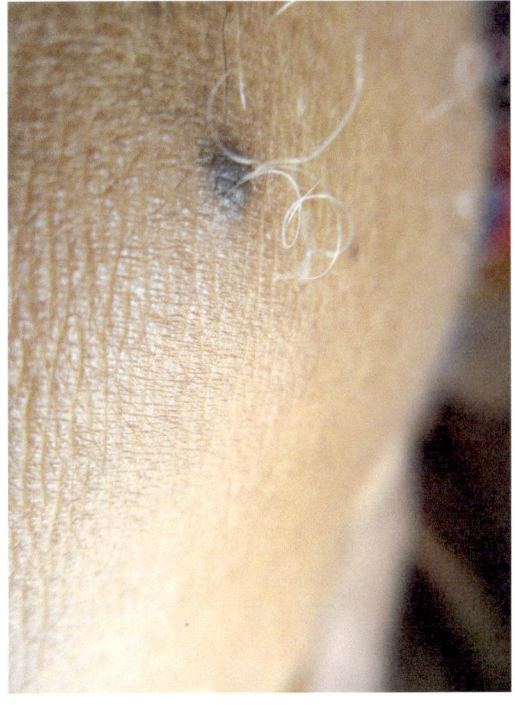

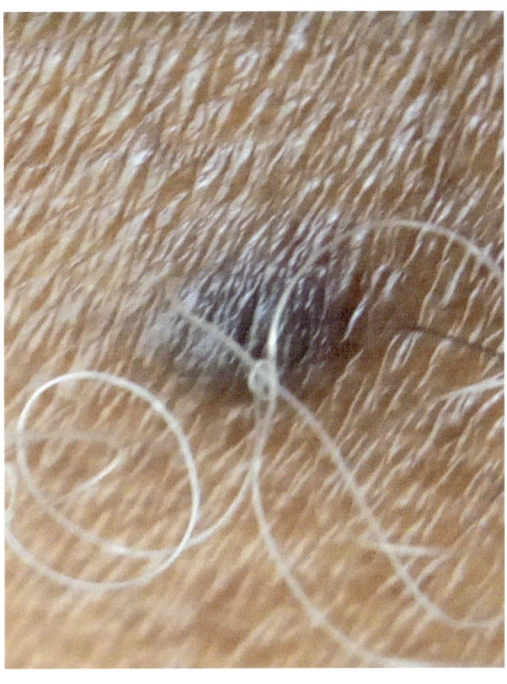

Fig. 9.9 A black spot on the anterior part of the left shoulder of an elderly male patient

Fig. 9.11 An enlargement of Fig. 9.10 shows the normally pigmented hair from the right side of the oval black spot

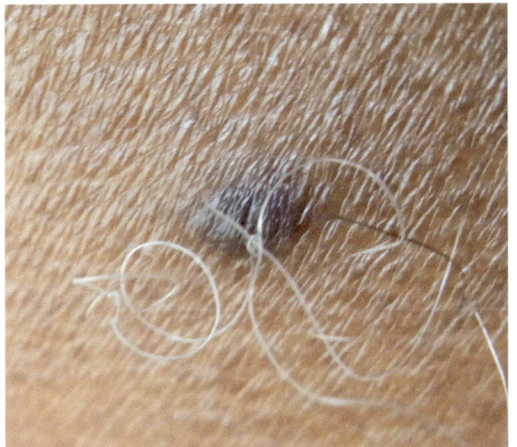

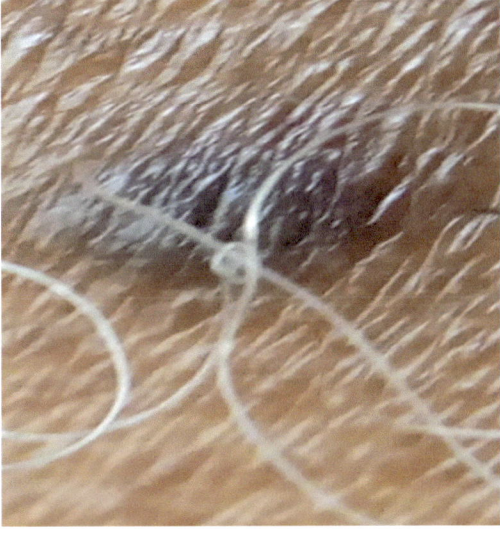

Fig. 9.10 The black spot on the left shoulder of the elderly male patient; a tuft of gray hairs and a single gray hair arise from the black patch

Fig. 9.12 A further enlargement of the single acquired melanocytic nevus

The black spot on this elderly patient's shoulder was not a presenting symptom but is documented because of the author's interest in recording it under this topic. The patient did not know the precise time he first noticed the black spot, for it had been there from the time he was a child. The spot does not itch or cause pain. He did not believe that it had increased in size, unless it was undetectable. The only concern that it caused him was having to remember not to injure it. That was why he had allowed hairs to grow through the black spot without clipping them—even after developing gray hairs and a tuft of gray hairs had arisen from it. This elderly man's nevi may be acquired as their time of onset most likely exceeded the time limit for congenital melanocytic nevi.

N.B.: The images in Figs. 9.10, 9.11, and 9.12 have been rotated 90° to the right, converting the original vertical axis of the oval nevus to transverse.

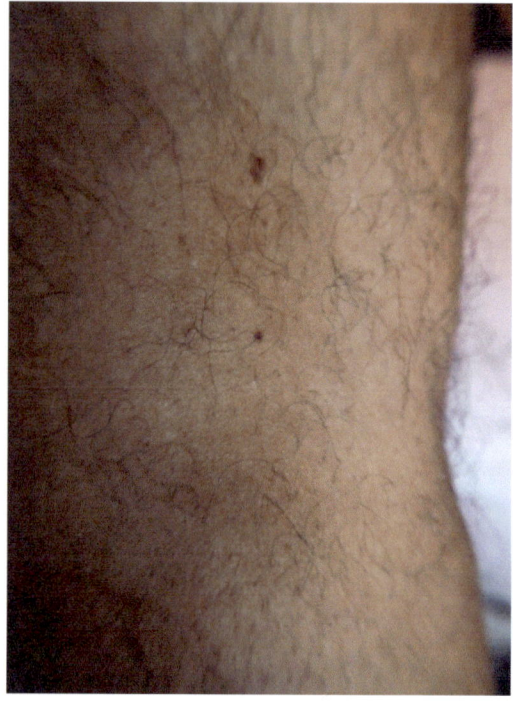

Fig. 9.13 Grayish-black macules on the same elderly patient

Diagnosis

Acquired melanocytic nevus with leukotrichia [4]

The same elderly patient had similar lesions on other parts of the body. They are shown in Figs. 9.13 and 9.14.

Figure 9.13: The history of the three black spots is that the patient noticed them in his adulthood. Like the one on the shoulder, they did not cause any symptoms. They caused him no bother as they are flat and on the same level as the normal surrounding skin. He has been having his bath and scrubbing the affected part with no fear of causing himself injury.

Examination showed three grayish-black macules on the medial surface of the left leg, just inferior to the left knee. The proximal lesion is the most prominent, measuring just 1 cm × 0.7 cm; it is roughly oval in shape and aligns with the longitudinal axis of the leg. The one that is posteroinferior to it is round, just as

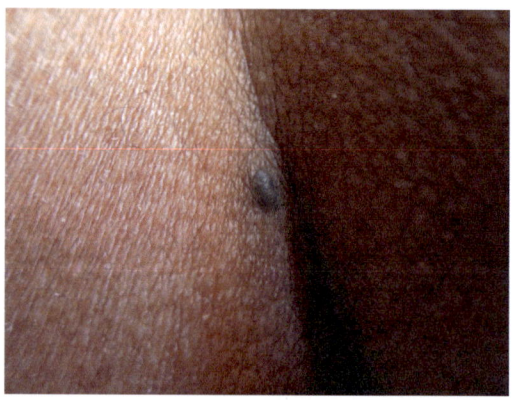

Fig. 9.14 A single, oval, jet-black, papule left lateral from the natal cleft

the one that is most inferior; they measure about 0.5 cm × 0.5 cm. A line connecting them would form a triangle.

The history about Fig. 9.14 is like that for Fig. 9.13; the only differences between the three are that the patient was certain that this was the most recent black spot on his body as he observed it accidentally just about 4 years earlier and that this one is raised from the skin. There was no history of increase in size over the few years and there was no history of weight loss.

Examination shows a 1 cm × 0.5 cm oval jet-black papule on the inner surface of the left buttock just lateral to the natal cleft.

Diagnosis

Acquired melanocytic nevi

Discussion

Melanocytic nevi may be congenital or acquired.

Synonyms of congenital melanocytic nevi include Mongolian spot, congenital dermal melanocytosis, and pigmented nevi. Congenital melanocytic nevi discussed briefly here are congenital dermal melanocytosis and they are found in the skin.

Congenital melanocytic nevi are seen in babies at birth or soon after birth; they are different from acquired melanocytic nevi that arise later in life. Some melanocytic nevi that arise beyond the time frame for congenital melanocytic nevi may have been inconspicuous during that period, only for the time of identification to place them as acquired melanocytic nevi.

With respect to acquired melanocytic nevi, the definite etiology is unclear, but exposure to ultraviolet radiation (principally of the sun), genetic factors, and growth factors is considered contributory to the development of this type of melanocytic nevi; however, whether genetic or environmental, no clear-cut etiological factor has been established. People with light skin pigmentation tend to acquire more numbers of melanocytic nevi than individuals with more intense skin pigmentation.

Compared with acquired melanocytic nevi, congenital melanocytic nevi pose a greater risk of the patient developing melanoma; this is more likely in patients with giant congenital melanocytic nevi in whom melanoma may develop in a part of the extensive lesion.

The acronym ABCDE (and *F*) is useful and easy for even nonmedical people to remember and apply.

A = *A*symmetry
B = *B*order for irregularity
C = *C*olor
D = *D*imension
E = *E*volution
F = "*F*unny looking"

The greater the changes or deviation from any of the already known *ABCDE* features of the patient's dermatological condition, the greater the cause for concern; in such cases the patient should seek specialist review by their dermatologist or any dermatologist.

The clinician must not assume that an adult presenting with melanocytic nevi means that they have acquired melanocytic nevi. The question about age at onset must be asked as the answer to that singular question may reveal the supposedly acquired lesion as congenital melanocytic nevi, especially if the response is at birth or during infancy.

During physical examination of the patient, the dermatologist or the young doctors working with them should not concentrate only on the lesions the patients usually present with but also examine palms and soles, in between the toes, and scalp. Dermatologists may need a topographic chart to document the precise location of melanocytic nevi when there are plenty. Distant and close-up photographs are also useful in noting the locations of the lesions and taking detailed view, respectively. A drawing by the doctor is better than nothing as it could clarify the description with just words.

Classification of congenital melanocytic nevi is frequently done using size as

Small: <1 cm
Intermediate: 1–3 cm
Large: >3 cm

Giant still falls under >3 cm although a congenital melanocytic nevus that is just a few centimeters larger than 3 cm ordinarily should not be in the same grouping as the extensive one described in an earlier chapter of this book.

The color of melanocytic nevi may range from normal skin color (nonpigmented), tan, brown, blue, and hyperpigmented to jet black. What is important is for the color of the lesion in the patient to be observed for any change. In Fig. 9.8, the patient's only lesion is jet black.

Asymptomatic melanocytic nevi that have become bothersome because of symptoms such as pruritus, pain, and bleeding should be examined further as there may be malignant transformation.

Significant changes that occur in a short time interval generally signal the need for investigations to rule out malignant change; the patient should be offered skin biopsy. Ordinarily, and in most cases, the lesions in a patient with congenital melanocytic nevi do not require investigations. However, in children who have multiple melanocytic nevi that are congenital and affect the skin on the posterior part of the scalp or skin over the spine, there are chances of the presence of neurocutaneous melanosis. MRI of the CNS may be carried out just in case the patient has benign nests of melanocytes in the central nervous system; if they are identified, they should be monitored with radiologic imaging as they could transform, over time, into central nervous system melanoma. Parents must be made aware of the risk of transformation to melanoma so that they do not relent in objective observation/ inspection of the lesions or fail to bring their children for scheduled appointments for follow-up care [5].

The patient and patient's close relatives are important in the management of congenital melanocytic nevi just as in other conditions that are long-term or life-long. Educating the patient or parent (if the patient is pediatric) is important as the patient may not come to hospital routinely for the condition to be reviewed, and the patient or parent may be the best person to observe changes in melanocytic nevi. The acronym "ABCDE and F" provides a simple means for them to assist the doctor in managing this condition.

Regarding the elderly patient with a solitary mole on the left shoulder, the development of a tuft of gray hairs right through the jet-black lesion is uncommon and is hereby reported. The diagnosis is acquired melanocytic nevus with leukotrichia [4].

Giant Congenital Melanocytic Nevus

Symptoms

The parents of this 6-month-old baby brought their daughter to the hospital with the main complaint of an extensive part of the body being covered by a black patch from birth.

When the baby was born, the mother was scared but although she and the father (who was also scared when he eventually saw the baby for the first time—for he was not there during the birth) had become a little accustomed to abnormal pigmentation of the baby's skin since she was, otherwise, normal, they still brought her to the teaching hospital for consultation. The parents were concerned that their baby looked "different" and were also worried that it may cause her negative effects in future.

The doctors in the general outpatient had not seen a case like this so they promptly referred the baby to the dermatologist.

The dermatologist took a detailed history and made the diagnosis.

Signs

Figure 9.15: The black lesion on the back of the baby's torso is, superiorly, from the junction between the upper third and middle third of the trunk. It extends, like a wide wrapping material, past the buttocks, and on to the thighs, but does not reach the knee joint skin flexures inferiorly. Three discrete, smaller, ovoid lesions are on the medial surface of the left leg; they are well delineated from normal skin.

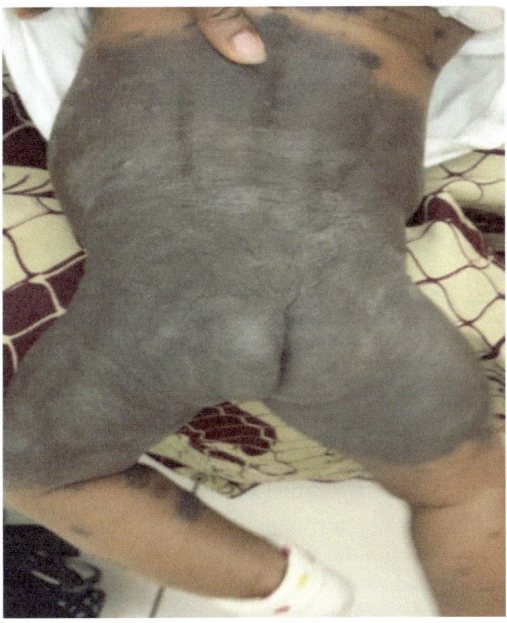

Fig. 9.15 Extensive black lesion on the back of the baby's torso

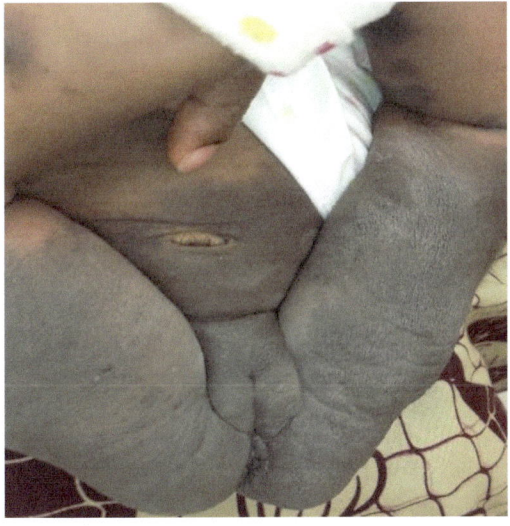

Fig. 9.16 An extensive black macule from above the umbilicus to the knees

Figure 9.16: The anterior part of the black lesion is equally extensive and has the upper border just superior to the umbilicus, runs through the perineum, and covers the two thighs up to the knees bilaterally.

It is like the baby is wearing a permanent corset that extends almost to the knees.

Diagnosis

Giant congenital melanocytic nevus

Treatment

This is challenging because it covers a significant part of the body. In much smaller melanocytic nevi, superficial removal procedures include curettage, laser, and dermabrasion. The question is "What is the purpose?" In cases like the one above, treatment does not provide significant improvement in color as the color reverts to the original intensity with time. Surgical removal is not exactly useful since the portion that can be removed successfully is unlikely to be the part that will become cancerous in the future—and in children, melanoma preferentially affects the nervous system. Emphasis is to support the patient psychologically, especially during adolescence, to accept the condition, and to live with it. The dermatologist should arrange for the services of clinical psychologists for suitable patients.

Etiology

In giant congenital melanocytic nevus, melanocytes proliferate and differentiate and continue to do so beyond the time they should have stopped. This is because mutation in NRAS gene causes altered protein (N-Ras protein) in the affected cells to be constitutively active.

Prognosis

The prognosis of giant melanocytic nevus is not good. The patient right from childhood (and especially from adolescence) needs psychological support. Patients must cope with the reality of living with this condition.

Follow-Up Care

Follow-up care could be extensive, but initially by pediatricians. Later, psychologists join to form a team that comanage the patient. If the parents or patients opt for surgical intervention, the plastic surgeon would be part of the team.

Discussion

Synonyms The lesion in the photograph above goes by other names, viz.: congenital giant pigmented nevus of the skin, congenital melanocytic nevus syndrome, giant pigmented hairy nevus, "bathing-trunk nevus," and giant congenital pigmented nevus.

Pathology Most cases of giant congenital melanocytic nevus are from mutation in the NRAS gene. NRAS refers to neuroblastoma RAS viral oncogene homolog. The NRAS gene is an oncogene. The gene directs the production of the N-Ras protein which regulates cell division. The N-Ras protein is a GTP-ase, converting GTP to GDP. In embryologic life, some somatic cells differentiate into melanocytes. In giant congenital melanocytic nevus, the cells proliferate and differentiate and continue to do so beyond the time they should have stopped. This is because mutation in the NRAS gene causes altered protein (N-Ras protein) in the affected cells to be constitutively active, therefore, staying turned on and relaying signals from outside the cells to their nuclei within the cells [6]. The signals relayed or transmitted by the N-Ras protein to the cell is thus for it to continue to proliferate and then differentiate into melanocytes. As an oncogene, there is a tendency for this gene to make the resultant giant congenital melanocytic nevus be predisposed to developing melanoma.

Presentation The condition may be symptomless or with minimal-to-mild symptoms like pruritus with or without dryness and dermatitis over the lesion. There may be hypertrichosis. The more significant symptom is psychological distress which could be of varying degrees.

Keloids

Symptoms

This patient, a middle-aged woman, came to the hospital to complain of multiple growths on her chest for at least 2 years. The growths were sometimes itchy and painful, with pain when she scratched due to the occasional itching. The growths were fewer at the beginning and had been developing gradually over the period. The patient did not know what caused them. She did not have thermal or chemical burns, scarifications, other forms of trauma, or any other significant exposure to her chest prior to the onset of the growths. She was not on "native," herbal, or traditional treatment prior to the onset of the growths. She was not aware of any innate aggravating or relieving factors but knew that paracetamol and Piriton® (chlorpheniramine maleate) were useful in reducing pain and itching, respectively, but the latter caused drowsiness that disturbed her work. She brought the complaint when she realized that she had not received a satisfactory response to treatment she received from healthcare practitioners in primary and secondary care facilities. She chose to come directly to the teaching hospital where she believed that she would be attended to by more senior doctors and, therefore, receive the best available medical services. She wanted this health challenge solved as it had become a cosmetic embarrassment to her, although the growths, thankfully, affected a part of the body that she could keep hidden for that length of time. She believed that this visit to the tertiary hospital would prove useful and be a way forward for her regarding this skin challenge, just as she feared that a further delay in escalating the treatment could worsen the condition and cause complications.

Signs

Figures 9.17 and 9.18 show multiple growths of various sizes and shapes but each with irregular margins. They show hyperpigmentation, hypopigmentation, and dyspigmentation. They are mainly discrete, but the large hyperpigmented lesion on the anterior surface of the left breast seems to be the result of a conglomeration of initially not-so-large growths. The growths were firm, rubbery, attached to the skin, and non-tender. There were no growths in any other part of the body. There was no axillary, supraclavicular, or infraclavicular lymphadenopathy. General examination did not show pallor or jaundice.

Diagnosis

Keloids

Figure 9.19: Growth on the hypogastric region (specifically suprapubic part) of the second patient. *The symptoms* of this woman in her late-30s were similar to the ones of the first patient, but the history was different. This patient had a single, large, very itchy growth that had lasted for about 10 years. The growth was not so large ab-initio but it was increasing in size. She had pain when she scratched it; occasionally she scratched to the point of wounding it. There were a few times that there was infection, and the experience had made her stop scratching vigorously in recent years. She remembered that prior to the onset of the rash she used to do close shaving of her pubic hair as frequently as she could. She used to wound herself in the process of ensuring a thorough shaving each time. Even when she developed the growths, she continued the shaving habit but made certain that she avoided the

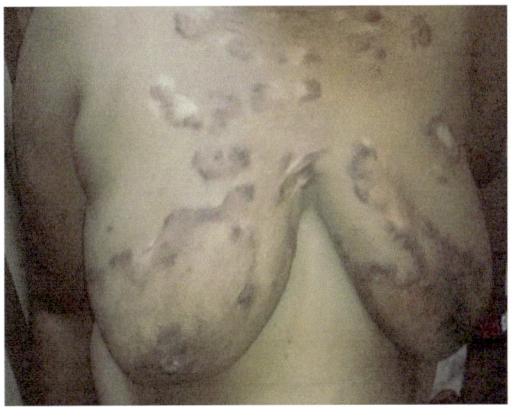

Fig. 9.17 Growths on the breasts and chest of the first female patient

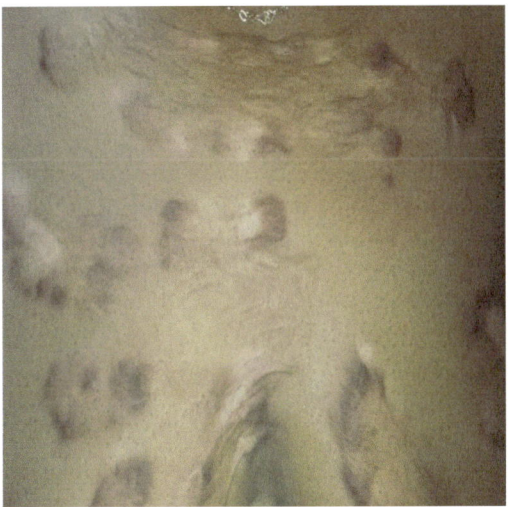

Fig. 9.18 Growths on the breasts and chest of the same patient

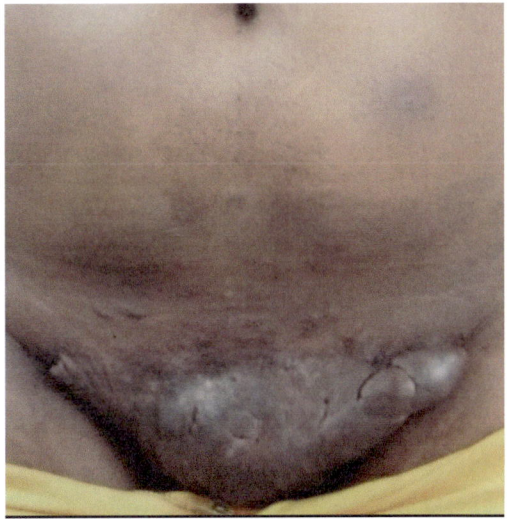

Fig. 9.19 Growth on the hypogastric region of the second patient

growth, paying attention to the skin surrounding the initial smaller growth. She did not have this growth in any other part of her body. She said that although she had been obese for many years, she was neither hypertensive nor diabetic. She was unmarried at the time and had not had any abdominal or surgical intervention. When referral was discussed, the patient mentioned that the growth was surgically removed about 5 years earlier, but there was a regrowth with the current one getting larger, over the years, than the initial keloid.

Signs

On examination, the patient was obese, with a BMI of 38 kg/m². The hyperpigmented 10.5 cm × growth had a transverse axis and was sausage-shaped with tapered right and left ends; the middle portion was heaped like a pile-up of a lobulated mass. The entire growth gave a semblance of irregularly shaped, firm, lobulated mass formed by spilled candle wax just before and at full hardening.

Diagnosis

Keloid

Treatment

The two patients were referred. The first was referred to the dermatologist to take over management. The second was referred to the dermatologist and plastic surgeon—the second patient was particular about her looks.

Etiology

Keloids are an overgrowth of scar tissue on parts of the body covered by skin. The basic pathology of keloids is excessive production of fibrous tissue most often occasioned by a variety of trauma.

In a minority of cases, a keloid may form unexpectedly, without any evidence of trauma.

Prognosis

The prognosis of keloids may be good or not so good; this depends on the size, location, patient's habits, recurrence, or form of intervention.

Follow-Up Care

Patients should be encouraged to keep the appointments for follow-up care. Keloids may recur even after apparently successful treatment. They should be advised to avoid what they may consider as microtrauma as even apparently inconsequential injuries in other people may result in keloids in keloid formers.

Discussion

Symptoms Symptoms of keloids include itching, heaviness, and pulling/constricting sensation, depending on the size and location. When keloids are large and over joints, they may restrict movement. Small keloids may be asymptomatic. Scratching of keloids should be avoided to prevent superficial or deep wounds that may become infected.

Treatment Treatment is keloid size-dependent and may be by intralesional steroid injections, cryotherapy using nitrous oxide (N_2O), surgical excision in one or more stages, laser application, or radiation therapy.

The patient with keloids on the chest and breast had been attended to by another doctor who had treated her with repeated doses of triamcinolone acetonide intralesionally. Triamcinolone acetonide is an acetonide (ester) form of triamcinolone. It is a synthetic glucocorticoid with both anti-inflammatory and immunosuppressive activity. The acetonide makes the corticosteroid more lipophilic allowing greater accessibility to the skin when injected. After ensuring a firm fit of suitable-size needle to syringe, it should be delivered gently and properly to avoid spillage/splash when injecting into a keloid. The drug tends to cause hypopigmentation of either the keloid, the surrounding skin, or both. Some of the lesions in this patient demonstrate hypopigmentation. Steroids not only cause hypopigmentation but also thinning of the skin as side effects. Methylprednisolone may be used as an alternative—but even with it, multiple injections should be avoided both in terms of sites and frequency.

Keloids tend to be commoner in people who are dark-skinned, especially people with Black skin. Among people with skin of color, some are more predisposed to developing keloids—they include those with a family history of keloids and those who have developed keloids in one or more parts of the body previously. The site may be anywhere that injury occurs, but the face and upper trunk (chest and upper back), shoulders, and ears (particularly earlobes) are the more common sites for keloids [7].

Keloids are like hypertrophic scars in the sense that they are not fine scars but overgrowths. The difference is that although hypertrophic scars grow above the skin they are limited to the size of the injury and consequent scar while keloids grow further above the skin and beyond the boundaries of the initial skin trauma.

The trauma preceding keloids may appear to be insignificant as in the patient with the suprapubic keloid who believed it was from repeated injuries during shaving. Other times they could be caused by skin injury during sports; domestic accidents, e.g., burns; etc. Ear piercing, tattoos, etc. also cause keloids in the predisposed. Infections and inflammatory reactions of the skin also cause keloids.

The size of keloids is variable, depending on the size of the antecedent skin trauma and the response of the patient's skin to the trauma. The site and/or size of keloids may make them aesthetic or cosmetic nuisance.

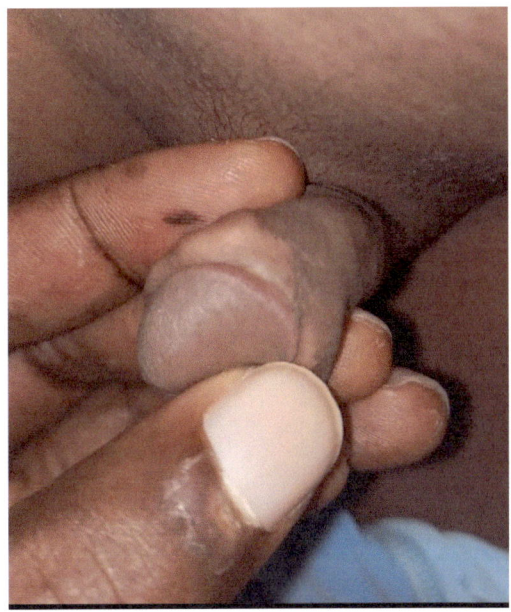

Fig. 9.20 Irregularity of the distal end of the penile shaft

Penile Calcinosis Cutis

Symptoms

The patient was a 9-year-old boy who was brought to the clinic by the father with the complaint of objects under the patient's penile skin. The first time it was noticed was when the boy was 8 years old. The father said that the first one was tiny and he pressed it and it came out with spontaneous healing of the site of extrusion. The son noticed two additional objects and one had grown to be larger than the other. The patient complained that he had pain on the skin over them, particularly the bigger one, when he touched them. There was no itching, skin discoloration, no painful urination, and no penile bleeding. He did not have them on any other part of the body. There was no history of penile or scrotal trauma recently or in the distant past. The boy was otherwise in good health and had no cause to receive an intravenous or intrapenile injection. The patient and the father were worried about the unusual objects developing on

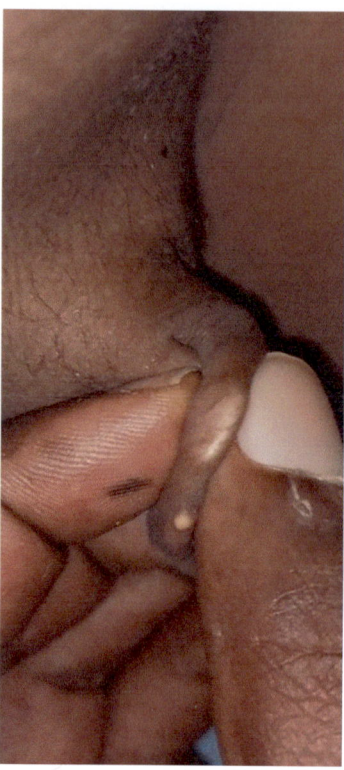

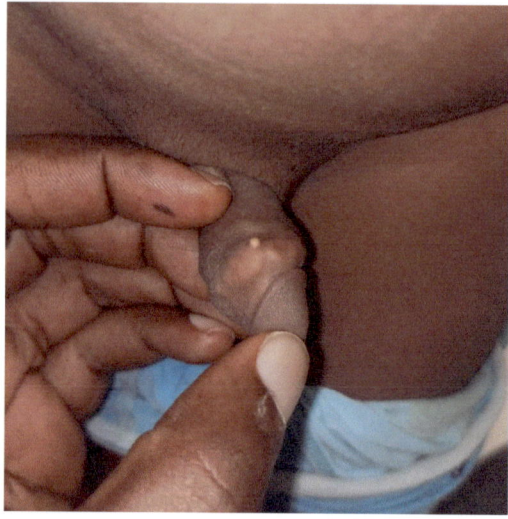

Fig. 9.22 Round off-white protrusion from the dorsal surface of the terminal end of the penile shaft

Fig. 9.21 Application of pressure to the distal end of the penile shaft shows ovoid subcutaneous growth

penile shaft bordering with the coronal sulcus; it was squeezed out with relative ease though with some pain, and it was yellow.

the patient's penis, did not know the cause, and were unaware of any other person having a similar condition. The father was concerned about the son's sexual performance in the future. Both the father and the patient expected to find the solution in the hospital.

Diagnosis

Penile calcinosis cutis

Treatment

Regarding the patient described in this case, the smooth, firm larger lesion was excised under local analgesia with plain lidocaine. The wound healed satisfactorily. As at the time of writing, there were no new growths.

Signs

On examination, the boy was circumcised. There were two subcutaneous penile nodules. Both were on the dorsal surface of the penis. The larger one was 2 cm × 1 cm, ovoid, firm, mobile, mildly tender, and on the distal half of the shaft. On palpation, the distal one was more superficial, spherical, 0.5 cm, soft, and at the distal end of the

Etiology

In calcinosis cutis, insoluble calcium salts are deposited in the skin and subcutaneous tissue.

Prognosis

The prognosis of penile calcinosis cutis is good; the same is true of scrotal calcinosis cutis.

Follow-Up Care

Both the patient and the father were glad that the boy underwent the procedure. The father brought the son to the clinic for scheduled follow-up appointments. The healing was satisfactory.

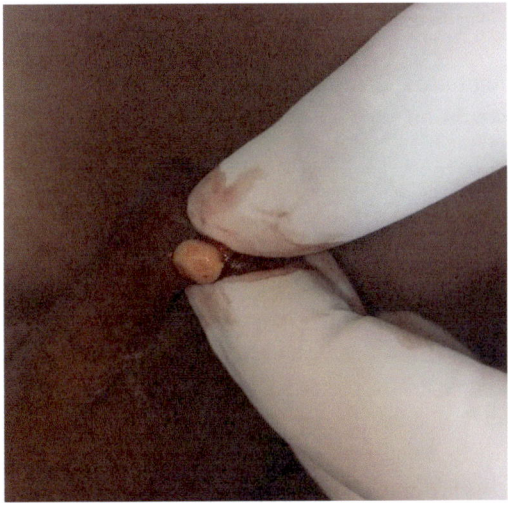

Fig. 9.23 Light yellow ovoid mass surgically extracted from the distal end of the penile shaft

Discussion

Deposition of calcium in the skin and subcutaneous tissue of the penis is uncommon; occurrence of these deposits is commoner in the scrotum. Calcinosis can affect other parts of the skin, e.g., the upper thighs and inguinal folds. Documented cases of penile calcinosis cutis in medical literature are not up to two dozen; it is possible that there are more cases that are either undiagnosed or undocumented. The lesions may be soft initially but eventually become firm or hard. They may be one or more; when they occur on the scrotum, the lesions tend to be more in number than the ones on the penis. A patient may have penile and scrotal lesions concurrently. Their sizes are variable but usually in the region of 2 mm. They have smooth outlines, and their degree of mobility during palpation is dependent on the depth.

Investigations Clinically, the diagnosis of calcinosis cutis of the penis or scrotum can be made from the history and physical examination findings. To establish the subtype of this disorder laboratory investigations may be carried out to demonstrate abnormal metabolism of calcium, phosphate, or both. Serum parathyroid hormone levels may be requested. After excisional biopsy, histopathological examination findings are useful in characterizing subtype.

There are five subtypes or mechanisms of these deposits, viz., idiopathic, dystrophic, metastatic, iatrogenic, and could be from calciphylaxis [8]. In idiopathic cases, there is neither evidence of trauma nor of metabolic disorder in the patient. In dystrophic lesions, there is tissue damage, but serum levels of calcium and phosphate are normal. Patients with metastatic calcinosis cutis show evidence of abnormal metabolism or calcium, phosphate, or both. In iatrogenic cases, the abnormal deposition is due to treatment the patient has undergone or is undergoing. In calciphylaxis, there is deposition of calcium in small blood vessels in the dermis and fatty tissue under the skin.

Treatment The treatment for penile calcinosis is excision. The patient and parents of minors should be reassured that the lesions do not recur, but they should also be informed that new ones may appear. The benign nature of this condition is a fact that the patient (or patient and patient's parents) should also be apprised of; this information gives them reassurance.

Neurofibromatosis Type 1 (von Recklinghausen's Disease)

Symptoms

Figure 9.24: The patient, a 34-year-old male farmer, said that he had grown with the growths from his childhood. He could not state the precise time they started. The growth had increased both in number and size as he grew older. The swellings were neither painful nor itchy. Describing the growths as present in virtually every part of his skin, he said that as he grew older and was currently in his adulthood, he felt embarrassed by people staring at him because the growths affected his face also. When he was a young child, precisely 23 years prior to this presentation, his father had taken him to a hospital where the largest growth was removed surgically. There was recurrence at the same site, and the growth was even larger than when it was

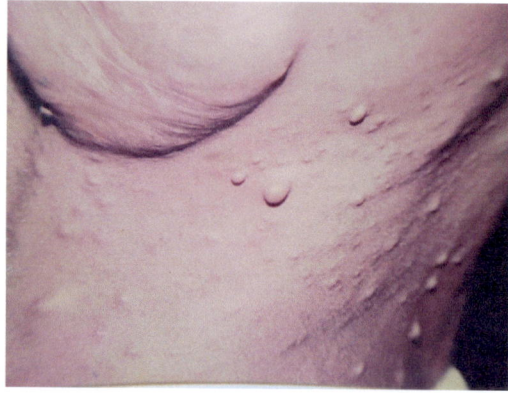

Fig. 9.24 Growths on the back of a 34-year-old male farmer. (Source: Reproduced with permission from *A Companion to Medical Students and Doctors*)

removed. There was no family history of this condition.

Signs

On examination, he had multiple soft, non-tender growths of various sizes and shapes from face to lower limbs. The predominant presentation was nodules. The largest of the growths was on the anterolateral surface of the left side of the chest; it was equally soft but was slightly overhanging. He also had hyperpigmented macules distributed on various parts of the body. He did not have axillary or inguinal freckles.

Symptoms

The second patient (in Fig. 9.25) was in his early 50s and presented with multiple, soft growths that were slightly darker than his unaffected skin. The growths which he had for most of his life were not painful or pruritic. He had become used to them and was able to function reasonably well. Over the years, they had increased in number and size but not to an alarming state. He was careful not to injure them. He did not like their number, size, or presence on his body. He was unhappy that he did not have smooth skin like almost everyone else had. Family history for the condition was negative.

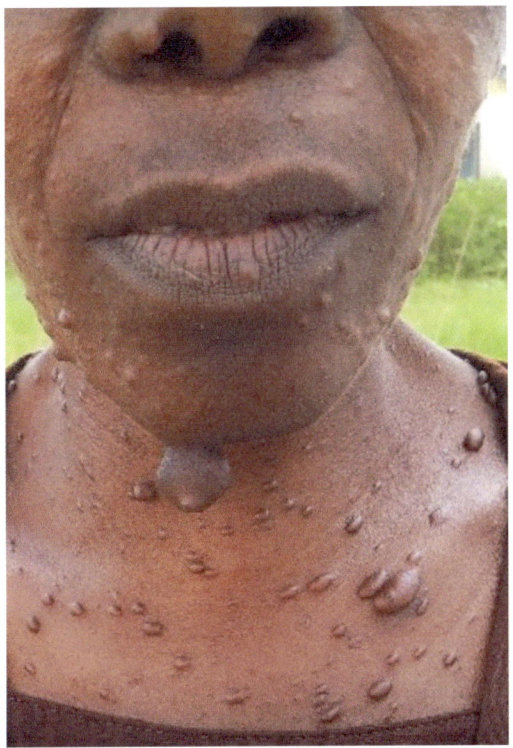

Fig. 9.25 A patient in his early 50s who presented with multiple, soft growths

Signs

Examination of the exposed part showed that the growths were multiple and varied in size and shape, with the shape of the ones on the neck and upper chest being principally ovoid; the growths tended to align with the natural cleavage lines of the neck and anterior chest skin. The growths on the face were mainly circular nodules though a significant number of them were ovoid; these did not follow any order. The largest growth was the flask-shaped one on the chin; it was almost pedunculated. As with the first patient, there were no axillary or inguinal freckles.

Going by the current criteria for clinical diagnosis of neurofibromatosis type 1, the diagnosis of neurofibromatosis when these patients were attended to is sustained. The criteria they met neurofibromatosis type 1 are six or more café au lait spots each of which measures at least 1.5 cm (15 mm) *and* one plexiform neurofibroma (the

first patient, i.e., in Fig. 9.24) *or* at least two typical neurofibromas (the second patient shown in Fig. 9.25).

Diagnosis

Neurofibromatosis type 1 (von Recklinghausen's disease)

Etiology

A genetic disease, neurofibromatosis type 1 is by autosomal dominant inheritance and so the deletion of only one neurofibromatosis type 1 gene is required for the disease to be expressed in the patient. In this disease, the synthesis of neurofibromin, a protein, is reduced. The protein is presumed to play the role of suppressing the development of tumor, and so its reduced synthesis allows this tumor to develop.

Prognosis

Prognosis cannot be generalized as it depends on the presentation in the patient. Patients who have just café au lait spots may have no challenges compared to patients with plexiform growths, lesions in internal organs, or malignant transformation.

Follow-Up Care

The specialist or the team who manage the patient with this disorder are the ones to determine the necessity and frequency of the patient's visits to the hospital follow-up care. It may be necessary to individualize follow-up care.

Discussion

Usual clinical presentation In childhood, neurofibromatosis type 1 first manifests as café au lait spots; the spots are multiple and increase in number and size. They may or may not be present at birth. These spots tend to become less conspicuous in adulthood as the color becomes less over time.

Inguinal and axillary freckles start to appear in childhood and adolescence.

Neurofibromas are cutaneous or subcutaneous growths; teenagers and adults manifest them, but older children may harbor these growths too.

Other features in neurofibromatosis type 1 include attention deficit hyperactivity disorder (ADHD), autism spectrum disorder, or learning disabilities; these conditions manifest right from childhood.

The neurofibromas can be superficial (cutaneous or subcutaneous), deep, or plexiform—the latter two are deep-seated with the depth increased in plexiform.

Complications Complications include local invasion by plexiform neurofibromas, peripheral neuropathy, and secondary hypertension—pheochromocytoma or renal artery stenosis may be responsible for secondary hypertension in this condition. Optic gliomas are the most common intracranial lesions of neurofibromatosis type 1.

Investigations Investigations are myriad. However, the actual ones chosen for the patient depend on the clinical presentation. Since the condition is not only dermal but affects internal organs, the history that the patient or parent provides and physical examination findings in the patient aid in determining which part of the body should be investigated. The following are investigation modalities that may be considered appropriate:

- Radiographs—These may be plain in patients with bony abnormalities or with contrast medium, e.g., in patients that require intravenous urography.
- Ultrasonography—This mode of investigation is useful when the growth is distinctly demonstrated to arise from the sheath of the nerve.
- Computed tomography (CT) scans—CT scanning helps in demonstrating neurofibromatosis type 1 lesions in nerve sheaths along the distribution and course of nerves in the brain, thorax (mediastinal), abdomen, paraspinal

sites, etc. The growths show solid, fusiform masses. In this form of neurofibromatosis, the lesions may also be spherical, plexiform, or dumbbell in shape.

- Magnetic resonance imaging (MRI)—For example, in patients with suspected nerve sheath tumors. Intradural neurofibromas are almost characteristically multiple in type 1 disease; however, in this condition, schwannomas—arising from the dorsal sensory root—are single while in type 2 they are multiple. Optic gliomas are also well delineated.
- Nuclear imaging—This mode of investigation complements the others when required. Radionuclide isotope bone scanning may be done on patients suspected to have neurofibromatosis type 1 growths within bone; it picks the lesions when and where present, but the findings may simulate other conditions—this method therefore has high sensitivity but relatively low specificity. When a neurofibroma is suspected to have undergone transformation into a malignant growth MRI, and positron emission tomography using fluorodeoxyglucose (FDG) which is taken up by the transformed growth provides images of the growth.

The two patients were not investigated or treated as they were attended to in a secondary care hospital in a rural area and during an outpatient medical outreach program in a primary care setting, respectively. They were referred to the nearest university teaching hospitals, but they did not return with any referral letter from the specialist to guide patient care in-between specialist follow-up consultations for review.

Treatment Management of the condition consists of adequate analgesia in patients who have pain, excision of the lesions surgically, use of radiotherapy, and psychotherapy to attend to the psychological component of the condition as there is no definite cure. Benefits of surgical treatment or radiation therapy should outweigh the risks. Complications arising from the presence of the growth in internal organs like the brain, liver, bile ducts, renal system, etc. are also treated according to their merit.

Follow-up care Annual checks (or other recommended checks for the index patient) are recommended for assessment of vision, hearing, etc. Evaluations depend on whether the patient is a child or an adult but should start from childhood. A child would require assessment of learning ability/difficulty and bone changes like scoliosis while an adult would require paying close attention to high blood pressure control or changes indicating malignant transformation of any of the lesions.

Melanoma

Symptoms

This patient complained of a small black spot on his right foot more than 3 years (but less than 4 years) prior to presentation in this hospital. He did not feel much concern about it but noticed that in the past year the growth had increased in size, become more painful, and occasionally bled with just slight trauma. The onset was gradual as he could not associate it with any trauma or severe illness at the time he first noticed it. The growth was only on the right foot, and he did not notice a similar development on the other foot or any other part of his body. The growth had made it inconvenient to wear shoes and he resorted to wearing flip-flops (called "slippers" locally); even with slippers, it was becoming difficult to move around, and he had to be constantly cautious not to hit his foot on anything so that there would not be bleeding.

He had gone to traditional healers for treatment for associates, and family members had suggested that he must have stepped on "something" with spiritual connotations although he knew that he did not step on any physical thing at the time. He was not satisfied with the proposed treatment and so he did not start it. He went to the primary care hospital in his community, but the healthcare providers there said that they did not know what the condition was although they provided him with dressing and an injection against tetanus. Over the period of this illness, the growth did not prevent him from conducting his work as a petty trader, but he knew that it would have been a great challenge if he was engaged in farming like people in his community. There was no past medical history of a similar growth anywhere in his body. Nobody in his family or the family he is from (his parents or siblings) had a similar growth. Coming to meet a doctor in a bigger hospital, he believed that he would receive appropriate treatment that would make him well.

Signs

The patient walked into the consulting room wearing flip-flops. He walked with caution but did not limp. He was not chronically ill-looking. He was mildly pale. He was afebrile. His vital signs were unremarkable.

Figure 9.26 shows the plantar surface of the foot of a 50-year-old man with an over 3-year, black growth with a brownish, fleshy portion

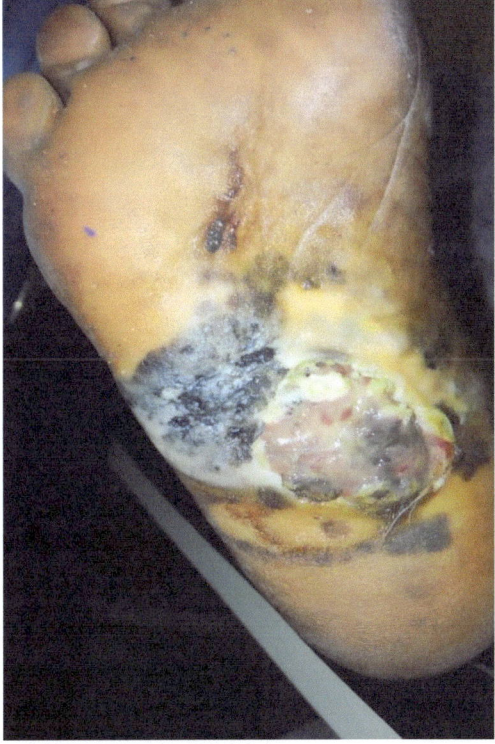

Fig. 9.26 The plantar surface of the foot of a 50-year-old man

medially. There was no bleeding or bleeding point, although the postero-medical aspect was reddish. The growth was asymmetrical and had irregular borders. At the time of taking the photograph, the growth was 8 cm in its widest diameter.

There was no significant regional lymphadenopathy.

Diagnosis

A presumptive diagnosis was melanoma, and the physician promptly referred the patient for specialist treatment, explaining the reason for the referral.

Treatment

The physician did not initiate treatment but promptly referred the patient to the dermatology department's clinic. The dermatologist was to initiate the treatment and co-opt other specialists as required.

Etiology

Malignant melanoma is a malignancy that originates from the transformation of melanocytes [9].

Prognosis

The prognosis of this malignancy is not good when the foot is involved; it is better in other locations of the lower extremity.

Follow-Up Care

Follow-up care plays a role in keeping the patient comfortable. If it is difficult for the patient to receive this care from the specialists in tertiary hospitals, the general practitioner should work in liaison with the specialists. The former would be

advised regarding when it is imperative to encourage the patient to go for their "check-up" while continuing to receive care. As mentioned, melanoma of the foot, especially for the patient who is not well informed or is not knowledgeable about the disease before its onset, is not good.

Discussion

Malignant melanoma is cancer of melanocytes or melanocyte precursors.

History When obtaining the history from a patient with lesions suspected to be melanoma, the physician should obtain information regarding the onset and duration of the lesion(s). It is important to know the number of lesion(s) identified by the patient and whether there has been an increase in the number or size of the lesions. Enquire from the patient if they noticed changes such as symmetry, bleeding, color, or ulceration before presenting in the hospital. Obtain a family history about similar growths, moles, or skin cancer.

Physical examination This should be a total body examination, to determine and document the number of lesions on the body as the patient may not have noticed all of them. Physical examination of the spots and growths should be comprehensive and include examination for superficial lymph node enlargement, abdominal examination, and eye examination. Most melanomas are in the skin, but because the eyes, mucosa, gastrointestinal tract, genitourinary tract, lymph nodes, and leptomeninges are other vulnerable sites, it is important to conduct comprehensive physical examination on patients as stated.

With respect to early melanoma lesions, *ABCD* is a mnemonic to characterize them, thus differentiating them from benign nevi. Features denoted by the mnemonic are *Asymmetry*—as they are usually asymmetrical; *Borders*—the borders are usually irregular; *Color*—which is deep black and may be a mixture of other colors; and *Diameter*—they are equal to or larger than 6 mm. Melanoma lesions may be in various parts of the body. Melanoma grows radially, followed by vertically. The first growth phase is growth in width, while the second growth phase involves growth in depth. Growth in depth is extension into the dermis and has a propensity for metastasis. Depth is a parameter for characterization of melanoma:

- Thin: 1 mm or less
- Moderate: 1–4 mm
- Thick: >4 mm

A general practitioner or family physician who has patients with a tentative diagnosis should refer the patients for investigations, diagnosis, and management or, if in the same center with the specialists, perform essential and basic investigations before referral to dermatologist, surgeon, and oncologist. The referring physician should inform the patients why they opt to refer their patient to other doctors and encourage them to accept the referral; if they are just given a referral letter with no explanations/counsel, some of them may not go because of financial considerations, long distance, or go much later at their convenience. It is essential to inform patients not to tamper with the lesions, especially the type and extent shown in the photograph.

Investigations Work-up on patients with melanoma involves laboratory investigations, imaging, and procedures. The doctor needs their results in making a diagnosis and determining steps to take in the management of certain patients.

- *Laboratory tests* include full blood count and liver function tests—transaminases, alkaline phosphatase, lactate dehydrogenase, total protein, and albumin.
- *Imaging* should cover ultrasonography of lymph nodes, chest radiography, CT scans of the chest, abdomen and pelvis, MRI of the brain, and positron emission tomography.

- *Procedures* include complete excisional biopsy, post-biopsy surgical excision, and sentinel lymph node biopsy (SLNB).

The investigations are important in determining the sites and extent of metastasis.

Histological examination findings in malignant melanoma are cell atypia—the cells are enlarged and have large nuclei that demonstrate hyperchromia and pleomorphism with prominent nucleoli; there are numerous mitotic figures and pagetoid growth pattern with an upward growth of melanocytes. Histological types of melanomas are as follows [10]:

- Superficial spreading
- Nodular
- Lentigo maligna
- Acral lentiginous
- Mucosal lentiginous

Most cases of malignant melanoma, approximately 70%, are the superficial spreading type.

One of the reasons for referring a patient for early and definitive diagnosis for expert management of melanoma is that the definitive treatment for melanoma at the early stage is surgical intervention. Surgery is wide local excision with SLNB and, if required, regional lymph node excision. When melanoma is at the advanced stage (with metastases), drugs are for adjuvant therapy.

Multiple-Choice Questions

1. Keloid: Which of the following statements is correct?
   A. It is a benign connective tissue tumor.
   B. It is synonymous with hypertrophic scar.
   C. It does not recur after surgical removal.
   D. It is not expected to respond to intralesional injections of steroids.
2. Which of the following statements about neurofibromatosis is correct?
   A. It is an autosomal recessive disorder.
   B. Café-au-lait spots are red patches of skin.
   C. The lesions are benign.
   D. It may undergo malignant transformation into a carcinoma.

3. A 53-year-old woman presents to you with skin lesions that you diagnose clinically as Campbell de Morgan spots (Capillary hemangioma). Which of the following is *not* a fitting association?
   A. Therapy—Observation by both the patient and you, the physician.
   B. Therapy—Commencement with ifosfamide on clinical grounds.
   C. Therapy—Laser therapy due to facial site.
   D. Therapy—Maceration of the lesion.

4. A 15-year-old high school student traumatized her right thumb while she was engaged in a phone discussion with a close friend and cleaning up her room at the same time during the weekend. Later, she consults you with a growth you diagnose as pyogenic granuloma. Which of the following statements is correct?
   A. The injury took place at least 3 months before the onset of the growth.
   B. Her presentation in hospital has no relationship with how she feels about the growth.
   C. The only reason she came is frequent severe bleeding.
   D. The injury took place within 2 weeks of onset of the growth.

5. Regarding melanoma, which of the following is *not* a type by histopathological classification:
   A. Maculopapular.
   B. Nodular.
   C. Acral lentiginous.
   D. Superficial spreading.

References

1. Cunliffe T. Cherry angioma (syn. Campbell de Morgan spots). The Primary Care Dermatology Society. Nov 24, 2024. Available from: https://www.pcds.org.uk/ clinical-guidance/cherry-angioma-syn-campbell-de-morgan-spot#:~:text=.

2. DeAngelis DD. Capillary hemangioma treatment & management. In: Ophthalmology. Medscape. Jan 23, 2023. Available from: https://emedicine.medscape. com/article/1218805-treatment.

3. Pierson JC. Pyogenic granuloma (lobular capillary hemangioma) workup. In: Dermatology. Medscape. Jan 6, 2025. Available from: https://emedicine.med-scape.com/article/1084701-workup#c7.

4. Kaur C, Thami GP, Kaur S. Nevomelanocytic nevus with leukotrichia. Case report. Indian J Dermatol Venereol Leprol. 2003;69(2):184–5. PMID: 17642876. Available from: https://ijdvl.com/ nevomelanocytic-nevus-with-leukotrichia/#:~:text=.

5. Mologousis MA, Tsai SY, Tissera KA, Levin YS, Hawryluk EB. Updates in the management of congenital melanocytic nevi. Children (Basel). 2024;11(1):62. https://doi.org/10.3390/children11010062. PMCID: PMC10814732 PMID: 38255375. Available from: https://pmc.ncbi.nlm.nih. gov/articles/PMC10814732/.

6. da Silva VM, Martinez-Barrios E, Tell-Martí G, et al. Genetic abnormalities in large to giant congenital nevi: beyond NRAS mutations. J Invest Dermatol. 2019;139(4):900–8. https://doi.org/10.1016/j. jid.2018.07.045. Epub 2018 Oct 22. PMID: 30359577. Available from: https://pubmed.ncbi.nlm. nih.gov/30359577/.

7. Chike-Obi CJ, Cole PD, Brissett AE. Keloids: pathogenesis, clinical features, and management. Semin Plast Surg. 2009;23(3):178–84. https://doi. org/10.1055/s-0029-1224797. PMCID: PMC2884925 PMID: 20676312. Available from: https://pmc.ncbi. nlm.nih.gov/articles/PMC2884925/.

8. Le C, Bedocs PM. Calcinosis cutis. In: StatPearls [Internet]. Treasure Island: StatPearls Publishing; 2023. Available from: https://www.ncbi.nlm.nih.gov/ books/NBK448127/.

9. Heistein JB, Acharya U, Mukkamalla SKR. Malignant melanoma. In: StatPearls [Internet]. Treasure Island: StatPearls Publishing; 2024. Available from: https:// www.ncbi.nlm.nih.gov/books/NBK470409/.

10. Smoller BR. Histologic criteria for diagnosing primary cutaneous malignant melanoma. Mod Pathol. 2006;19:S34–40. Available from: https://www.nature. com/articles/3800508.

Carbuncle

Symptoms

The patient with this condition was a young man who complained of "a big boil" in his left armpit. The boil was initially small but increased in size within 5 days and had become painful enough for him to be almost constantly aware of its presence; the pain also limited the range of movement of his left upper limb and therefore restricted his daily activities. He remembered shaving his armpits with a razor blade 4 days prior to the appearance of the painful swelling. Associated symptoms were fever and chills. He came to the hospital because of the complaints and the fact that despite the boil breaking he barely had relief and did not like the sight of pus and blood that discharged from it.

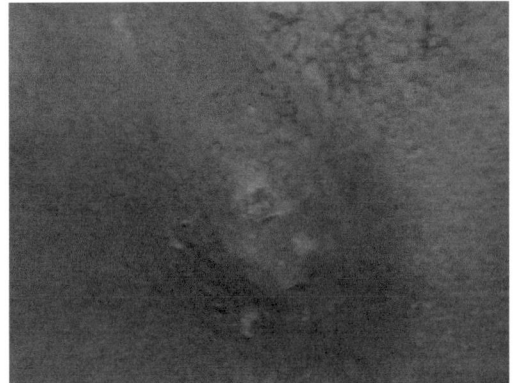

Fig. 10.1 The axilla of a young man who complained of "a big boil" in his left armpit

Signs

On examination of the left axilla, the solitary ovoid swelling was approximately 4 cm × 3 cm and was located at almost the center of the axilla. It was mainly nonmobile, hyperemic, and tender, with a pustular point located at the inferolateral part of the swelling, from where serosanguineous fluid discharged. There was loss of superficial layer of the skin as evidenced by wet flakes on the tender swelling and surrounding its base. The surrounding skin was wet. He had a little axillary hair growth (apparently, he had avoided shaving in the past approximately 10 days).

Supplementary Information The online version contains supplementary material available at https://doi.org/10.1007/978-3-031-97503-5_10.

Diagnosis

Carbuncle

Treatment

Systemic antibiotics to which *Staphylococcus aureus* is sensitive should be administered orally as they are effective and more convenient than via the parenteral route that is usually unnecessary, except in patients with diabetes mellitus or with a depressed immunological status. If the cause is methicillin-resistant *Staphylococcus aureus* (MRSA), then antibiotics that are effective against MRSA should be prescribed for the patient.

Etiology

The etiological agent of carbuncle is usually *Staphylococcus aureus*; it may be methicillin-resistant *Staphylococcus aureus* (MRSA).

Prognosis

Prognosis of carbuncle is good especially in patients whose skin condition is not recurrent. Small carbuncles usually heal without leaving a scar—unlike the large, multiple, or deep ones.

Follow-Up Care

As insinuated in the abstract, the management of carbuncles needs provision of follow-up care. This may entail keeping a record of the patient's fasting blood glucose and, occasionally, glycosylated (glycated) hemoglobin (HbA1c).

Discussion

Usual clinical features Since carbuncle is an aggregate of furuncles (boils), it is larger and tends to be deeper-seated and more inconveniencing as symptoms include painful large swelling; contained pus, discharging pus, or discharged pus; and occasional fever with or without chills. Carbuncle is an infection with interconnection of follicles beneath the skin surface [1]. It is immovable in any direction, and the inflammatory process is responsible for associated tenderness on palpation. Initially, the swelling is small but quickly increases in size; it has a hyperemic base and the immediate surrounding skin (a feature that may not show in the dark skinned); it develops more than one punctum; pus develops within the swelling and is best seen at the tip of each punctum—the purulent points form at the same time or soon after the first. Eventually, there is skin rupture at the point of least resistance and yellowish material is discharged. Spontaneous discharge causes alleviation of pain especially if much pus is released. When the patient interferes and opens a carbuncle prematurely, only little pus is released, and there may be associated bleeding manifesting as bloody or serosanguineous discharge; the rest of the carbuncle may form a firm swelling.

A patient may have just one or a few carbuncles but many in diabetes mellitus and in immunosuppression from disease, e.g., HIV infection or iatrogenic immunosuppression, e.g., immunosuppressant therapy or chemotherapy. Carbuncles may be recurrent.

Carbuncles may develop almost anywhere there is hair on the body; therefore, non-glabrous areas like the trunk (front and back), gluteal skin, thighs, axillae, groin, nape, etc. are common sites for carbuncles.

Investigations Carbuncle is essentially a clinical diagnosis. In multiple or recurrent cases, investigations should be carried out to identify the underlying cause. Microscopy and culture of discharge from a spontaneously discharging carbuncle or from incision and drainage define the causative organism; antibiotic sensitivity results may confirm continuation of the antibiotic prescribed empirically or may redirect treatment towards using another antibiotic to which the etiological agent is most sensitive.

Treatment Systemic antibiotics to which *Staphylococcus aureus* is sensitive should be administered orally as they are effective and

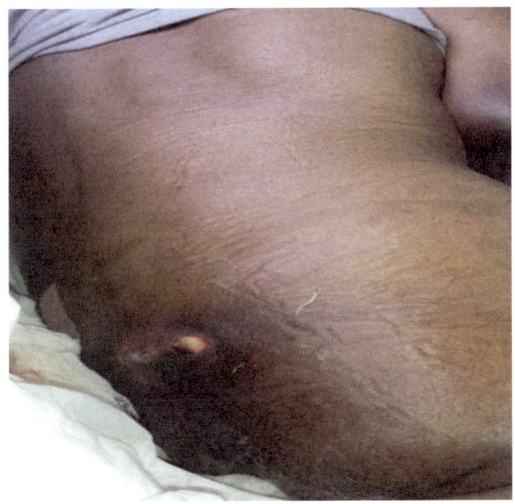

Fig. 10.2 The lower back of a patient with a pressure injury

titioners. The injury took place nearly 4 months earlier. Unfortunately, from weakness of the lower limbs, he developed an inability to sit on the bed and became "bed-bound." He needed comprehensive help by members of his immediate family and extended family members to gather the funds and get an assistant to bring him to the hospital and be available to attend to some of his social and other needs while on admission.

He was managed by the orthopedic surgery team, but the team promptly invited the medical team and dermatologist to join in the care of this patient as he was admitted with a discharging wound on the lower back. The patient said that the wound was there for 6–8 weeks.

Signs

The patient had paraplegia and paraparesis. He had a transverse ulcer measuring 6 cm × 1.5 cm at the lumbosacral area. The ulcer was deep and was filled with off-white to yellowish slough with a discharge that soiled the gauze at the time of wound inspection before carrying out wound dressing.

The dermatologist was to give advice regarding the skin as his management progressed.

Diagnosis

Pressure injuries

Treatment

His treatment was not primarily by the dermatologist, who was to provide advice and adjunctive care. The treatment he received consisted of thorough care of the wound with wound dressings, and there were plans to carry out debridement of necrotic and devitalized tissue. Wound swab was taken for microbiological examination, and he was placed on a broad-spectrum antibiotic based on local sensitivity studies while awaiting the results of the microscopy, culture, and sensi-

more convenient than via the parenteral route that is usually unnecessary. If the cause is MRSA, then antibiotics that are effective against MRSA should be prescribed for the patient.

Concomitant treatment of HIV should take place if the patient is positive to HIV. Patients with diabetes mellitus should be advised and encouraged to adhere with their treatment to bring their blood glucose level within the normal range. If control remains difficult despite confirming the patient's adherence to prescribed medications, dose adjustments or review of the drugs may be required.

Incision and drainage may be required if appropriate antibiotic therapy was not commenced promptly and enough time elapsed for significant pus to form [2].

Pressure Injuries

Symptoms

This middle-aged man with spinal injury from a fall from a height at a building construction site spent some time at home in an attempt to observe the expected improvement by not-orthodox prac-

tivity studies. He was also placed on metronida-zole against anaerobic infection.

Etiology

Protracted exertion of pressure on the bony prominences from prolonged immobility. It is important to note that immobility of just 2 h for certain people can provide the nidus for the development of pressure injury; these are bedrid-den people and patients undergoing surgery [3].

Prognosis

The prognosis is not good. The condition requires long-term care as there may be a recurrence of pressure injury after it might have healed or the patient may develop it at another site.

Follow-Up Care

The patients tend to increase in weight unless they have comorbidity that is catabolic in nature, thus causing weight loss. The patients tend to require emotional and psychological support, and this should be provided. The follow-up care may overlap the in-patient care. Following discharge, the follow-up appointments should be planned, as far as it is reasonably practicable, to be on a day and time frame that all physicians concerned are available to attend to the patient who may return for the follow-up care in a wheelchair.

Discussion

The skin is the largest organ in the body. Its mul-tiple functions can be summarized as presenting a barrier that protects the internal parts of the body from the deleterious effects of the external environment.

This topic was chosen to demonstrate not only the uniqueness of the skin but also the intercon-nectivity it provides various parts of the body. This high level of relatedness extends to medical practice as neither the physician nor the patient should consider all skin disorders as primarily skin diseases. Though some simple conditions may be expressed only in the skin, many diseases that affect the skin are not limited to the skin. Because they are not limited to the skin, they are linked to other medical specialties and the spe-cialists therein. It is therefore common experi-ence in medical practice for dermatologists to need the input of other specialists and other spe-cialists to need the services of dermatologists. There are conditions that affect the skin and need the input of plastic surgeons, orthopedic sur-geons, hematologists, and pathologists in other subspecialties, psychologists, psychiatrists, fam-ily physicians, etc. The management of pressure injury is one of them, especially when it is not anticipated and prevented, or when it occurs, and it is not done aggressively and promptly.

Pressure injuries go by other names, viz.:

- Decubitus ulcers
- Pressure ulcers
- Pressure sores
- Bed sores

The currently preferred name is pressure injuries.

Pathology The basic pathology of pressure injuries is poor vascularization of the skin with resultant devitalization of the affected skin at various stages. This usually occurs in areas where there are bony prominences making appli-cation of sustained external pressure and shear-ing to the skin overlying such areas lead to reduction in the blood supply to the skin. The cause of pressure to the skin is not always a bony prominence as it could be a medical device or some other device.

Risk factors The risk factors for this condition include uncontrolled diabetes mellitus, smoking, alcohol and drug use, and peripheral vascular dis-ease which may have negative impact on the macrovasculature and microvasculature. Other risk factors are reduced mobility, obesity, and exposure of the skin to wetness/dampness of clothing and bedding occasioned by incontinence of urine or feces. Additional factors that predispose people to pressure injuries are serious medical conditions like cardiovascular or neurological diseases, hypotension, dehydration, and malnutrition. In the hospital setting, patients undergoing surgical operations while under anesthesia for many hours are at a greater risk of developing pressure injuries [4].

The common factors among these and other risk factors are usually advancing age and reduced mobility. Individuals who are advanced in age tend to have reduced mobility.

Preventive measures Since pressure injuries can occur in the conscious and the unconscious, adequate care must be provided for anybody who spends prolonged periods in the sitting or lying positions.

Regarding the conscious, they should be encouraged to move or assisted to move or change positions at will. Spatial arrangements of the room or house should be such as can give an older person with visibility and mobility challenges a sense of safety to stand and walk without fear or risk of trips, slips, and falls. There should be access to the toilet so that they can go there and return without calling for help every time they need to urinate or defecate. This paragraph is inserted because every effort at avoiding limitation to chair, wheelchair, or bed is a measure of prevention because of anticipation of pressure injury development; this is preferred to prevention of decubitus ulcer when the person is already wheelchair bound or bedridden.

When a patient of any age is comatose for a long time or must lie on the bed for other reasons though they are conscious, e.g., paraplegic patients from spinal injuries, proper nursing care is paramount as care by various specialists in medicine for the primary reason for patient's hospitalization can be complicated by the patient developing pressure injury as an inpatient.

If an older person is a resident in an assisted living facility, there must be a total commitment to implementation of pressure sore prevention plan by the personnel of the facility.

Pressure injuries can occur at home, hospital, or assisted living facility, making the three short paragraphs above necessary to prevent occurrence.

Stages of pressure injuries The stages of this condition are as follows:

Stage 1 pressure injury = Non-blanchable erythema of intact skin
Stage 2 pressure injury = Partial-thickness skin loss with exposed dermis
Stage 3 pressure injury = Full-thickness skin loss
Stage 4 pressure injury = Full-thickness skin and tissue loss
In addition, there are unstageable pressure injury and deep pressure injury.

In unstageable pressure injury, there is full-thickness skin and tissue loss that is obscured.

In deep pressure injury, the injury demonstrates persistent non-blanchable deep red, maroon, or purple discoloration.

Investigations Investigations that are required for patients with pressure injuries depend on the extent of the injury. As earlier indicated, the injury does not have to entail obvious ulceration. The earlier the stage of the injury, the less complicated the investigations are. The investigations may be laboratory, radiological, or histopathological. The following are examples:

- Full blood count (FBC), i.e., complete blood count (CBC)
- White blood cell differential counts
- Erythrocyte sedimentation rate (ESR)
- Urinalysis

Depending on the health status of the patient or development of complications, further investigations may include any of the following:

- Serum transferrin
- Serum proteins
- Blood culture

- Urine culture
- Stool microscopy for white blood cells
- Plain radiography
- Magnetic resonance imaging
- Tissue or bone biopsy
- Bone scan

Management Management of pressure injuries may be medical or surgical.

In the early stages, the following are useful:

- Reduction of pressure
- Thorough care of the wound
- Satisfactory control of infection
- Adequate debridement of necrotic and devitalized tissue

Most pressure injuries are superficial, and they heal by secondary intention.

When surgical intervention is required, the patient must be prepared and certified fit for reconstruction of the injury.

It must be remembered that some patients that develop pressure injuries already have comorbidities, some of which are serious. Even when the patient's pressure injury is set for reconstruction, the specialists who attend to other comorbidities should certify that the planned surgical intervention does not aggravate that/those condition(s) or vice versa.

Complications It is better to manage the patient's condition and limit it to Stage 1 or Stage 2. If the patient develops an ulcer, any of the following may complicate pressure injuries.

- Anemia
- Osteomyelitis
- Sepsis
- Pyarthrosis
- Autonomic dysreflexia
- Malignant transformation

As mentioned in the earlier part of this topic, multidisciplinary care may be the way to go for certain patients; this means that a psychologist, psychiatrist, family physician, chaplain, etc. may be required even if the request is made by the patient or patient's relatives—if the services of nonmedical personnel do not complicate the patient's medical care.

Systemic Lupus Erythematosus (SLE)

Symptoms

The two photographs are of a middle-aged woman. She had recurrent oral/tongue ulcers with no dysphagia or odynophagia though she could not tolerate spicy foods. There were no active tongue lesions currently. The photographs demonstrate two features of systemic lupus erythematosus (SLE).

Signs

Figure 10.3 shows two rashes on the frontal scalp and parieto-occipital scalp. Both are irregularly shaped macules, of the same pigmentation as unaffected scalp. The anterior scalp demonstrates

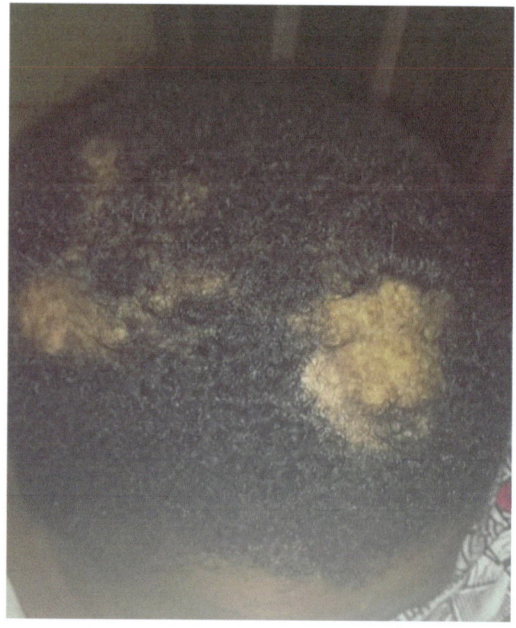

Fig. 10.3 Two rashes on the frontal scalp and parieto-occipital scalp

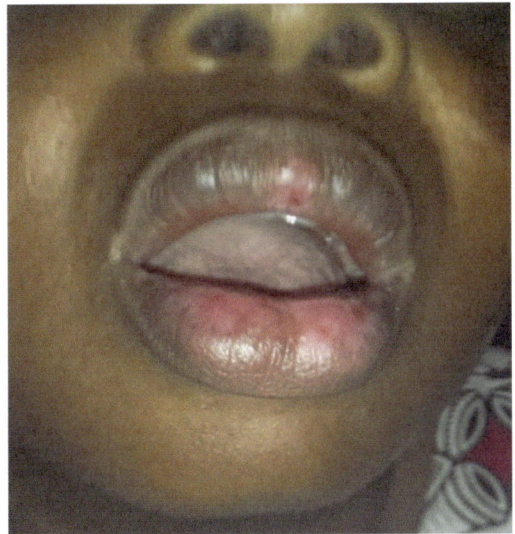

Fig. 10.4 The right malar area with an indistinct macule; the lip soreness

a greater degree of alopecia than the posterior one. They are chronic cutaneous discoid rashes.

Figure 10.4 shows the right malar area with an indistinct hypopigmented, vertically disposed ovoid macule while the lips demonstrate soreness with hyperemic patches—muco-cutaneous oral lesions. The lip lesions were signs of previous oral ulcers.

Diagnosis

Systemic lupus erythematosus (SLE)

Treatment

Cure is not available, but management consists of control of the patient's symptoms and ensuring that flare-ups are minimal in severity and frequency. Useful tips for patients include lifestyle modification with simple things like appropriate diet and difficult ones like avoidance of exposure to sunlight in tropical weather. Severe cases of SLE require anti-inflammatory agents, e.g., corticosteroids and high-potency immunosuppressant, non-biologic disease-modifying antirheumatic drugs (DMARDs) like azathioprine, methotrexate, and hydroxychloroquine in conjunction with

the newer drug, Belimumab—a monoclonal antibody and B-lymphocyte-stimulator-specific inhibitor. Hydroxychloroquine plays a principal role in the management of all SLE patients on a long-term basis. Less severe cases make do with mild immunosuppressants and short courses of NSAIDs.

Etiology

Systemic lupus erythematosus is a result of autoantibody response to nuclear and cytoplasmic antigens.

Prognosis

The prognosis depends on factors like the time of commencement of treatment, the extent of the injury, the age of the patient, and the nutritional and general health status of the patient.

Follow-Up Care

For patients with pressure injuries, follow-up care is essential, and this fact must be communicated very clearly to the patient and the patient's family members or caregivers.

SLE is a chronic inflammatory disease that can affect any organ system in the body, has a predilection for females from child-bearing age, and runs a relapsing and remitting course.

Clinical presentation Because the condition can affect any part of the body, symptoms can be from/in any of the organs/systems in the body apart from constitutional symptoms like fever, arthralgia, weight changes (loss or gain), and fatigue. Inasmuch as symptoms are myriad, the classic presentation is the triad of fever, joint pain, and rash.

- *Fever* may be from an acute bacterial infection; since SLE patients are considered immune-compromised, there should be a high index of suspicion of an infective process when there is fever. The febrile illness may precipitate SLE flare just as SLE and infection may occur at the same time. While most such infections are bacterial, atypical infections and opportunistic ones may occur.

- *Joint pain* of SLE may be arthralgia or from arthritis. The joint affectation is usually polyarticular and symmetrical. The degree of joint swelling and concomitant joint pain may not match; moreover, the joint pain tends to affect both small and large joints. SLE patients on corticosteroid or cytotoxic drug therapy are predisposed to developing avascular necrosis, especially of the neck of the femur. There may be myalgia also.
- *Rashes*—With respect to *rashes*, the features of these skin manifestations of SLE are malar rash, photosensitivity, and discoid lupus. The malar rash is characteristically erythematous (in the light-skinned), over the cheeks and nasal bridge but not involving the nasolabial folds—the so-called butterfly rash. Discoid lupus is not a feature in all patients with SLE; it is a chronic lupus rash. Photosensitivity is a third feature of the rashes. An SLE patient may also present with urticaria and telangiectasias. The patient also had alopecia of the scalp. Alopecia is not a specific skin manifestation of SLE, tends to involve the temporal region, and causes patchy hair loss.

Fatigue may be from drug reactions—just like fever may be. Vitamin D supplementation may improve fatigue and reduce disease activity. Weight loss may reflect the active disease process while weight gain could be from nephritic syndrome and anasarca, side effect of corticosteroid therapy, etc. There may be dermatological features like malar rash and discoid lupus while in another patient there may be myocarditis or pericarditis as cardiac manifestations or neuropsychiatric features like seizures or psychosis [5]. They may also present with renal problems like acute nephritic disease—the patient with acute nephritis may have hematuria and blood pressure check may show elevation of the blood pressure; other features may be of acute or chronic renal failure—with symptoms and signs of uremia and fluid overload; adult nephrotic syndrome patients have dependent edema and hyperlipidemia. There may be hematologic presentation clinically with anemia, thrombocytopenia, leukopenia, or lymphopenia as laboratory manifestations. A positive family history of autoimmune disease makes the diagnosis of SLE more probable [6].

A person is classified as having SLE when there is biopsy-proven lupus nephritis with antinuclear antibody (ANA) or anti-double-stranded DNA (anti-dsDNA) antibodies, in the alternative the presence of four of the diagnostic criteria which must include a minimum of one clinical and one immunologic criterion.

Investigations Relevant investigations are laboratory and radiological (radiographic and advanced imaging techniques).

- Laboratory: Useful simple laboratory tests include full blood count and differential count (which should demonstrate thrombocytopenia, hemolytic anemia), urinalysis with microscopy (which should show proteinuria, urinary cellular casts), and serum creatinine which should be deranged—all being features of cytopenias and renal dysfunction [7]. Additional laboratory tests that the physician should request are ESR, C-reactive protein (CRP) level, autoantibody tests, liver function tests, creatine kinase assay, complement levels, and spot protein/spot creatinine ratio. The doctor should also request tests that are not available in peripheral medical facilities but are affordable for the patient and the patient referred to carry them out in other centers.
- Radiological: If the clinical features suggest that radiological and other imaging tests promise to assist in making a diagnosis, such tests should be carried out, e.g., joint radiography in arthritis, arthralgia, or avascular necrosis; chest radiography or MRI in pleural effusion, interstitial lung disease, or pulmonary hypertension; echocardiography in cases of pericarditis or myocarditis; and brain MRI in seizures.

Procedures Procedures may also be carried out in suspected cases to assist in arriving at a diagnosis; such procedures include lumbar puncture, arthrocentesis, and renal biopsy.

Kaposi Sarcoma

Symptoms

The symptom was a growth on both feet for about one-and-a-half years in a 33-year-old female patient who was HIV-positive. The growth on the right foot was significantly more severe than the one on the left foot. The lesions grew gradually, and the pain increased as the growths increased. This patient developed Kaposi sarcoma lesions on the lower limbs bilaterally. A doctor in a secondary-care medical facility referred the lady to a dermatologist in the nearest teaching hospital. The lesions prompted investigations including biopsy for histopathological examination and HIV screening that led to the diagnoses of Kaposi sarcoma and HIV infection. The specialist was to commence treatment for this patient but, being financially incapacitated and a single dose of the medication costing the equivalent of $200, treatment could not be commenced until about 15 months after diagnosis. However, during this period she, on an out-patient basis, received supportive therapy for the sarcoma and HAART for HIV infection. It was after she was able to obtain funds from various sources of assistance that she returned to the hospital for hospitalization to receive treatment with monitoring. Thankfully, there was enough financial support to commence the treatment and see it to the last dose of the medication. This does not happen for many patients who are in dire need of treatment for certain conditions and is a source of frustration for many doctors and other hospital personnel who attend to such patients directly.

Please note that photographs were not taken at the first presentation of this patient and that all photographs were taken during the treatment. Note also that though both feet were involved, the lesions on the right foot were significantly more than those on the left foot; that is why the right foot was chosen to demonstrate the positive response to treatment although the treatment commenced significantly later than it should have been.

As at the time the patient was admitted for commencement of treatment, she had become wheelchair bound not just because of her poor health condition but because of the extent of the lower limb lesions which were significantly painful, preventing her from walking.

Signs

At the first presentation following referral to the teaching hospital, there was serosanguineous discharge from parts of the foot lesions. She was treated with antibiotics and dressing of the lesions and encouraged to take HAART regularly.

Figure 10.5 is a photograph concentrating on the lesions on the right foot of this patient. Note

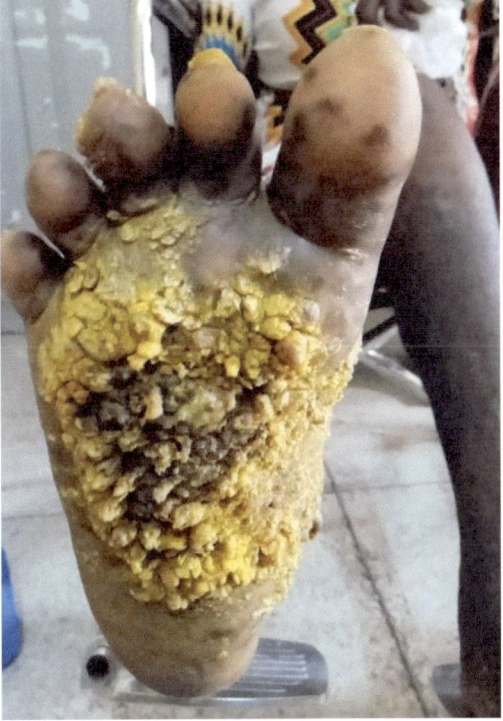

Fig. 10.5 The lesions on the right foot of the patient

multiple yellowish, nodular, and polyp-shaped lesions covering most of the sole of the foot. The lesions were approximately 1 cm. wide 2–3 cm. long (i.e., from the base). They were firm. A close inspection of the central part of the lesions shows that the base and that part are hyperpigmented. Initially, the lesions were of the color of the sole of the foot, but the patient continued using Savlon® brand of cetrimide/chlorhexidine solution to apply to the lesions which eventually took up the color of the antiseptic agent. Distributed unevenly on the remainder of the sole of the affected right foot are multiple, hyperpigmented plaques (which in a two-dimensional photograph look like hyperpigmented macules) of various sizes and shapes which extend to the toes. Only about 10% of the surface of the right sole has normal pigmentation. The lesions on this foot gave the sole a distorted anatomy.

Comparison should be with similar photographs after further doses of the cytotoxic drug and not with the initial photograph, Fig. 10.5 above, which is a close-up image for describing the lesions. Note that the patient was still using a wheelchair at this point.

At this time, she was beginning to wear slippers—soft rubber open-top and open-tip foot-

wear. The lesions were regressing especially centrally and medially. By this time, the patient had received the third dose of cytotoxic drugs intravenously.

The lesions of Kaposi sarcoma were hyperpigmented plaques extending from about the upper one-fifth of the legs to the dorsi of both feet. The plaques were thick. The right foot (sole) lesions necessitated application of crepe bandage. At this stage of treatment, the patient was still wheelchair bound.

Figure 10.10 was taken during the fourth dose of intravenous cytotoxic drug therapy. When compared with the photograph with crepe bandage, the hyperpigmented plaques are less. By

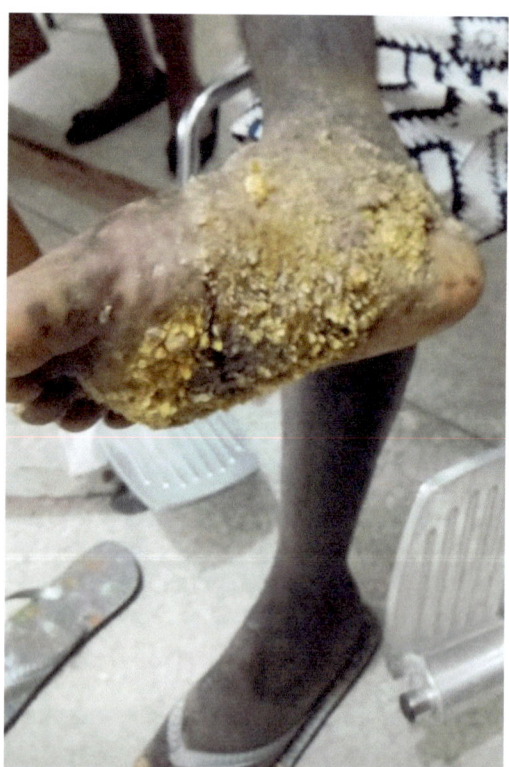

Fig. 10.7 The patient still using a wheelchair

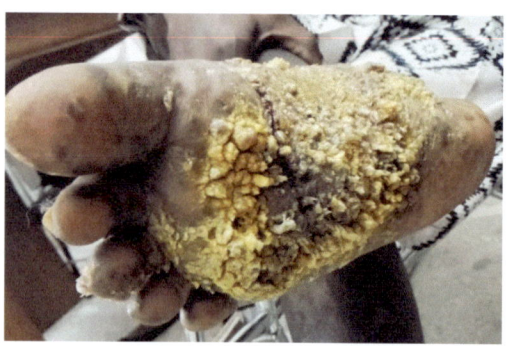

Fig. 10.6 The foot lesions after the second dose of pegylated liposomal doxorubicin intravenously

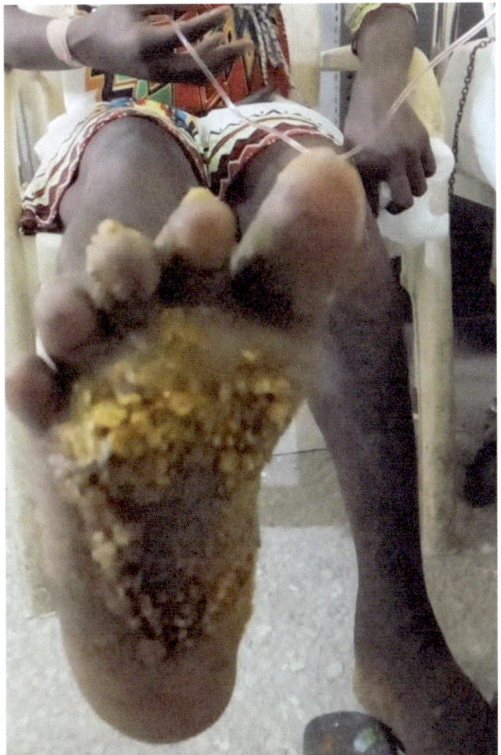

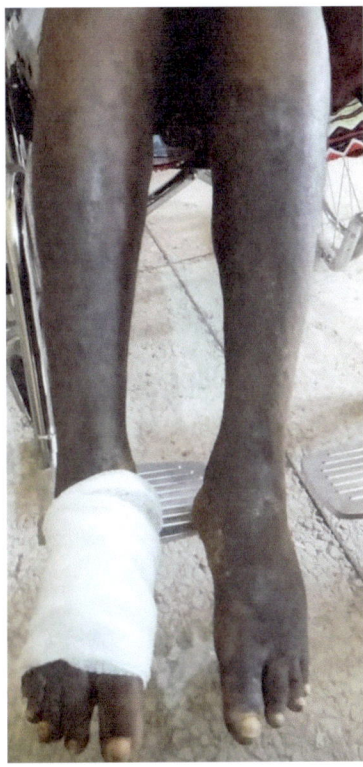

Fig. 10.8 The patient with regressing foot lesions. Note the intravenous line set up for her intravenous medication

Fig. 10.9 The legs and feet of the same patient

this time, the patient had quit using a wheelchair and was sitting on a normal plastic chair with an armrest and able to use a cane to walk. She was able to wear the soft rubber slippers on which she was resting her feet and the left one just beside her left foot.

There was significant resolution of the hyperpigmented plaques. The skin of the legs was of normal pigmentation although the skin of the left ankle and dorsum of the left foot was still hyperpigmented. The skin of the affected parts was still rough, lichenified, and of irregular surface. This patient was able to walk without a cane at this point though she walked slowly with evidence of some pain.

Figure 10.12, the photograph of the medial surface and sole of the right foot, shows remarkable improvement with the original lesions having reduced to just plaques with the same pigmentation as normal sole of the foot.

This patient complained of multiple growths on both feet (tops and soles) for more than 6 months. There was associated pain, but the pain was bearable as he only took analgesics purchased over the counter when the need arose. He had stopped wearing footwear that are designed to cover a person's feet for they no longer fitted him; that was why he was only able to wear the simple footwear shown in the photograph with difficulty.

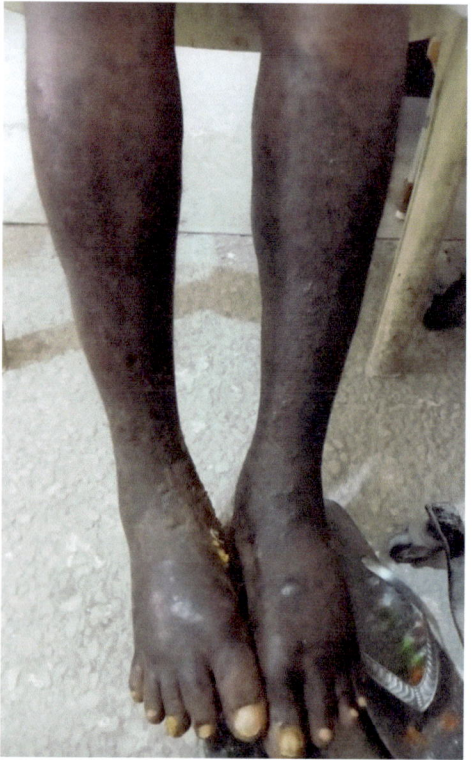

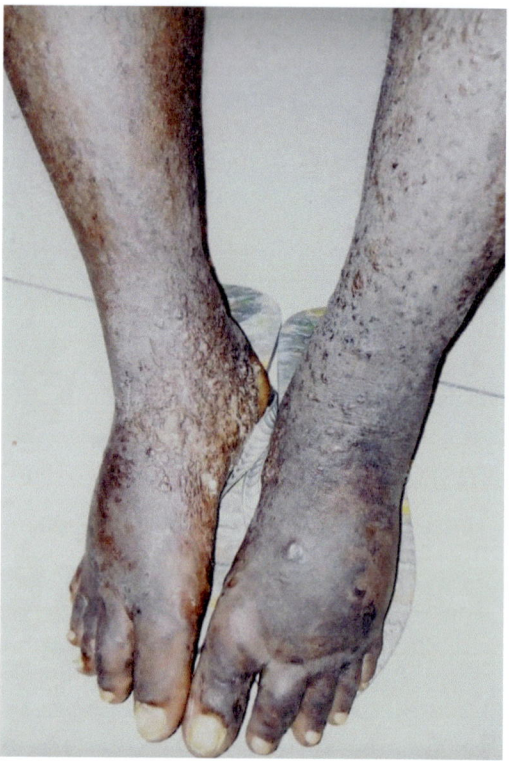

Fig. 10.10   Status at fourth dose of intravenous cytotoxic agent

Fig. 10.11   The legs and dorsi of feet after the sixth dose of pegylated liposomal doxorubicin

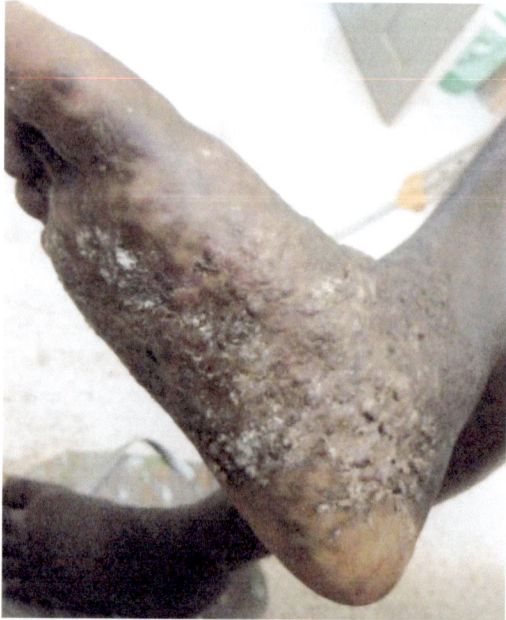

Fig. 10.12   The medial surface and sole of the right foot

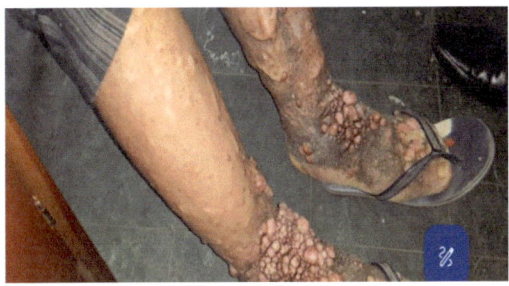

Fig. 10.13 The legs and feet of another adult male patient

Signs

On examination, the patient had firm nodules that made it difficult for him to wear shoes. The toes of his feet did not fit the design of the flip-flops; this meant that he was unable to fit the space between his big toes and second toes around the vertical plastic that connected the sole of the flip-flops with the two wings/arms at the top of the footwear. The nodules are multiple and, on the surface, appear to be discrete but link with one another at the level of the skin. The nodules are of diverse sizes with the largest about 2 cm × 1 cm and are ovoid or circular; the lesions that are smaller in size are in the majority. There is no evidence of bleeding, ulceration, or crusting. There is also no evidence of discharge. The dorsi of both feet are hyperpigmented up to and slightly superior to the ankle on the right and further up the distal part of the leg on the left. The pigmentation of the barely affected part of the right leg shows that this patient has Black skin of moderate pigmentation; when this observation is extrapolated to the left leg, that leg is significantly hyperpigmented because of the dermatological disease process.

Diagnosis

Kaposi Sarcoma

This diagnosis was made on the basis of clinical presentation. The patient attended an outpatient medical outreach that was free to all patients. He was referred to the nearest teaching hospital. The author does not know if he went, for he did not return to give a feedback (or return with any document from the teaching hospital) before the 1-week medical outreach for his community ended.

Treatment

The first patient was treated with pegylated liposomal doxorubicin intravenously [8]. Adjunctive treatment was started and continued for many months prior to commencement of the cytotoxic agent.

Etiology

The etiological agent of Kaposi sarcoma (KS) is the Kaposi sarcoma-associated herpesvirus (KSHV). It is the human herpesvirus 8 (HHV8) [9]. The virus infection triggers this angioproliferative neoplasm of endothelial origin.

Prognosis

Without association with HIV-AIDS, the prognosis is good, about 70%. Since Kaposi sarcoma is recognized as an AIDS-defining cancer and sub-Saharan Africa carries a disproportionately heavy burden of HIV-AIDS, Kaposi sarcoma is a common cancer in this region of the world with high numbers of this cancer still being recorded [10]. Prognosis of Kaposi sarcoma in sub-Saharan Africa, where people with Black skin are indigenous, is unlikely to be good until HIV-AIDS is contained.

Follow-Up Care

Follow-up care for patients with Kaposi sarcoma is better if the patients can attend to follow-up care with HIV-AIDS at the same time. This is because many patients must make arduous trips to and from hospitals, and even when they live in the towns and cities, the clinics have heavy loads of patients with consequent extended wait times.

Multiple-Choice Questions

1. Carbuncle: Which of the statements below is correct?
   A. It is synonymous with folliculitis.
   B. It runs a chronic course.
   C. It has the tendency to recur in some patients.
   D. It usually affects the big toe.

2. Which of the following is a correct relationship pertaining to carbuncle?
   A. Etiology—Parasite.
   B. Presentation—Asymptomatic.
   C. Pathophysiology—Aggregation of small abscesses.
   D. Treatment—Topical antiseptics.

3. A 39-year-old male with BMI 29 kg/m^2 presents with a second episode of carbuncles in 4 months. Which of the following conditions is *not* a risk factor?
   A. Diabetes mellitus.
   B. Hypertension.
   C. Kidney disease.
   D. Herpes zoster.

4. A 43-year-old obese woman with BMI 38 kg/m^2 presents to you with a history of bilateral inframammary rash of 1 month which has become worse in the previous 2 weeks. Which of the following statements is correct?
   A. Intertrigo is primarily a fungal infection.
   B. If she is obese the symptoms are unlikely to recur after treatment.
   C. Superimposed fungal or bacterial infection is expected to occur.
   D. The treatment of choice is a fluorinated corticosteroid cream.

5. Which of the following relationships about systemic lupus erythematosus (SLE) is correct?
   A. Sex predilection—Male.
   B. Truncal distribution—Photosensitive SLE.
   C. Other common sites—Blood cell lines.
   D. Diagnostic criteria—Clinical findings are of overriding importance.

References

1. Troxell T, Hall CA. Carbuncle. In: StatPearls [Internet]. Treasure Island: StatPearls Publishing; 2023. Available from: https://www.ncbi.nlm.nih.gov/books/NBK554459/.

2. Hee TG, Jin BJ. The surgical treatment of carbuncles: a tale of two techniques. Iran Red Crescent Med J. 2013;15(4):367–70. https://doi.org/10.5812/ircmj.2992. PMCID: PMC3785916 PMID: 24083015. Available from: https://pmc.ncbi.nlm.nih.gov/articles/PMC3785916/.

3. Bansal C, Scott R, Stewart D, Cockerell CJ. Decubitus ulcers: a review of the literature. Int J Dermatol. 2005;44(10):805–10. [PubMed] [Reference list].

4. Zaidi SRH, Sharma S. Pressure ulcer. In: StatPearls [Internet]. Treasure Island: StatPearls Publishing; 2024. Available from: https://www.ncbi.nlm.nih.gov/books/NBK553107/#:~:text=.

5. Justiz-Vaillant AA, Gopaul D, Soodeen S, Arozarena-Fundora R, Barbosa OA, Unakal C. Neuropsychiatric systemic lupus erythematosus: molecules involved in its imunopathogenesis, clinical features, and treatment. Molecules. 2024;29(4):747. https://doi.org/10.3390/molecules29040747. Available from: https://www.mdpi.com/1420-3049/29/4/747#:~:text=.

6. Ulff-Møller CJ, Simonsen J, Kyvik KO, Jacobsen S, Frisch M. Family history of systemic lupus erythematosus and risk of autoimmune disease: Nationwide Cohort Study in Denmark 1977–2013. Rheumatology. 2017;56(6):957–64. https://doi.org/10.1093/rheumatology/kex005. Available from: https://academic.oup.com/rheumatology/article-abstract/56/6/957/3037983?redirectedFrom=fulltext#google_vignette.

7. Hepburn AL, Narat S, Mason JC. The management of peripheral blood cytopenias in systemic lupus erythematosus. Rheumatology (Oxford). 2010;49(12):2243–54. https://doi.org/10.1093/rheumatology/keq269. Epub 2010 Sept 7. PMID: 20823093. Available from: https://pubmed.ncbi.nlm.nih.gov/20823093/#:~:text=.

8. Udhrain A, Skubitz KM, Northfelt DW. Pegylated liposomal doxorubicin in the treatment of AIDS-related Kaposi's sarcoma. Int J Nanomedicine. 2007;2(3):345–52. PMCID: PMC2676669 PMID: 18019833. Available from: https://pmc.ncbi.nlm.nih.gov/articles/PMC2676669/#:~:text=.

9. American Cancer Society. What causes Kaposi sarcoma? April 19, 2018. Available from: https://www.cancer.org/cancer/types/kaposi-sarcoma/causes-risks-prevention/what-causes.html.

10. Motlhale M, Sitas F, Bradshaw D, et al. Epidemiology of Kaposi's sarcoma in sub-Saharan Africa. Cancer Epidemiol. 2022;78:102167. https://doi.org/10.1016/j.canep.2022.102167. Available from: https://www.sciencedirect.com/science/article/pii/S1877782122000728.

Medications in Dermatology

Mechanisms of Drug Action and Drug Use in Dermatology

Tetracyclines Tetracyclines are the antibiotic class that are most frequently used in the treatment of bacterial and inflammatory dermatological conditions. The mechanism of action of tetracyclines is multipronged [1]. That is why this class of drugs is useful in treating conditions that may not be primarily of bacterial origin. Tetracyclines do the following and more:

- Suppress chemotaxis and migration of neutrophils.
- Inhibit phospholipase A2.
- Inhibit activation of mast cells.
- Scavenge reactive oxygen species (ROS).
- Inhibit metalloproteinases.
- Inhibit expression of nitric oxide synthase.
- Inhibit inflammation-stimulating products from bacteria.

Tetracyclines may be low-dose tetracycline (a first-generation tetracycline), the easier-to-take doxycycline and minocycline (which are second-generation tetracyclines), or sarecycline (a third-generation tetracycline). Tetracyclines are useful in treating patients with acne vulgaris, rosacea, hidradenitis suppurativa, and bacterial skin infections that are caused by bacteria that are sensitive to tetracyclines. Gastrointestinal disturbances may prevent drug adherence of patients who are on tetracycline or doxycycline; minocycline and sarecycline may or may not be taken with food [2]. Patients may be on these drugs for up to 3 or 4 months.

Clindamycin Clindamycin binds to the 50S subunit of ribosomes in bacteria. It interferes with transpeptidation, inhibits the early stage of elongation of the protein chain, and consequently inhibits protein synthesis.

Macrolides, Penicillins, and Cephalosporins These are other classes of antibiotics that are used in dermatology.

Corticosteroids Steroidal anti-inflammatory agents used in dermatology are essentially corticosteroids. These steroids are available for topical use as lotions, creams, ointments, and solutions; they are also available as injections to be injected into skin lesions as intralesional injections. They exert anti-inflammatory and antipruritic effects. Topical corticosteroids suppress the migration of polymorphonuclear leukocytes (neutrophils) and reverse the increased permeability of capillaries which are features of inflammation. Examples are hydrocortisone 1% cream, betamethasone cream, methylprednisolone injection, and triamcinolone acetonide injection—the latter is a fluorinated corticosteroid. Hydrocortisone is mild and is useful in acute urti-

I. Ukot, *Understanding Diseases in Skin of Color*, https://doi.org/10.1007/978-3-031-97503-5_11

caria from, e.g., insect bites. Betamethasone is more potent and is effective in conditions like neurodermatitis (lichen simplex chronicus), psoriasis, and contact dermatitis; application of potent corticosteroid creams should be avoided in cases of significant area of skin coverage for prolonged periods as cutaneous absorption in such cases could cause elevation of blood pressure or blood glucose in the patients. Their local effects on the skin from long-term application include skin atrophy, striae, bruising, and telangiectasias. The creams pose a greater risk than the intralesional injections as patients, in some countries, can purchase them over the counter from the same or a different sale outlet without prescription and use the drugs for long periods. The injections are administered by qualified medical personnel.

Retinoids Vitamin A is retinol; retinoic acid is one of the metabolites of vitamin A. Retinoids are derivatives of vitamin A or molecules that are structurally or functionally like vitamin A. Retinoids are molecules that bind to retinoic acid receptors in the skin; the direct binding of the ligand with the receptor leads to activation of the receptor with the result that genes that are sensitive to retinoic acid are transcribed. Retinoids cause reduction of epithelial cell turnover rate and enhance differentiation of these cells [3]. Retinoids are used in the management of acne, post-inflammatory hyperpigmentation, psoriasis, photoaging, keratosis pilaris, and Kaposi's sarcoma. Of the six classes of retinoids, tretinoin which is all-trans retinoic acid is available in resource-poor countries; an example is isotretinoin. When all-trans retinoic acid is applied topically, there is induction of collagen synthesis. Tretinoin also blocks degradation of collagen, and this property makes it useful in photoaging; the cream is applied before exposure to ultraviolet radiation under sunshine. In acne, the effects of treatment with retinoids are increased follicular turnover, increased shedding of corneocytes from the stratum corneum, increase in proliferation and differentiation of cells, and reduction in the formation of microcomedones. Tretinoin therefore exerts positive

effects on the epidermis and dermis. Tretinoin may cause skin irritation and local dryness and should not be used during pregnancy and in patients who are hypersensitive to the drug.

Moisturizers Moisturizers are preparations that moisten the skin. There are three types of moisturizers—humectants, emollients, and occlusives. Moisturizers have water phase and oil phase. Humectants provide the stratum corneum with water, and this is important in improving skin hydration in dry skin or in areas of the skin with dry lesions. Examples of the components of humectants are glycerol, hyaluronic acid, and urea [4]. Emollients fill inter-corneocyte cluster gaps (the spaces between clusters of corneocytes [present in the stratum corneum]); in this way they help in achieving suppleness and elasticity of the skin. Emollients contain saturated and unsaturated hydrocarbons. Examples of the components of emollients are fatty acids, cholesterol, and fatty alcohols. Occlusives prevent trans-epidermal water loss by forming a hydrophobic barrier on the surface of the skin [5]. Occlusives contain oils and waxes. Examples of the components of occlusives are petroleum jelly, zinc oxide, beeswax, and mineral oil. Emollients and occlusives are therefore mostly lipid based with a small fraction composed of the water phase of these moisturizers. Moisturizers are useful adjuncts in the treatment of dermatitis (e.g., atopic, seborrheic, contact), but the patient should commit to using them for long periods (or continuously) as recommended by the physician. Some patients may develop skin irritation from constituents of humectants and emollients; with regard to occlusives, oiliness of the patient's skin may be unacceptable to those who are particularly conscious of the appearance of their skin.

Antihistamines Histamine is a vasoactive compound that is present in mast cells in granular form. Mast cells are in the skin. When mast cells degranulate, the released histamine leads to extravasation of fluid into surrounding tissue with the result of edema; the other effect of histamine is dilatation of small blood vessels. The combination of vasodilatation and tissue edema with irritation of nerves in the skin produces itching. Antihistamines that are used in dermatology are mainly H1-receptor blockers. The human H1-receptor is a member of the G-protein coupled receptors. H1-blockers are antihistamines that bind the same receptors that histamine binds but tend to keep the receptors in an inactive state; they produce a result opposite to what histamine produces and are effectively inverse agonists of histamine. Second-generation HI-receptor blockers are preferred as they are generally non-sedating. The patient may not have complete relief when antihistamines are used as the pruritic skin condition may also be due to non-histamine vasoactive agents. In susceptible individuals, there may be drowsiness and sedation when non-sedating antihistamines are used. The drugs include cetirizine; levocetirizine, e.g., Xyzal®; loratadine; desloratadine; and fexofenadine; they are essentially for systemic use. The drugs are available as injections for severe conditions that require rapid relief. There are also oral preparations for adult and pediatric age groups. First-generation H1-receptor blockers also have topical preparations, and these should be used when the lesions are few or small—they act locally and should preferably be used for short periods. Second-generation HI-receptor blockers are effective in allergic conditions and are superior to the first-generation H1-receptor blocker by their high selectivity of the H! receptors, and longer duration of action, coupled with low penetration into the central nervous system [6]. The allergic conditions for which they should be used include skin conditions like acute urticaria, chronic idiopathic urticaria, papular urticaria, dermographism, and others.

Keratolytics Keratolytic drugs like anthralin and salicylic acid remove scales from thick skin lesions making other topical agents accessible to the lesions. Dermatological conditions that improve with keratolytics include warts, seborrheic keratosis, acne, psoriasis, and dandruff.

Coal tar Coal tar is an antipruritic and an inhibitor of deregulated proliferation of the epidermis and infiltration of the dermis. Coal tar-containing shampoos are useful for the treatment of scalp psoriasis.

Non-steroidal anti-inflammatory drugs (NSAIDs) Ultraviolet radiation stimulates the enzyme cyclooxygenase-2 (COX-2) expression in the epidermis; normally, it is not present in the skin. Polyamines are aliphatic compounds that possess more than two amino groups; these molecules are implicated in the development of non-melanoma skin cancers. NSAIDs block the induction of ornithine carboxylase leading to inhibition of the synthesis of polyamines. Prostaglandins are synthesized from the fatty acid, arachidonic acid. Prostaglandins are unsaturated carboxylic acids. Prostaglandin E2 stimulates keratinocytes to proliferate. NSAIDs promote apoptosis of keratinocytes. NSAIDs that are selective cyclooxygenase-2 (COX-2) inhibitors have better safety profiles even in patients that need to use them beyond a few days. Analysis of data from three large longitudinal cohort studies, however, asserts that rather than reduce the risk of developing skin cancers the use of COX-2 inhibitors is associated with a moderate risk of developing basal cell carcinoma. NSAIDs are useful in acne, psoriasis, urticarial vasculitis, sunburns, and erythema nodosum. They may be useful in the prevention and treatment of non-melanoma skin carcinomas.

Difluoromethylornithine Difluoromethylornithine (DFMO), a fluorinated analog of ornithine. It is an irreversible suicide inhibitor of the enzyme ornithine decarboxylase [7]. The enzyme catalyzes the synthesis of polyamines. Polyamines are implicated in the genesis of non-melanoma skin cancers. The drug is known to provide chemoprophylaxis against skin cancers. It goes by the name Eflornithine; it is available as a cream for use in dermatology for patients with abnormal hair growth in conditions like hirsutism and hypertrichosis. It is also a drug used (as oral and intravenous preparations) to treat human African trypanosomiasis (sleeping sickness) caused by *Trypanosoma brucei* gambiense and *Pneumocystis carinii* pneumonia.

Vitamin E Vitamin E (commonly called alpha-tocopherol although it incorporates tocotrienols and tocopherols other than α-tocopherol) is a lipid natural antioxidant associated with cell membranes; it protects the cell membranes including those of the skin from reactive oxygen species which are highly reactive compounds derived from diatomic oxygen, e.g., alpha-oxygen, peroxyl radical, and hydroxyl radical. Vitamin E is a scavenger of lipid peroxyl radicals, therefore protecting the lipid environment. In dermatological conditions, it is used as an anti-inflammatory agent. Serum levels of vitamin E may be low in conditions like acne, vitiligo, psoriasis, and atopic dermatitis justifying their inclusion in the management of these conditions.

Immunomodulators Immunomodulators are anti-inflammatory drugs and prevent cell proliferation. They are direct cytotoxic agents, doing so by inhibition of intracellular cell adhesion molecules (ICAMs) and induction of apoptosis [8]. They are analogs of thalidomide. Nonsteroidal immunomodulators include macrolactams, e.g., tacrolimus. Unlike topical corticosteroids, topical tacrolimus does not reduce collagen synthesis. It is useful in treating atopic dermatitis, psoriasis, mucosal erosive lichen planus, and corticosteroid-induced rosacea. It may be used in combination with clobetasol propionate ointment to treat resistant cutaneous lupus erythematosus in adult patients. Other examples of macrolactam immunomodulators include pimecrolimus and cyclosporine.

Contact sensitizers Contact sensitizers are also nonsteroidal immunomodulators. Two examples of contact sensitizers are squaric acid dibutyl ester and diphenylcyclopropenone. The mechanism of action of squaric acid dibutyl ester is extravasation and recruitment of activated autoreactive T cells. The mode of action of diphenylcyclopropenone is cytokine release and T-cell activation.

Immunostimulators Immunostimulators are another group of nonsteroidal immunomodulators. An example of immunostimulators is imiquimod; it is a synthetic drug. It enhances the synthesis of cytokines and therefore improves natural immune response. Imiquimod is used in the management of common warts, genital warts, actinic keratosis, keloids, and molluscum contagiosum. In keloids, it enhances the production of collagenase which breaks down the excessive collagen tissue in the disease [9]. Imiquimod also has antiviral and antitumor effects.

Miscellaneous immunomodulators There is a miscellaneous group of immunomodulators. They are topical agents and injectable drugs. The topical agents include anthralin, zinc, calcitriol, calcipotriol, and interferon-alpha. The injectable drugs are recombinant intralesional injections, an example of which is intralesional Bacillus Calmette-Guérin (BCG).

Calcipotriol Calcipotriol is a synthetic vitamin D3 analog. The drug binds to keratinocyte vitamin D receptors to exert its immunomodulatory effect. While it inhibits keratinocyte proliferation, it enhances their differentiation. It does not cause photosensitization, children tolerate it, and it does not cause skin atrophy. The side effect of skin irritation precludes its application on the face and should not be prescribed for patients with lichen simplex chronicus or atopic eczema—as they are already very pruritic conditions. It is used in the treatment of vitiligo.

Calcitriol Calcitriol is a miscellaneous immunomodulator. It is a metabolite of vitamin D3. It is tolerated better than calcipotriol and so may be used in the treatment of psoriasis of the face, neck, and flexural parts of the skin. It is not recommended for children less than 15 years of age. Vitamin D analogs like calcitriol prevent thinning of the skin; the foams and solutions are beneficial in, e.g., scalp psoriasis.

Anthralin Anthralin is also in the group of miscellaneous immunomodulators. Among other effects, it inhibits the synthesis, repair, and replication of DNA in cells like keratinocytes, fibroblasts, and lymphocytes. It has antimitotic activity. It is useful in treating alopecia areata and lichen planus that is not extensive.

Zinc sulphate Zinc sulphate for topical administration is another drug in the miscellaneous group of immunomodulators. It inhibits the release of inflammatory cytokines from keratinocytes; the cytokines are interleukin-1 (IL-1) and interleukin-6 (IL-6). It may be used in combination with erythromycin to treat acne and in combination with clobetasol to treat lichen planus, chronic eczema, or eczematous psoriasis.

Calcineurin inhibitors Calcineurin inhibitors suppress the synthesis of pro-inflammatory cytokines. The drugs bind to macrophilin-12 which is an intracellular protein; this takes place in the cytoplasm of the targeted cells. An example of calcineurin inhibitors is tacrolimus. These drugs are useful in treating atopic dermatitis, psoriasis, and vitiligo; they regulate the synthesis of melanin and cause the restoration of keratinocyte and melanocyte calcium homeostasis.

Leukotriene modifiers Arachidonic acid and leukotrienes are here discussed prior to leukotriene modifiers.

Arachidonic acid is a polyunsaturated omega-6 fatty acid. The metabolism of this molecule is important in diseases that are related to leukotrienes. Leukotrienes are potent smooth muscle constrictors. Leukotriene modifiers modify the amounts of this molecule and reduce the response of patients in whom there is hyperresponsiveness to leukotrienes. When arachidonate 5-lipoxygenase (commonly referred to as 5-lipoxygenase) acts on arachidonic acid, it produces the intermediate called 5-HPETE. This is the 5-lipoxygenase pathway, and it entails enzymatic breakdown of arachidonic acid to 5-*hydroperoxyeicosatetraenolic* acid (5-HPETE). Further metabolism of this intermediate leads to synthesis of leukotriene A4 and eventually leukotrienes B4, C4, D4, and E4.

Leukotriene B4 is implicated in the recruitment of inflammatory cells, e.g., neutrophils and T helper-2 cells into the skin in allergic and inflammatory skin conditions. Later, the cysteinyl leukotrienes induce proliferation of keratinocytes and skin fibrosis.

There are two types of leukotriene modifiers: leukotriene receptor antagonists and leukotriene synthesis inhibitors. *Leukotriene receptor antagonists* antagonize/block cysteinyl leukotrienes (leukotriene A4, B4, C4, D4, and E4) at their receptors. The receptors are present in smooth muscles of the bronchi and in the skin. Eosinophils, mast cells, and basophils synthesize cysteinyl leukotrienes. Examples of second-generation cysteinyl leukotriene antagonists are montelukast, zafirlukast, and pranlukast. *Leukotriene synthesis inhibitors* interrupt the 5-lipoxygenase pathway and consequently block the synthesis of all leukotrienes. They significantly reduce the synthesis of leukotrienes. An example of leukotriene synthesis inhibitors is zileuton. Leukotriene modifiers are also anti-inflammatory agents and have corticosteroid-sparing effects. These drugs are useful in the management of atopic dermatitis, acute and chronic urticaria, dermographism, bullous skin diseases, psoriasis, and other inflammatory skin diseases.

Antifungals Antifungal drugs can be categorized into three major classes: allylamines, azoles, and hydroxypyridones. They are available for oral and topical use in skin infections.

Allylamines Squalene epoxidase is an enzyme that is involved in the synthesis of ergosterol. Ergosterol is an essential constituent in fungal cell membrane; it is a sterol. Allylamines inhibit the enzyme. Inhibition of enzymatic conversion of squalene to ergosterol results in the accumulation of squalene within the fungal cell and eventual fungal cell death. Allylamines are effective in the treatment of dermatophytosis caused by *Trichophyton*, *Microsporum*, and *Epidermophyton*. Allylamines gain access into hair follicles and the stratum corneum. Examples of allylamines are terbinafine and naftifine.

Azoles Azoles inhibit a cytochrome P450-dependent enzyme. The enzyme is lanosterol 14-alpha-demethylase. The enzyme converts lanosterol to ergosterol. Instability of the cell wall results in fungal cell death. Azoles may be imidazoles or triazoles. *Imidazoles*: Effective topical imidazoles include clotrimazole, miconazole, econazole, oxiconazole, ketoconazole, and sertaconazole. Clotrimazole, miconazole, and econazole treat dermatophyte infections and candida (yeast) infections. Oxiconazole treats tinea capitis, tinea corporis, tinea cruris, and tinea pedis. Ketoconazole is a broad-spectrum antifungal that treats dermatophyte infections and seborrheic dermatitis. Sertaconazole is not only fungistatic like the others but also anti-inflammatory; it also effectively treats tinea pedis interdigitalis. *Triazoles*: Fluconazole and itraconazole and first-generation triazoles; there are second-generation triazoles and they include voriconazole, efinaconazole, and albaconazole. Fluconazole is used in the treatment of dermatophyte infections and cutaneous candidiasis. Itraconazole is taken orally for the treatment of onychomycosis; it is available for pulse therapy. Absorption is expected to be increased by concomitant intake of whole milk. Efinaconazole and albaconazole are useful for treatment of onychomycosis.

Hydroxypyridones Hydroxypyridones are another group of antifungal drugs. They are broad-spectrum antimicrobials that have antidermatophyte, anticandidal, anti-inflammatory, and antibacterial effects. They do not affect ergosterol synthesis but inhibit the transportation of essential compounds across the cell membrane of fungal cells; part of this is by chelating polyvalent cations and thus inhibiting enzymes that are metalloproteins. They are weak acids. Depending on the concentration of these compounds, they may be fungistatic or fungicidal. Examples are ciclopirox and ciclopirox olamine—the former is the free acid, and the latter is the salt; in both cases the active component is ciclopirox. This drug is effective for the treatment of pityriasis versicolor, tinea corporis, tinea pedis interdigitalis, tinea cruris, cutaneous candidiasis, and scalp seborrheic dermatitis and seborrheic dermatitis on other parts of the body.

Griseofulvin Griseofulvin is an old antifungal agent. It was isolated from *Penicillium griseofulvum*. *Stachybotrys levispora* is one of other sources from which griseofulvin can be isolated. Both organisms are fungi. Griseofulvin may no longer be used in some practice settings. In dermatophytosis, dermatophytes infect essentially the upper layer of the epidermis (the stratum corneum). The drug arrests mitosis in fungal cells and makes the superficial layer of the epidermis resistant to infection by these fungi. It achieves this by preventing the synthesis of the microtubule mitotic spindle in the metaphase. The drug is fungistatic to dermatophytes. Griseofulvin is the drug of choice for treating pediatric patients especially in resource-poor countries as it is cheaper than most antifungal drugs. The dose is 10 kg/kg body weight/day for about 4 weeks. It has an affinity for and is deposited in new keratin formed by keratinocytes. It effectively treats tinea infections.

Antiviral drugs Antiviral agents that are used in dermatology as anti-herpesvirus drugs include acyclovir, valacyclovir, famciclovir, and penciclovir. The targets of these drugs are mainly herpes simplex virus and less of Varicella-Zoster virus.

Acyclovir is an acyclic purine nucleoside analog. It is a synthetic nucleoside. It is converted to acyclovir triphosphate. The host (human) and the virus have DNA polymerases. Acyclovir triphosphate inhibits the enzyme that the virus initiates, i.e., viral DNA polymerase, but hardly does that to the human equivalent enzyme. When acyclovir is ingested, its active form (acyclovir triphosphate) prematurely terminates the DNA viral chain in its early stages of formation; the result is truncation of synthesis and replication of the viral chain. Acyclovir is used for the treatment of varicella, mucocutaneous herpes simplex, herpes zoster, and initial and recurrent episodes of genital herpes. For topical use, it is available as an ointment. It can be taken orally as oral suspension in children and tablets and capsules for older patients. Injections of the drug come as solutions or powder to be reconstituted for administration of the injection; the injection is useful in severe cases like eczema herpeticum and disseminated herpes simplex.

Valaciclovir (also spelt as valacyclovir) is a nucleoside analog. It is a DNA polymerase (enzyme) inhibitor. Valaciclovir is a prodrug of acyclovir. Valaciclovir is converted to acyclovir which is further converted to acyclovir triphosphate; this enzymatic conversion is by the process of phosphorylation. The active agent against herpes viruses is acyclovir triphosphate. It is acyclovir triphosphate that inactivates DNA polymerase in the virus. The inactivation is by competitive inhibition of the enzyme. Acyclovir triphosphate stops elongation of viral DNA chain, and the molecule is an obligate DNA chain terminator.

Famciclovir is a prodrug of penciclovir—a diacetyl ester prodrug of 6-deoxypenciclovir. To yield penciclovir, the two acetyl groups in famciclovir are removed. The first cleavage takes place in the intestinal wall after taking the drug orally; this is done by esterases. The second cleavage occurs in the liver, and it is by oxidation by oxidases. The result is the active antiviral, penciclovir.

Penciclovir is an acyclic guanine nucleoside analog, i.e., an acyclic derivative of guanine. Penciclovir triphosphate can be incorporated into the extending viral chain, unlike acyclovir triphosphate.

Cidofovir is a nucleoside analog of deoxycytidine monophosphate. Cidofovir diphosphate is a competitive inhibitor of deoxycytosine-5′-triphosphate. DNA polymerases employ the substrate to gain access into viral DNA. What cidofovir diphosphate does is competitively inhibit DNA polymerases from using their normal substrate (deoxycytosine-5′-triphosphate) and replaces the substrate [10]. Rather than incorporating deoxycytosine-5′-triphosphate into the DNA of the infecting virus, the enzyme incorporates cidofovir diphosphate which is useless in building the DNA chain for eventual replication [10]. This is the mode of action of this antiviral drug. Cidofovir is active against

human papillomaviruses (HPV) and herpes simplex virus (HSV). The drug can, therefore, be used to treat herpes simplex skin lesions. In HIV patients with recalcitrant molluscum contagiosum skin lesions, the cream with a higher concentration of cidofovir is required compared with 1% required in condyloma acuminata (genital warts).

Foscarnet, *Vidarabine*, and *Idoxuridine* are other effective anti-herpesvirus agents.

A to Z of Medications in Dermatology

Acyclovir
Albaconazole
Alpha-tocopherol
Anthralin
Azathioprine
Azelaic acid
Bacillus Calmette-Guérin
BCG
Belimumab
Benzoyl peroxide
Benzyl benzoate emulsion 10–25%
Benzylamines
Betamethasone
Bichloroacetic acid
Butenafine
Calamine lotion
Calcipotriene
Calcitriol
Cantharidin
Catechins ointment
Cetirizine
Chloroquine
Ciclopirox
Ciclopirox olamine
Cidofovir
Clarithromycin
Clindamycin
Clofazimine
Clotrimazole
Coal tar shampoo
Co-cyprindiol
Cyclosporine
Desloratadine

Diamino diphenyl sulfone
Diphenylcyclopropenone
Doxycycline
Econazole
Efinaconazole
Eflornithine
Erythromycin
Famciclovir
Fexofenadine
5-Fluorouracil
Fluconazole
Foscarnet
Fusidic acid 2% cream
Glycerine
Glycerol
Hyaluronic acid
Hydrocortisone
Hydroxychloroquine
Idoxuridine
Imiquimod
Interferon injections
Iodine
Isotretinoin
Itraconazole
Ivermectin
Ketoconazole
Lactic acid
Levocetirizine
Loratadine
Malathion
Methylprednisolone
Miconazole
Minocycline
Minoxidil
Montelukast
Moxidectin
Mupirocin
Naftifine
Omalizumab
Oxiconazole
Penciclovir
Permethrin cream
Pimecrolimus
Platelet-rich fibrin matrix
Podofilox

Podophyllin
Podophyllotoxin
Pranlukast
Rifampicin
Salicylic acid
Sarecycline
Selenium sulfide
Sertaconazole
Squaric acid dibutylester
Sulfur ointment
Tacrolimus
Terbinafine
Tetracyclines
Tretinoin
Triamcinolone acetonide
Trichloroacetic acid
Urea
Valacyclovir
Vidarabine
Vitamin D3
Xyzal®
Zafirlukast
Zileuton
Zinc sulphate

Multiple-Choice Questions

1. Scabies: Which of the statements below is correct?
   A. A tick causes it.
   B. Transmission is characteristically by physical contact with an infected individual.
   C. It is hardly pruritic.
   D. It responds to treatment with 25% benzyl benzoate emulsion.
2. Miliaria: Which of the statements below is incorrect?
   A. It is caused by sweat retention.
   B. It has keratin plugging of sweat pores as a feature.
   C. It may be accompanied with irritation of skin.
   D. It should be treated with antibiotics.

3. With respect to treatment of tinea capitis, which of the following associations is correct?

   A. Griseofulvin—No longer recommended for treating children.

   B. Itraconazole—First-line treatment.

   C. Nystatin—Drug of choice.

   D. Terbinafine—More effective treatment of *Trichophyton* infection.

4. Which of the following is a correct association pertaining to tinea corporis?

   A. Tinea incognito—Corticosteroid therapy of lesions.

   B. Advancing border of rash—Absence of vesicles.

   C. Mild presentation—Immunocompromise.

   D. Concentric rings in rashes—*Trichophyton tonsurans.*

5. A 22-year-old female university (college) student presents with sparse lesions of folliculitis. Which of the following treatments would you prescribe?

   A. Topical antibiotic.

   B. Oral antibiotic.

   C. Phototherapy.

   D. Local moist heat.

References

1. Ghangurde AA, Ganji KK, Bhongade ML, Sehdev B. Role of chemically modified tetracyclines in the management of periodontal diseases: a review. Drug Res (Stuttg). 2017;67(5):258–65. https://doi.org/10.1055/s-0043-100633. Available from: https://www.thieme-connect.com/products/ejournals/abstract/10.1055/s-0043-100633.

2. Rupert J, Hughes P. Sarecycline (Seysara) for the treatment of acne. New drug reviews. Am Fam Physician. 2020;102(4):245–6. Available from: https://www.aafp.org/pubs/afp/issues/2020/0815/p245.html.

3. Hansen LA, Sigman CC, Andreola F, Ross SA, Kelloff GJ, De Luca LM. Retinoids in chemoprevention and differentiation therapy. Carcinogenesis. 2000;21(7):1271–9. https://doi.org/10.1093/carcin/21.5.271. Available from: https://academic.oup.com/carcin/article-abstract/21/7/1271/2896292?redirectedFrom=fulltext.

4. Danby SG, Draelos ZD, Gold LFS, et al. Vehicles for atopic dermatitis therapies: more than just a placebo. J Dermatol Treat. 2022;33:685. https://taylorandfrancis.com/knowledge/Medicine_and_healthcare/Clinical_nutrition/Humectants/

5. Purnamawati S, Indrastuti N, Danarti R, Saefudin T. The role of moisturizers in addressing various kinds of dermatitis: a review. Clin Med Res. 2017;15(3–4):75–87. https://doi.org/10.3121/cmr.2017.1363. PMCID: PMC5849435 PMID: 29229630. Available from: https://pmc.ncbi.nlm.nih.gov/articles/PMC5849435/.

6. Linton S, Hossenbaccus L, Ellis AK. Evidence-based use of antihistamines for treatment of allergic conditions. CME Rev. 2023;131(4):412–20. Available from: https://www.annallergy.org/article/S1081-1206(23)00524-0/fulltext.

7. El-Sayed ASA, George NM, Yassin MA, et al. Purification and characterization of ornithine decarboxylase from *Aspergillus terreus*; kinetics of inhibition by various inhibitors. Molecules. 2019;24(15):2756. https://doi.org/10.3390/molecules24152756. Available from: https://www.mdpi.com/1420-3049/24/15/2756.

8. Guerra-Espinosa C, Jiménez-Fernández M, Sánchez-Madrid F, Serrador JM. ICAMs in immunity, intercellular adhesion and communication. Cells. 2024;13(4):339. https://doi.org/10.3390/cells13040339. PMCID: PMC10886500 PMID: 38391953.

9. Betarbet U. Keloids: a review of etiology, prevention, and treatment. J Clin Aesthet Dermatol. 2020;13(2):33–43. Available from: https://jcadonline.com/keloids-scars-treatment-review/.

10. Verhees F, Legemaate D, Demers I, et al. The antiviral agent cidofovir induces DNA damage and mitotic catastrophe in HPV-positive and -negative head and neck squamous cell carcinomas in vitro. Cancers (Basel). 2019;11(7):919. https://doi.org/10.3390/cancers11070919. PMCID: PMC6678333 PMID: 31262012. Available from: https://pmc.ncbi.nlm.nih.gov/articles/PMC6678333/.

Answers and Notes for MCQs

Chapter 1

1. (**C**) Protection the human body from deleterious effects of ultraviolet radiation is one of the functions of the skin. Other functions of the skin are prevention of loss of tissue fluids, regulation of body temperature, and production of cholecalciferol.

2. (**B**) In albinism, there is congenital deficiency of tyrosinase. Tyrosinase converts tyrosine to dopaquinone—this is the first step in the synthesis of melanin. In the absence of this enzyme, the normal chain of reactions towards production of melanin does not take place in albinism. This means that in the situation of reduction or total absence of tyrosinase, the pigment-producing cells (melanocytes) do not produce melanin. Melanin is photoprotective to skin by absorbing ultraviolet radiation from the sun. The absence of melanin in albinos subjects them to sunburn. The absence of pigment (melanin) is not only from the skin but also from the iris, retina, optic nerve, and hair. Other features are nystagmus and intolerance of sunlight. Patients with albinism are prone to developing squamous cell carcinoma.

3. (**D**) Histological findings in vitiligo are total absence of melanocytes because these pigment-producing, deep-seated cells are absent ab-initio. There is total loss of pigmentation of the epidermis irrespective of the prevailing skin color of the patient; the affected parts of the skin are white. In vitiligo, there is a predilection for perioral and periocular distribution of the lesions initially; other parts that are involved in the initial stages are forearms, hands, and feet. The clinical presentation of vitiligo is depigmented macular rashes and patches of skin. They are well-demarcated, circular, oval, or linear rashes with variable sizes from millimeters to centimeters. The disease is associated with autoimmune diseases, especially of the thyroid gland.

4. (**B**) In an 18-year-old female who presents in your clinic following the observation by her younger sister that she has "a couple of whitish rashes" on her back, the layer of the skin where the pathology of pityriasis versicolor occurs is stratum corneum. The etiological agent of pityriasis versicolor is a yeast. The yeast is Malassezia, and three species are implicated, viz., *Malassezia furfur* (*Pityrosporum orbiculare*), *Malassezia sympodialis*, and *Malassezia globosa*. The macules are usually hypochromic, not achromic, in the dark-skinned; they are multiple, irregularly shaped, of assorted sizes, with tendency to coalesce. The macules have tiny scales. Predisposing factors include warm, humid environments, and use of corticosteroids or skin lubricants. Immunosuppression and malnutrition are also predisposing factors though many patients with pityriasis versicolor do not have these two conditions. The treatment of pityriasis versicolor is effectively achieved with antifungal agents to which the yeast is susceptible; these include clotrimazole, econazole, ketoconazole, terbinafine, and naftifine. Depending on the extent of the body surface

I. Ukot, *Understanding Diseases in Skin of Color*, https://doi.org/10.1007/978-3-031-97503-5

that is covered, topical drugs may be used or oral drugs prescribed.

5. (**A**) Considering the 15-year-old secondary school (high school) student who, 8 weeks earlier, moved into the school residential facility for students and recently observed sleeplessness from pubic hair itching and itching of axillary hair which is worse at night but also elicits a distracting and embarrassing urge to scratch during classes, the diagnosis is most likely phthiriasis pubis. Pediculosis pubis (or phthiriasis pubis), the parasitic infestation *Pthirus pubis* causes, preferentially affects the hairs on the pubic region. Much less commonly, the crab lice may infest hair on the mustache, axilla, eyebrows, anterior chest wall, or beards. The causative organism is called crab louse because when viewed under the microscope it is reminiscent of the shape of a crab. This parasitic infestation is frequently transmitted by sexual contact or direct bodily contact. The infection may be transmitted by fomites like clothing, towels, and bedding used by an infested individual.

Chapter 2

1. (**C**) Erythrasma is a dry, slightly scaly, macular rash with a tendency to expand. It is an intertriginous skin disease that is aggravated by a warm, humid environment. The lesions of erythrasma are pruritic. The causative organism is the Gram-positive bacterium, *Corynebacterium minutissimum*. Predisposing factors for the development of erythrasma include excessive sweating, obesity, diabetes mellitus, depressed immunity, and advancing age. The affected skin examined under Wood's lamp (produces ultraviolet light) is fluorescent, showing coral red in erythrasma. Topical and oral drugs are effective for treatment, e.g., topicals: benzoyl peroxide, mupirocin cream, fusidic acid, or clindamycin cream; and oral drugs: erythromycin, clarithromycin, or tetracycline. Erythrasma may coexist with candidal intertrigo.

2. (**D**) Cutaneous candidiasis is one of the differential diagnoses of erythrasma. Others include tinea corporis, tinea cruris, tinea pedis, allergic contact dermatitis, irritant contact dermatitis, and seborrheic dermatitis. Healthy lifestyle and exercise help to counter obesity or prevent its development and, therefore, have a beneficial effect on treatment and/or prevention. Predisposing factors for erythrasma include hyperhidrosis, diabetes mellitus, obesity, advanced age, immune compromise, poor hygiene, and warm climate. First-line treatment of erythrasma consists of topical antibiotics (e.g., mupirocin, clindamycin, erythromycin, and fusidic acid) or the antifungal, miconazole. Ozonated olive oil is also effective for treatment. Oral antibiotics (e.g., erythromycin, clarithromycin, or the combination of amoxicillin and clavulanic acid) are second-line therapy for erythrasma.

3. (**A**) Furuncle is a small abscess; it involves both skin and subcutaneous tissue. Purulent material is from a single opening in a furuncle. Common sites for furuncles are rich in hair follicles—these include the axillae, neck, and gluteal region. Superficial folliculitis is a tender pustule that affects the hair follicle. Furuncle is also seen in deep folliculitis.

4. (**D**) Patients with tuberculoid leprosy have sparse macular lesions with paresthesia; some of the rashes may be large. Having active cellular immunity, the immune response is satisfactory in tuberculoid leprosy patients, and they show a strongly positive result to lepromin test. The causative organism of leprosy is a Gram-positive acid-fast bacillus, *Mycobacterium leprae*. Its incubation period may exceed 5 years. In indeterminate leprosy, normal sensation may be a feature of the hypopigmented macules. Leonine facies are a feature of lepromatous leprosy.

5. (**B**) *Mycobacterium leprae*, a naturally extremely slow-growing Gram-positive acid-fast bacillus, is cultured in Dubos-Lowenstein-Jensen medium and thyroxine sodium. The causative pathogen in leprosy, *Mycobacterium leprae*, is specific, and no other *Mycobacterium* is implicated in the etiology of this disease.

The presentation of leprosy is dependent on the response of the host to the etiological agent. In tuberculoid leprosy, the host's cellular immunity is still robust with resultant few skin manifestations and mild asymmetric peripheral nerve involvement. Patients with tuberculoid leprosy produce a positive response to skin tests that use antigens from killed *Mycobacterium leprae*.

Chapter 3

1. (**C**) In some patients, the lesions have lasted so long and given them so little concern symptomatically that they consider them to be normal; this explains why in rural practice in some developing countries some patients with extensive pityriasis versicolor do not complain of it when they consult a doctor with other symptoms. Pityriasis versicolor is caused by *Pityrosporum orbiculare*. The lesions are scaly—the scales are tiny. Most times pityriasis versicolor affects the upper part of the trunk. It responds satisfactorily to treatment with 2.5% selenium sulfide.

2. (**C**) Tinea capitis is caused by *Microsporum* and *Trichophyton*. It is characterized by broken hairs and scaly areas of the scalp. It manifests as pseudo-alopecia. Tinea capitis has a predilection for older children, not newborn babies.

3. (**C**) In an 11-year-old girl brought to your clinic on account of a second rash on the body with rashes that are almost round and pruritic, skin scrapings demonstrating dermatophyte would best enable you to sustain a tentative diagnosis of tinea corporis. Close bodily contact with a cousin on a recent visit having similar rashes is a lead but not the best of the available options for this question. The positive history of carbuncle 1 month earlier is not related to this patient's current dermatological condition. Blood culture to rule out bacterial secondary infection is not indicated in this case and could be a misdirection of the resources of the medical facility.

4. (**B**) In this 39-year-old factory supervisor with a 9-month history of interdigital rash between two toes who presents to the clinic with a 6-week complaint of itchy rashes in the groin area, infection at the two sites is most likely occupational. The requirement of wearing safety boots and socks/stockings for many hours and wearing coveralls in a factory setting with warmth and moisture in the affected part of the body makes this worker (and others) prone to developing tinea cruris and tinea pedis. In this patient, infection by transfer from the interdigital clefts (e.g., via towel) to the groin is likely; this is auto-inoculation (self-inoculation). Treatment should not terminate on disappearance of the rashes but should continue till 10–14 days thereafter. This ensures elimination of the dermatophyte. The etiological agent is a dermatophyte, but it could be *Candida albicans*, a yeast causing the initial intertrigo between toes. To avoid recurrence, the doctor should give the patient adequate information on foot/footwear care, use and maintenance of underwear, as well as correct use of towels so as not to transfer the infection from one part of the body to another.

5. (**D**) With respect to tinea cruris, the use of appropriate fitting cotton underwear (undergarment) that enables aeration of the groin assists in keeping that part of the body dry and clean. The underwear should be well ironed and changed frequently. Moreover, towels used for infected interdigital clefts and toes should not be used to dry other parts of the body. Close bodily contact with other people should be avoided to prevent spreading the skin disease or acquiring it. The etiology of moniliasis is *Candida* species (e.g., *Candida albicans*); the etiological agent of tinea cruris is a dermatophyte, especially *Trichophyton rubrum* and *Epidermophyton floccosum*. Infection is at the stratum corneum, not the dermal layer of the skin. Grayish-white macule or plaque is more in keeping with candidal intertrigo. Tinea cruris is groin ringworm (jock itch) and has the characteristics of other tinea infections—central healing and clearing area and an active periphery/border.

Chapter 4

1. (**B**) Herpes zoster virus is one of the herpes viruses that cause infection in humans. The infection (also called Shingles) is a reactivation of chickenpox. In herpes zoster infection, there is no sex predilection. Herpes zoster lesions are vesico-papules along the dermatome of peripheral nerves, quite painful, especially when extensive. The pain may persist as post-herpetic neuralgia after healing. The lesions are usually unilateral, but in extensive cases, they may be bilateral. They may break up and form crusted superficial ulcers. Herpes zoster is sometimes a manifestation of a depressed immunity, and so HIV infection should be suspected and the patients investigated when they present with herpes zoster infection, especially with extensive lesions. Prednisolone is a useful therapeutic agent. Antivirals like acyclovir and valacyclovir are useful in treatment.

2. (**D**) Among individuals that have herpes zoster (shingles), the population requiring treatment are the immunocompromised, persons that are over 50 years, and any patient who presents with severe disease that may become protracted. Treatment is usually conservative and incorporates the commonly available and affordable calamine lotion; wet dressings with Burow's solution, i.e., 5% aluminum triacetate which is applied for 30–60 min four to six times daily; and non-steroidal anti-inflammatory drugs. The etiology of herpes zoster (shingles) is Varicella zoster virus (VZV) and not Herpes simplex virus (HSV). The disease progression after a prodrome of pain and paresthesia is macules > papules > vesicles. The vesicles become crusted and eventually resolve. The most common site of herpes zoster lesions is thoracic dermatome.

3. (**C**) Warts are caused by the human papilloma virus (HPV); the virus is infective to squamous epithelium of genitals and skin. Warts demonstrate hyperkeratosis. They are small, firm, rough, painless, pigmented skin growths (verrucae vulgaris), but they can appear to be confluent, in clusters, and increase in size (mosaic warts). They are contagious and the venereal variety is not always acquired by sexual contact as warts are acquired by direct skin contact with infected individuals. They can spread from one site to another in the same person and can spread from person to person. De novo, they are unusual in the elderly. HPV is associated with the development of cancer of the genitals, mouth, and throat. Warts can be removed by cryotherapy, surgical excision, electrocautery, or chemical cautery e.g., with podophyllin.

4. (**C**) A 26-year-old sexually active female who presents to you with genital rashes and fever has herpes genitalis if, on examination, she also has inguinal lymphadenopathy and vaginal discharge. Further examination of a female patient with primary herpes genitalis is expected to show cervical lesions that are ulcerated or vesicular. If the rashes are in the form of cauliflower growth, it is genital warts caused by the epidermotropic human papilloma virus (HPV). Painless vulvar ulcer tilts the diagnosis towards syphilis. Intense pruritus vulvae is a feature that is more in keeping with trichomoniasis. In males who present with herpes genitalis, penile ulceration occurs and is sequel to painful, hyperemic, vesicular lesions; the ulceration may also occur on the perineum or anus.

5. (**D**) With respect to genital warts, painless, pruritic growths are characteristic. While human papilloma virus (HPV) is the etiological agent, it is not limited to HPV-6 as HPV-11 also causes genital warts (condyloma acuminatum); they cause low-risk benign HPV lesions. In >90% cases of genital warts, the etiological agents are the two types—6 and 11. Warts at the external urinary meatus hardly cause urinary retention. Flat lesions of the penile meatus may cause bleeding. It is common to have multiple warts. Descriptions of genital warts include papular, plaque-like, cauliflower, filiform, pearly, fungating, verrucous, lobulated, and smooth.

Chapter 5

1. (**B**) Onchocerciasis of the skin presents with rashes that are pruritic and papular; over time there is associated scarring and lichenification of the affected skin. Leopard skin is sequel to patchy depigmentation of the skin of the legs in patients with onchocerciasis of the skin. Though a specific test, skin snip microscopy is not useful for early or mild disease as the *Onchocerca volvulus* microfilariae concentration is not high enough and may be missed; it is an invasive procedure necessitating taking skin snips that are up to 3–5 mg, immersing the specimens in NaCl immediately and examining them under the microscope to pick up emerging microfilariae. Enzyme-linked immunosorbent assay (ELISA) is more sensitive than skin snip microscopy; it is also less invasive; the same applies to polymerase chain reaction (PCR).

2. (**A**) Features of lichenified onchodermatitis (LOD) are pruritic, raised, discrete, hyperpigmented papulonodular plaques that are associated with lymphadenopathy; they may be confluent and may feature excoriation. Patients who present with multiple, solid papules each with dimension >1 mm have acute papular onchodermatitis; this patient with eye involvement would have gone beyond this stage of skin disease. Palpable, firm, movable, nontender nodule over a bony prominence describes the subcutaneous nodules that contain adult *Onchocerca volvulus*, and this skin presentation is onchocercomata (onchocercomas). Wrinkling and dryness of the skin describes atrophy, a significant abnormality, in onchodermatitis.

3. (**B**) In a 5-year-old child with scabies, pruritus may be severe enough to result in sleepiness during classes at school. This is because the intense pruritus is worse at night when the mite tends to migrate towards the skin surface. The mites hardly infest the face and so scabies is hardly a presentation in the face, especially in adults. The eruptions are not large blisters but thin and superficial burrows; they cause itching rather than pain. When

there is pain, it is usually due to secondary bacterial infection by *Staphylococcus aureus* or *Streptococcus pyogenes*, in which case the patient develops impetigo and may proceed complications like sepsis, acute glomerulonephritis, or acute rheumatic fever.

4. (**B**) In a 27-year-old otherwise unemployed commercial sex worker positive for HIV, presentation with extensive pruritic and eczematous rashes is usual of scabies. In adults, facial, palmar, and plantar rashes are atypical; rather, this is more in keeping with scabies in the pediatric age group. This patient is expected to have mild, if any, itching. The patient is prone to having fungal skin infection concomitantly.

5. (**C**) Topical corticosteroids are useful in short courses for treating patients who suffer from intense pruritus—which may lead to insomnia and severe scratching with excoriations and Koebner's phenomenon. Hydrocortisone 1%, though having the lowest potency, is useful even in pediatric patients. The repeat course of Ivermectin treatment is 7–10 days after initial treatment; each dose is 200 μg/kg/day. Permethrin: This neurotoxin comes as a lotion 5% cream. The lotion is applied to the entire body and rinsed off 8–12 h later; it paralyzes and subsequently kills the ectoparasite—*Sarcoptes scabiei* var hominis—"var" refers to variety, the human variety. Two courses are advised but not mandatory as one course suffices. Crotamiton 10% lotion or cream is not the best treatment option for scabies as the therapy is fraught with failures.

Chapter 6

1. (**C**) "Exclamation mark" hairs are not pathognomonic of alopecia areata as they are also a feature of trichotillomania. The distal end of an exclamation mark hair in alopecia areata is usually frayed while in trichotillomania it is usually blunt. Alopecia areata does not affect the texture of the skin. Hair loss is partial. The lesions in alopecia areata are usually round or oval. Treatment of alopecia may be with

intralesional steroids; psoralens are for treatment of vitiligo.

2. (**A**) Paronychia may be fungal or bacterial in etiology. It causes swelling of the area surrounding the nail. The nail fold may become bulbous and slightly painful when it is a fungal infection or more painful if it has a bacterial etiology. There is the likelihood of a positive history of engagement in work involving putting the hands in water frequently or for prolonged periods.

3. (**D**) Surgical excision of hidradenitis suppurativa lesion is the preferred method for treatment when fistulas, sinus tracts, abscesses, or scars develop; this should be done early for best results. Predilection of hidradenitis suppurativa is for the skin that bears apocrine glands. The disorder affects the terminal portion of follicular epithelium. The parts of the skin that bear apocrine glands include the axillae, inframammary area, between the glutei, and in the groin; these are the common sites of hidradenitis suppurativa. Finasteride is useful for medical treatment of this condition in the initial stages; other drugs include spironolactone and triamcinolone acetonide administered as an intralesional injection.

4. (**C**) Abnormality in pigmentation and/or shape of nail is a feature of onychomycosis. Non-dermatophyte molds are part of the etiological agents of onychomycosis; others include yeasts and dermatophytes. Not only the nail plate is involved but also the nail matrix in onychomycosis. Itraconazole is one of the drugs used for treating patients with onychomycosis, but the course of therapy lasts longer than for other conditions, i.e., 6 to 8 weeks for fingernail infection and 12 weeks of daily administration for toenail infection.

5. (**B**) For a 25-year-old artisan who presents with a painful 3-day bulbous swelling of the lateral and medial nail folds, and a small area of fluctuance of the surface of the skin of the medial nail fold, the most appropriate investigation is Gram staining microscopy with culture and sensitivity studies on discharge; in this patient where there was no drainage but evidence of purulent collection, an aspirate is the most logical specimen from the swelling. Fungal studies using KOH and microscopy are useful in chronic paronychia—in this patient, the infection is acute and most likely bacterial. If herpetic whitlow is suspected, Tzanck smear is required—the index patient, although presenting with pain and within 3 days of onset, is unlikely to have a viral infection which does not form a pustule unless there is a bacterial secondary infection. Blood sugar level and glycated (glycosylated) hemoglobin (HbA1c) does not seem to be the most appropriate test for this patient because the history would have pointed to diabetes mellitus; however, in patients with diabetes mellitus, fasting blood glucose and, from time to time, HbA1c should be checked for diabetic control. Patients who have repeated episodes of acute paronychia should be investigated for diabetes mellitus. Scaping of the medial end of the nail plate for fungal studies is not warranted in this patient because the infection is not onychomycosis that requires specimen from the nail plate for mycological studies.

Chapter 7

1. (**A**) Pimples (acne vulgaris) usually has its onset at puberty. It manifests as papules, pustules, and nodules. It may be complicated by scar formation. The face, upper chest, and upper back are common sites of acne vulgaris.

2. (**D**) Miliaria crystallina presents as tiny, pinhead, vesicles that are fragile. In miliaria profunda, there are papular rashes; the blockage of sweat glands is at the junction between the epidermis and dermis. The result is leakage of sweat into the papillary dermis. In miliaria rubra, the tiny papules are erythematous (reddish, "rubra") in individuals with skin color that makes the color obvious. Obstruction of sweat glands is in the epidermis. The papular rashes are pruritic. Miliaria pustulosa presents

as pustular eruptions in patients with miliaria rubra. The pus-forming rash may simulate impetigo contagiosa, but it is not synonymous.

3. (B) Leakage of sweat into the epidermis or dermis, a result of ductal obstruction, explains the clinical presentation of the distinct types of miliaria. Sweat ductal blockage does not prevent sweat production in the affected eccrine sweat glands. Miliaria pustulosa, especially when extensive, may progress to heat exhaustion if not adequately and time-ously treated. In miliaria crystallina, the site of blockage of sweat is close to the pores on the surface of the skin (at the sub-corneal layer, i.e., just below the stratum corneum). The inflammation is therefore minimal, and the patient is frequently asymptomatic. This is different in miliaria with leakage at deeper layers of the skin.

4. (C) In nodulocystic acne, the nodules exceed 5 mm in diameter as well as have associated comedones and inflammatory lesions; scar-ring is also a feature. Mild acne presents as comedones and a few papulopustules. In com-edonal acne, there is absence of inflammatory papules and nodules. In moderate acne, there are inflammatory papules; other features are comedones and pustules.

5. (A) The release of bradykinin contributes to the development of urticaria. This vasoactive substance is not the sole agent; others include histamine, leukotriene C4, and prostaglandin D2. These are released from mast cells and basophils in the dermis. Exercise is one of the predisposing factors for developing urticaria in susceptible individuals. Other predisposing factors are environmental factors like cold or heat; foods like certain sea foods; and medica-tions to which the individual is allergic; insect bites and stings; emotional stress; body care products like creams, lotions, perfumes, hair dyes, etc. especially if recently introduced and used; dust, mold, plants, and dander from pets; and skin contact with rubber, latex, nail polish, or use of jewelry that incorporate nickel. In urticaria the wheals blanch, are raised, and palpable. Pruritus is a characteris-tic of urticaria. Acute urticaria cases have a history of less than 6 weeks while chronic or recurrent urticaria have duration exceeding 6 weeks. Educating the patient on identifying and avoiding the offending allergen (and they could be multiple) is important, and being a preventive measure should not be made the last line of management of urticaria—it should be top on the list of management measures.

Chapter 8

1. (B) Dandruff is seborrheic dermatitis of the scalp in its mild form. Areas of the body that are involved in seborrheic dermatitis are the face, scalp, and trunk. The specific parts are rich in sebum. Seborrheic dermatitis is a pap-ulosquamous disorder. Seborrheic dermatitis is associated with the commensal yeast *Malassezia furfur*. This and other species are lipid dependent and split fat using the enzyme lipase, releasing free fatty acids that trigger skin inflammation. Using fluorinated steroids is not advocated. Low-potency corticosteroids are recommended for application topically, but even these should not be used for extended periods as they may cause thinning of the skin and telangiectasias. Examples of recom-mended low-potency topical steroids are hydrocortisone, mometasone furoate, and desonide.

2. (D) Patients with psoriasis obtain some relief from their symptoms by regular applica-tion of moisturizers. The main topical agents are corticosteroids, coal tar, and anthralin. In psoriasis, the cell line that undergoes hyperp-roliferation is keratinocyte. Exposure to sun-light daily is a simple modality of treatment. Psoriasis occurs in children and teenagers also.

3. (C) Pitting may occur in nail psoriasis just as there may be subungual hyperkeratosis, ony-cholysis, or oil-drop sign. Plaque psoriasis is a usual form of psoriasis. It is difficult to treat

as it resists treatment. It is not a life-threatening disease. Distribution of psoriatic lesions is symmetrical over the body. The face is more commonly involved in pediatric patients than in adults. Psoriasis is a complex, multifactorial, and chronic inflammatory disorder of the skin. Implicated factors are environmental, immunologic, and genetic. It frequently affects skin on the scalp, elbows, knees, glans penis, lumbosacral area, and the cleft between the glutei. The most common dermatologic form of psoriasis is psoriasis vulgaris (chronic inflammatory psoriasis). Dermatologic varieties of psoriasis include plaque psoriasis, guttate psoriasis, pustular psoriasis, erythrodermic psoriasis, nail psoriasis, scalp psoriasis, and inverse psoriasis. Non-dermatologic forms include psoriatic arthritis, conjunctivitis, or blepharitis. Psoriasis is principally a clinical diagnosis.

4. (**A**) The lesions of lichen planus are usually polygonal. This shape is part of the physical descriptive characteristics of lichen planus—the "six *P*s," viz., *p*ruritic, *p*olygonal, *p*lanar, *p*urple *p*apules, and *p*laques. Though some patients with lichen planus are asymptomatic, most patients have severe pruritus which is an important feature of the disease. Wickham's striae are found on the mucosa of the mouth, and these lesions on the buccal mucosa are lacy, reticular, white plaques. Intralesional corticosteroids should be used when lichen planus lesions are few; an example is triamcinolone acetonide at the lower concentration preparation, or higher concentration for hypertrophic lichen planus. For pruritus of the skin lesions, antihistamines are useful when taken orally. Topical antipruritic drugs that contain lidocaine, phenol, menthol, or camphor are also effective for treatment. Corticosteroids may also be applied topically.

5. (**C**) Regarding the 25-year-old man with a deep tone of Black skin, the presentation of lichen planus is not purple lesions; rather they are light gray plaques. The rashes cover a significant portion of total skin area making him feel distraught and embarrassed, occasioning the specific request for expeditious resolution of the lesions.

Chapter 9

1. (**A**) Keloid is a benign connective tissue tumor that usually follows trauma. The trauma may be as mild/minor as ear piercing.

2. (**C**) Neurofibromatosis is an autosomal dominant disease with multiple benign skin growths. Café-au-lait spots are brownish patches of the skin. Surgical removal of all neurofibromatosis lesions in a patient is not a recommended treatment.

3. (**B**) Ifosfamide is a drug, the use of which is associated with the development of Campbell de Morgan spots (Capillary hemangioma). The dermatological condition is also associated with drugs such as alkylating agents (class of antineoplastic drugs), e.g., the nitrogen mustards like cyclophosphamide and chlorambucil. Other drugs associated with their etiology are cyclosporine and tamsulosin. Curettage, carbon dioxide laser therapy, and cryotherapy are treatment modalities. Treatment is usually not required unless there is infection, a cosmetic embarrassment when the lesion is present in a conspicuous site, or the growth erodes into the epidermis or it undergoes maceration.

4. (**D**) Regarding the 15-year-old high school student who traumatized her right thumb while she was engaged in a phone discussion with a close friend and cleaning up her room at the same time during the weekend, the injury took place within 2 weeks of onset of pyogenic granuloma; this is the usual presentation. It is unlikely to be pyogenic granuloma if the growth occurred at least 3 months after the trauma. Her presentation in hospital has a direct relationship with how she feels about the growth; at least the negative cosmetic appearance of the growth and the restriction imposed by the thumb during writing and typing are enough to justify her coming to the

hospital to seek treatment. The only reason she came for consultation cannot be frequent severe bleeding; she could have bleeding, but it would be mild and not severe, just as the bleeding may be one of the reasons for consultation but not the primary reason.

5. (C) Regarding melanoma, maculo-papular is not a type by histopathological classification. The types are superficial spreading, nodular, lentigo maligna, acral lentiginous, and mucosal lentiginous.

Chapter 10

1. (C) Carbuncle is an acute bacterial infection. It commonly affects the nape and the axilla. When recurrent, the patient should be evaluated for diabetes mellitus. When there is not only recurrence but also not responding adequately to antibiotic treatment, running a chronic course, and with foul-smelling purulent discharge in the axilla, hidradenitis suppurativa should be suspected and the patient evaluated in greater detail.

2. (C) A carbuncle is an aggregation of small abscesses from bacterial infection of multiple hair follicles. A carbuncle is usually one but in an individual with suppressed immunity carbuncle may be multiple or recurrent. Common sites are axillae, groin, nape, gluteal area, and thighs. A carbuncle is symptomatic and there is usually pain. Treatment is by drainage, but before it forms, much pus systemic antibiotics may suffice when treatment is started early.

3. (B) Hypertension is not a risk factor for a second or further episode of carbuncles in this obese 39-year-old man. Diabetes mellitus, kidney disease, obesity, poor hygiene, and herpes zoster are risk factors. A patient with herpes zoster should be investigated for the likelihood of positive HIV status.

4. (C) In this obese 43-year-old woman who presents to you with a history of bilateral inframammary rash of 1 month which has become worse in the previous 2 weeks, superimposed fungal or bacterial infection is expected to occur. Intertrigo is a condition that primarily affects areas of the body that have skin folds due to combination of heat, poor aeration with trapping of moisture, and friction. Parts of the body that are prone to intertrigo include folds such as inframammary, infrapannicular, interdigital, genitocrural, axillary, and infragluteal. Being obese, the symptoms are likely to recur after treatment. The treatment of choice is not necessarily a fluorinated corticosteroid cream; treatment should be based on history, physical examination, and investigation of the patient. Apart from the duration that is clearly indicated in this case, history taking should include the following, among others: Is this the first episode? If it is not the first, how many? What time interval? Is there a relationship with weather? Is there a history of hyperhidrosis? Is this patient diabetic? Is there immunocompromise or immunosuppression? What inner clothing is used and what care is given to it? Is there involvement of other intertriginous areas? If the feet are involved how many interdigital clefts are involved? Did the foot condition precede the inframammary condition? Does the patient's occupation require using covered footwear for many hours? How does the patient keep, use, and maintain socks, and stockings? How does the patient use a towel? How dry is the towel in-between use? Is there a possibility of nosocomial transfer of infection? On physical examination, is there evidence of chronicity, or inflammation? With respect to investigation, findings show no growth, normal skin flora, fungal growth, bacterial growth, or fungal and bacterial growth. If it shows yeast, prescribe an antifungal that, e.g., *Candida albicans* in candidal intertrigo is expected to be susceptible to. If there is bacterial growth, treat the patient based on antibiotic sensitivity results. Do not fail to provide the patient with current information on preventive measures.

5. (C) Apart from the skin, blood cell lines are commonly affected in systemic lupus erythematosus (SLE). The results are anemia (red

blood cells), leukopenia and lymphocytes (white blood cells), and thrombocytopenia (platelets, thrombocytes). There is a female preponderance with systemic lupus erythematosus with more than 90% occurrence in females. Exposed parts of the body, e.g., face and upper limbs, are the sites when photosensitive SLE predominates. While clinical findings are important in making the diagnosis of SLE, they are not of overriding importance. Laboratory investigations utilized for diagnosing SLE include full (complete) blood count with differential white blood cell count, erythrocyte sedimentation rate (ESR), liver function tests, serum creatinine, autoantibody tests, creatine kinase assay, urinalysis, and urine microscopy, and complement levels. Imaging studies are useful in assessing involvement of organs like the heart, joints, and brain. In SLE, the autoimmune disorder features inflammation in multiple systems and autoantibodies are produced. Multiple factors associated with SLE include environmental, hormonal, immunoregulatory, ethnic, genetic, and epigenetic factors.

Chapter 11

1. (**D**) *Sarcoptes scabiei*, a mite, causes scabies. Scabies is very pruritic, especially at night. Transmission can be by fomites. It commonly affects the buttocks, interdigital clefts, and penis. It responds to treatment with 25% benzyl benzoate emulsion.
2. (**D**) Miliaria may be accompanied with an irritating sensation on the skin but not classical pruritus. It occurs in many people who sweat excessively. The rashes are small pin-head sized. Management may involve use of a cooling topical agent like calamine lotion, also wearing of light cotton clothing, and avoiding tight clothes made from synthetic material. Frequent cool baths may help just as exposure to a cool indoor environment, e.g., with air conditioning may soothe the skin.
3. (**D**) *T*erbinafine is more effective for treating tinea capitis caused by *Trichophyton* species;

the same applies to itraconazole. With respect to treatment of tinea capitis, griseofulvin is still used for treating even pediatric patients. The drug is available in liquid and tablet forms and is affordable; duration of treatment may be longer compared with using newer antifungals. Headache is a side effect that some patients may feel uncomfortable with. Griseofulvin produces the highest cure rate for tinea capitis. Tinea capitis caused by *Microsporum* species responds better to griseofulvin. Itraconazole is not a first-line treatment of tinea capitis; it should not be prescribed for patients with features of heart failure. Nystatin is not used to treat tinea capitis or any tinea infection; tinea capitis is caused by dermatophytes and these fungi are resistant to nystatin. Yeasts, e.g., *Candida albicans*, are sensitive to nystatin. The opposite is true for griseofulvin that is active against dermatophytes but not against yeasts.

4. (**A**) When a patient treats tinea corporis with topical corticosteroids, they are prone to developing tinea incognito with chronicity and aggravation of the initial features, often making diagnosis a difficulty. This may be prevented by encouraging the general populace to present dermatological conditions to the hospital without prior treatment. This advice is beneficial for other dermatological and non-dermatological conditions; misdiagnosis, late presentation, and diagnosis of more severe conditions can be prevented. In countries where a wide variety of over-the-counter drugs are available for purchase without physicians' prescription, it is a big challenge to the health of the population. Tinea corporis exhibits a central healing area and a peripheral advancing border of ongoing pathology. The advancing border has vesicles as well as papules, scales, crust, or bullae. Patients with immune compromise, especially HIV-positive patients, have severe presentation with deep abscess formation; the patients also tend to have disseminated disease. *Trichophyton concentricum* is the cause of tinea imbricata which causes rashes with concentric rings. Other dermatophytes that cause tinea corporis

are *Trichophyton rubrum*, *Trichophyton tonsurans*, *Trichophyton verrucosum*, *Trichophyton mentagrophytes*, and *Trichophyton interdigitale*. Of the *Microsporum* genus, *Microsporum canis* and *Microsporum gypseum* are known etiological agents.

5. (**A**) With few lesions of folliculitis in this 22-year-old female university student, topical antibiotic would be the recommendation. Examples include mupirocin 2% ointment, fusidic acid 2% cream, and clindamycin 2% gel 12 hourly over the lesions. Oral antibiotics are systemic antibiotics; they are more appropriate in extensive cases. When features of systemic presentation are present, e.g., fever, cellulitis, or lymphadenitis, systemic antibiotics are warranted. Phototherapy requires the equipment unless the patient can obtain the portable one and can invest the time required for each session. Local moist heat must be applied for 15–20 min. Applying antibiotic cream does not take any appreciable time.

Index

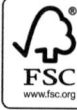

MIX
Papier aus verantwortungsvollen Quellen
Paper from responsible sources
FSC® C105338

If you have any concerns about our products,
you can contact us on
ProductSafety@springernature.com

In case Publisher is established outside the EU,
the EU authorized representative is:
Springer Nature Customer Service Center GmbH
Europaplatz 3, 69115 Heidelberg, Germany

Printed by Libri Plureos GmbH
in Hamburg, Germany